E. New

AGING AND MENTAL HEALTH

POSITIVE PSYCHOSOCIAL APPROACHES

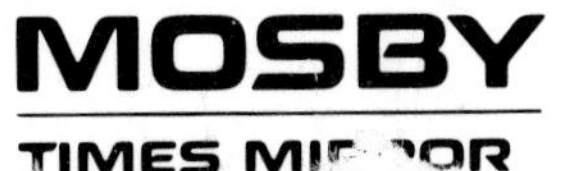

AGING & MENTAL HEALTH

POSITIVE PSYCHOSOCIAL APPROACHES

ROBERT N. BUTLER, M.D.

Research and Practicing Psychiatrist, Psychoanalyst,
and Gerontologist; Faculty, Washington School of Psychiatry,
Howard University School of Medicine, Washington Psychoanalytic Institute,
Washington, D. C.

MYRNA I. LEWIS, ACSW

Mental Health Specialist, Parkside–Arthur Capper Community
Mental Health Team, Washington, D. C.;
Private Individual and Group Psychotherapy Practice

with 26 *illustrations*

SAINT LOUIS

THE C. V. MOSBY COMPANY

1973

Second printing

Printed in the United States of America

International Standard Book Number 0-8016-0916-X
Library of Congress Catalog Card Number 72-92507

Distributed in Great Britain by
HENRY KIMPTON, LONDON

COVER

The great Russian novelist and teacher Leo Tolstoi telling stories to his grandchildren. Tolstoi's creative work has extended understanding of the nature and flow of human life from childhood to old age. Family life, faith, war and peace, human liberty, poverty and power, love and death were among his great literary themes. (Courtesy The Trustees of the British Museum.)

To our

GRANDPARENTS

FOREWORD

Many older persons are already deeply indebted to Dr. Butler for the significant contributions he has made to the field of aging. The number of indebted persons will increase sharply as the result of the decision by Dr. Butler and Ms. Lewis to author *Aging and Mental Health: Positive Psychosocial Approaches.*

Physicians, clergymen, social workers, nursing home personnel, and all others who deal with emotional crises that confront older persons will benefit from reading this discussion. Hopefully, many older persons who are not working in the field of aging will also read the book. From it, they can derive knowledge and insights that, if heeded, can contribute to the prevention of mental illness in the latter years of life.

As I have had the privilege of meeting with thousands of older persons in the last two years I have identified, among others, the following three messages that they are endeavoring to convey to society:

1. We want to make our own decisions regarding our own lives; we don't want other persons to make the decisions for us.
2. We want to continue to be involved in life; we don't want to be put on the shelf.
3. We want to be treated with dignity.

This affirmative approach to old age is the theme that runs throughout *Aging and Mental Health: Positive Psychosocial Approaches.* The "losses" that older persons experience are confronted in a frank and realistic manner. At the same time the authors demonstrate how these losses can contribute to the strengthening rather than the deterioration of mental health in old age.

Older persons want to approach life affirmatively. The chief obstacle to such an approach is the impact of ageism, which the authors so effectively identify and analyze. Those who give expression to ageism assume that growing old consists of a series of defeats. The authors believe that society has the capability, by rejecting ageism, of making it possible for the aging process to be characterized by a series of victories.

Far too often, for example, it is assumed that when an older person enters a nursing home he does so in preparation for death. It is clear, however, that many can be rehabilitated, both physically and mentally, if their care is approached with that objective in mind. Then it becomes possible for them to return to their own homes, often to become involved in constructive activity on behalf of society, and to experience the satisfaction that comes from a realization that the last days of life are indeed proving, in many respects, to be the best days.

The emphasis these authors place on the importance, both for the older person and for society, of continued involvement in life is one that needs to be underlined. Unfortunately, the trend in our nation is in the direction of more and more institutions' requiring retirement at a given age. In addition there is a trend in the direction of lowering the age for compulsory retirement. This means that our society must provide counseling, training, and placement services that will enable those who will be or have been forced to retire to have an opportunity for systematic, meaningful involvement in, for example, community service activities. Noninvolvement leads to rapid mental and physical deterioration. Noninvolvement deprives society of services that older persons are uniquely equipped to render.

It is hoped that the leadership provided by the authors of this book, as well as other leaders in the field of aging, will lead to a decision on the part of many educational institutions to help prepare persons to work in the field of aging. Far too many physicians and clergymen, for example, try to avoid ministering to the needs of older persons. Many medical and theological schools, by ignoring the importance of studies in the area of aging, share responsibility for such attitudes—attitudes that are in direct conflict with the concept of the dignity and worth of each individual, irrespective of age.

I believe that Dr. Butler and Ms. Lewis have made a contribution that will lead to replacing despair with hope in the lives of many older persons.

Arthur S. Flemming, *Chairman*
White House Conference on Aging

PREFACE

Much about old age is not known, but infinitely more is known than is applied. This text is being written at a time of some progress in the struggle for quality mental health care of the elderly. Isolated instances of fine care can be found in mental hospitals, medical centers, community mental health centers, nonprofit homes for the aged, and even commercial homes. But progress is still inadequate in most parts of our country. Little basic education on the nature of old age and its problems is offered in the professions of medicine, nursing, social work, and the varied mental health specialties.

Students who are otherwise humane and interested in people are likely to be uninterested, repulsed, or frightened by the thought of working with the elderly. Educators, professionals, and lay people alike react in a similar manner. Why? Part of the answer lies in a familiar national prejudice we have called *ageism*. Ageism is a systematic stereotyping of and discrimination against people because they are old, just as racism and sexism accomplish this in relation to skin color and gender. Old people are categorized as senile, rigid in thought and manner, garrulous, and old-fashioned in morality and skills; and a multitude of other labels are applied. Ageism allows the younger generations to see older people as different from themselves; thus they subtly cease to identify with their elders as human beings. Mental and physical health problems can be more easily ignored, as can the frequently poor social and economic plight of older people. However, an added factor in ageism causes uneasiness. Unlike racists and sexists, who never need fear change in their skin color or gender, ageists are at least dimly aware that if they live long enough they too will end up being "old"—the object of their own prejudice—and the ageists' attitudes turn into self-hatred. Where does ageism come from? There are many cultural influences, ranging from a productivity-minded society that places little value on the nonproducers to a thinly disguised attempt to avoid the personal realities of human aging and death. The traditional buffers of religious beliefs are in a process of challenge and change. No generally accepted ethical or philosophical system has yet evolved to deal with human life and death as a whole. So the individual fills the frightening vacuum with a self-protective prejudice that makes old people its victims. As is often the case with prejudice, the victims tend to believe the negative definition of themselves, and old people may accept and expect the treatment they receive—hardly a condition for sound mental health.

Ageism plays an important role in the generally negative opinion about mental health care in old age. In this text we hope to dispel some of the traditional diagnostic and treatment myths. We shall be discussing normal healthy aging versus mental illness in old age, age-related problems versus lifelong problems, and endogenous (inside—i.e., personality) versus exogenous (outside

—i.e., environmental) problems. Contrary to popular belief older people can change, they can use treatment, and they often do improve as a result of care. Individual and group psychotherapy should always be considered rather than automatically ruled out. "Senility" is an overused and inaccurate term. Old people need freedom—encouragement to move in new directions; autonomy and independence are precious commodities for them. "Identity" needs to be flexible so that individuals are not trapped in a fixed role or view of themselves. The physical, social, cultural, and economic aspects of people's lives will be considered intricately woven into their mental conditions.

In providing information about old age, we do not espouse such fields as geriatric psychiatry, geriatric psychology, and geriatric social work. Mental health specialties must of course include the significant emotional aspects of old age, but we feel this information should be part of a core therapy of the life cycle of man rather than a separate entity. Some specialization is inevitable; some research foci are desirable; but excessive specialization is fragmentation, pure and simple, and more comfortable for the provider of mental health care than for those receiving services. Mental health specialists should be responsible for persons of all ages, races, socioeconomic classes, and diagnostic categories if they are to function in a flexible, useful manner. The swing toward specialization has focused attention on particular problem areas, but now we see the need for a gathering together: a focusing on the individual from birth through death in a coherent manner. Old people are first of all people, like everyone else, with old age being a developmental stage of their ongoing lives. We seem to forget that people are alive until they actually die.

The mental health specialists we will be referring to include all of the people who contribute to the mental health care of the elderly in various settings. Nurses aides, nursing assistants, technicians, and paraprofessionals are as vital to care as psychiatrists, social workers, psychologists, and registered nurses. All function interdependently and even in some cases interchangeably. Homemakers and community aides and physical, recreational, and occupational therapists are included, as well as administrators and the nonpsychiatric staff of treatment institutions. Clergymen, policemen, and lawyers are surprisingly involved in the lives of mentally ill old people. The elderly receive psychiatric care in public clinics and hospitals, foster care homes, nursing homes, and health maintenance facilities. If they can afford it, they go to private practitioners, private hospitals, and counseling agencies. A myriad of services closely affect the mental health of old people—welfare agencies, food stamp programs, Social Security and Medicare, health insurance companies, churches, public transportation, police protection, and pharmacists. The absence, presence, and style of functioning of any of these can greatly influence emotional well-being or cause stress.

We are particularly concerned about the training institutions and programs that produce mental health specialists—schools of medicine, social work, or nursing, departments of psychology, and mental health training courses. Negative predilections about the elderly may become solidified as students see the problems of old age given short shrift in classroom curricula. We have heard and seen grossly inaccurate material presented by otherwise well-trained educators. Nobody wants the field work placements in old age homes or training duty on geriatric wards. Old people are written off as untreatable and depressing. Research, when it is done, is too often aimed at lengthening life rather than making life satisfying, dignified, or at least bearable. In our view, the study of late life is a natural and valuable part of an understanding of human beings. Treatment of mental health problems of older people is not only mandatory, but often productive.

In our writing, we have aimed for a down-to-earth, practical approach which, nonetheless, points to an ideal not yet attained. We have made a deliberate effort to write in a straightforward style, avoiding jargon while at the same time introducing the basic terminology of the field. We hope that both professional and lay readers will find the book useful in their understanding of old people.

We acknowledge first the many elderly people with whom we have collaborated in care and research. Through their questions, and those of medical, social work, and nursing students, as well as allied health professionals, we have been forced to think through our understanding of the nature of older people and their problems.

Certain people have directly contributed to this book. Jean Jones, Librarian of the American Psychiatric Association, was a great aid to us. Helen Zeidler has served as research assistant. Monte Vanness, Cindy Hamilton, and Nancy Schwartz have typed the manuscript.

We are especially indebted to Dr. William A. Reid and to Shirley Ford, Magnolia Burton, and Irving Williams, of the Parkside–Arthur Capper Community Mental Health Team in Washington, D. C.

We wish to give special recognition to the contributions of the Committee on Aging of the Group for the Advancement of Psychiatry: Drs. Charles M. Gaitz, Alvin I. Goldfarb, Lawrence F. Greenleigh, Maurice E. Linden, Prescott W. Thompson, Montague Ullman, and Jack Weinberg.

We are grateful to our critical readers: Frances M. Carp, Ph.D., Institute of Urban and Regional Development, Berkeley, California; James Carter, M.D., Department of Psychiatry, Duke University Medical Center, Durham, North Carolina; Arlene Hynes, Librarian, St. Elizabeths Hospital, Washington, D. C.; Hobart C. Jackson, M.S.S., Administrator, Steven Smith Home for the Aged, Philadelphia, Pennsylvania, and Chairman, National Caucus on the Black Aged; Jean Jones, Librarian, American Psychiatric Association, Washington, D. C.; Leslie S. Libow, M.D., Mt. Sinai City Hospital Center, Elmhurst, New York; Marjorie F. Lowenthal, Professor and Director, Adult Development Research Program, Langley Porter Neuropsychiatric Institute, San Francisco, California; Robert Morris, Ph.D., Professor of Social Planning, Florence Heller Graduate School, Brandeis University, Waltham, Massachusetts; Dorothy V. Moses, R.N., Professor of Nursing, School of Nursing, San Diego State College, San Diego, California; Bernice L. Neugarten, Ph.D., Professor and Chairman, Committee on Human Development, University of Chicago, Chicago, Illinois; Helen Padula, ACSW, State of Maryland Department of Mental Hygiene, Baltimore, Maryland; Ollie A. Randall, Ph.D., Social Work, New York, New York; William A. Reid, M.D., Psychiatrist and Director, Parkside–Arthur Capper Community Mental Health Team, Washington, D. C.; George Roby, M.S.W., Division Chief, Adult Services, Washington, D. C.; Sheldon S. Tobin, Ph.D., School of Social Work, University of Chicago, Chicago, Illinois; Montague Ullman, M.D., Director, Community Mental Health Center, Maimonides Medical Center, Brooklyn, New York; Arthur Waldman, M.A., Administrator, Philadelphia Geriatric Center, Philadelphia, Pennsylvania; Jack Weinberg, M.D., Clinical Director, Illinois State Psychiatric Institute, Chicago, Illinois; and George Wolfe, M.S., Social Work, Takoma Park, Maryland.

Robert N. Butler
Myrna I. Lewis

CONTENTS

PART I

The nature and problems of old age

1

WHO ARE THE ELDERLY?

The presenting psychiatric symptoms of three elderly people are discussed briefly in the following paragraphs.

Mr. K is a black man, age 66. He has come to a psychiatric hospital on his own, stating that he is depressed and has recently felt almost uncontrollable impulses to harm others. Occasionally he worries that he is being followed, his phone tapped, his food tampered with. He appears in poor health and underweight, although dressed neatly and appropriately. He lives with a 68-year-old widowed sister in two rented rooms; he was married and separated years ago and has only occasional contact with his children, who have moved away. He has been employed regularly all his life in a variety of jobs, from service station attendant to cook in a hamburger shop. Two years ago he was forced to stop work because of ill health, but his sister is still employed as a housekeeper. Income is minimal. He responds to a black nursing assistant at the hospital with an outpouring of his feelings of anger and bewilderment but becomes passive and vague in the presence of both black and white male resident physicians.

Are Mr. K's psychiatric symptoms due to his personality characteristics and early history? Or could a physical disease condition be affecting his personality? What part may be played by malnutrition? Is he underweight because he is either physically sick or psychologically unable to care for himself, or is it because he has almost no money for food from month to month? Is his depression an acute reaction to physical illness or a lifelong response to social conditions? Why does he speak to the nursing assistant but turn silent at the sight of doctors? Why does he seem to have so little retirement income?

Mrs. P, white, age 88, has become disoriented and wanders out on the streets at night. After neighbors called the Community Mental Health Center, a psychiatrist–social worker team made a home visit. Mrs. P's husband died fifteen years previously, and she has been living alone in a home they purchased fifty years ago in the central part of the city. Her income is higher than that of most widows. The home was orderly but badly in need of repair. The heat had been turned off by the gas company. Mrs. P's hearing had deteriorated. She expressed a terror of intruders and had armed herself with a stick and a kitchen knife. She determinedly announced she would never leave her home.

Why is she living alone in a big house and why has she allowed the home to deteriorate and the gas to be shut off? Is her disorientation caused by poor health, isolation due to hearing loss, or lack of a proper diet? Is her fear of intruders exaggerated or realistic in her neighborhood? What has she been doing with her money, since she appears to have very little food? Should she be moved forcibly to a nursing institution, or is there some way to help her remain at home?

Mr. H is a white man, age 70. He has contacted a private psychiatrist because he is feeling suicidal. He is well off financially, lives with his wife, but feels increasingly upset and self-destructive. He retired as a college professor earlier in the year. His health is good but recently he has panicked because he feels his memory is failing.

Is Mr. H overreacting to a minor memory change? If so, why is this so upsetting to him? Or does he perhaps have an undiagnosed chronic brain syndrome? Are suicidal thoughts rare for a man his age?

Each of these elderly persons came to the attention of mental health personnel with psychiatric symptoms. But, as is obvious, evaluation of the symptoms requires an understanding of the person's entire life situation—his physical status, personality, family

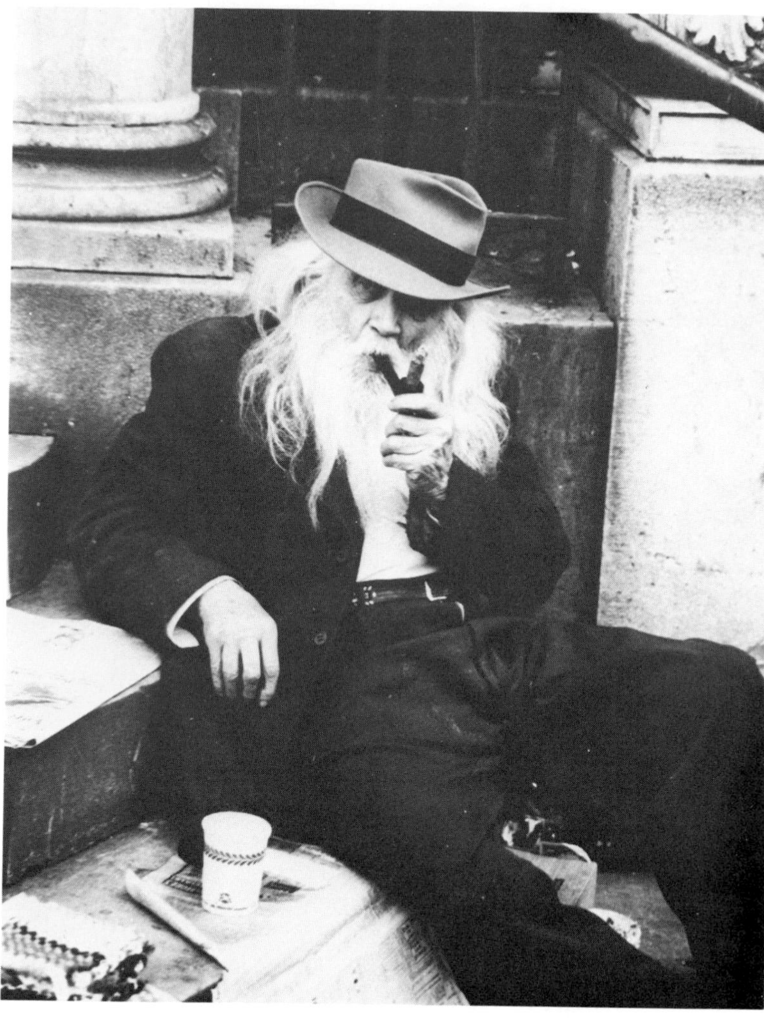

What is old age?
Photo by David Spilver.

history, racial background, income, housing, social status, educational level. Realistic and appropriate treatment is greatly facilitated by a fairly sophisticated understanding of both social and psychological phenomena. We shall therefore in this chapter give an overview of the environmental realities of the elderly in order to provide a general background for our later discussion of the more specific aspects of mental health care of the elderly.

WHAT AGE IS CONSIDERED "ELDERLY"?

Aging, of course, begins with conception. The selection of age 65 for use as the demarcation between middle and old age is an arbitrary one, borrowed from the social legislation of Chancellor Otto von Bismarck in Germany in the 1880s. This definition of old age has been adhered to for social purposes—as a means for determining the point of retirement or the point of eligibility for various services available to the elderly. But the age of 65 has little relevance in describing other aspects of functioning such as general health, mental capacity, psychological or physical endurance, or creativity. Gerontologists have attempted to deal with this unreliable concept of "oldness" after 65 by dividing old age into two groups: early old age, 65 to 74 years, and advanced old age, 75 and above. But the obvious point is that age is a convenient yet frequently inaccurate indicator of a person's physical and mental status and must not be relied on with too much zeal for evidence about human beings.

NUMBER OF ELDERLY IN THE UNITED STATES

Total elderly population

In the United States there are now some 20 million people who are age 65 or older. In this group of elderly persons 10 million are over 73 years of age; 1 million are 85 or over. And more than 106,000 are over 100 years of age. All of these totals have risen dramatically during this century. In 1900 the average human life-span was 47 years, and only 4% of the population were 65 and older.* The high rate of infant mortality was a substantial influence in the low life expectancy. Today with improved public health measures, especially in sanitation, and with a reduction in infant mortality, the average life expectancy has increased to 71 years. The elderly now represent nearly 10% of the population and the percentage is expected to increase further in response to new medical discoveries, improved delivery of health care, and the presently declining birth rate.

Men versus women

A marked difference exists between the life expectancies of men and women. Older women numbered more than 11 million in 1970, compared to more than 8 million men. For every 100 persons over 65, 57 are women and 43 men. Women outlive men every place in the world where women no longer perform hard physical labor and where adequate sanitation and a reduced maternal mortality are present. In the United States in 1970 there were 105.5 females per 100 males in the total population. More

*The sharp increase in survival has had many profound social consequences; for example, when marriage was made a sacrament in the ninth century A.D. the prospect of marriage lasting into the couple's forties was small. The concepts of retirement and late-life leisure were rudimentary at best.

Table 1-1. Number of females per 100 males by age

Age in years	Females per 100 males
Under 25	98.4
25 to 44	104.7
45 to 64	109.1
65 and over	138.5
65 to 74	128.8
75 and over	156.2

Source: Herman B. Brotman, Administration on Aging, Department of Health, Education, and Welfare.

boy babies were born than girls, and boys continue to outnumber girls until age 18. At this point a shift occurs. In the older population, where women outnumber men by 3 million, there are 135 women for every 100 men. The ratio changes from 120 per 100 for ages 65 to 69 to more than 160 per 100 at age 85 and over.

The life expectancy of a baby boy born in the United States in 1970 is 67 years and that of a baby girl is 74 years, seven years longer. In 1970, for people who are already 65 years old, life expectancy is fifteen additional years, again with a differential between men (thirteen years) and women (sixteen years).*

Black versus white

The number of the black elderly has risen from 1.2 million in 1960 to 1.6 million in 1970. They now constitute 7.8% of the total black population. Black people have a lower life expectancy than white, resulting, we can safely assume, from the generally lower socioeconomic status accorded to blacks in the United States. Table 1-2 shows death rates by age, race, and sex. Although comprising more than 10% of the total population, black people make up only 8% of the older age group. The effects of institution-

*One must remember that the individual's life expectancy at birth is not the same as when he reaches 65.

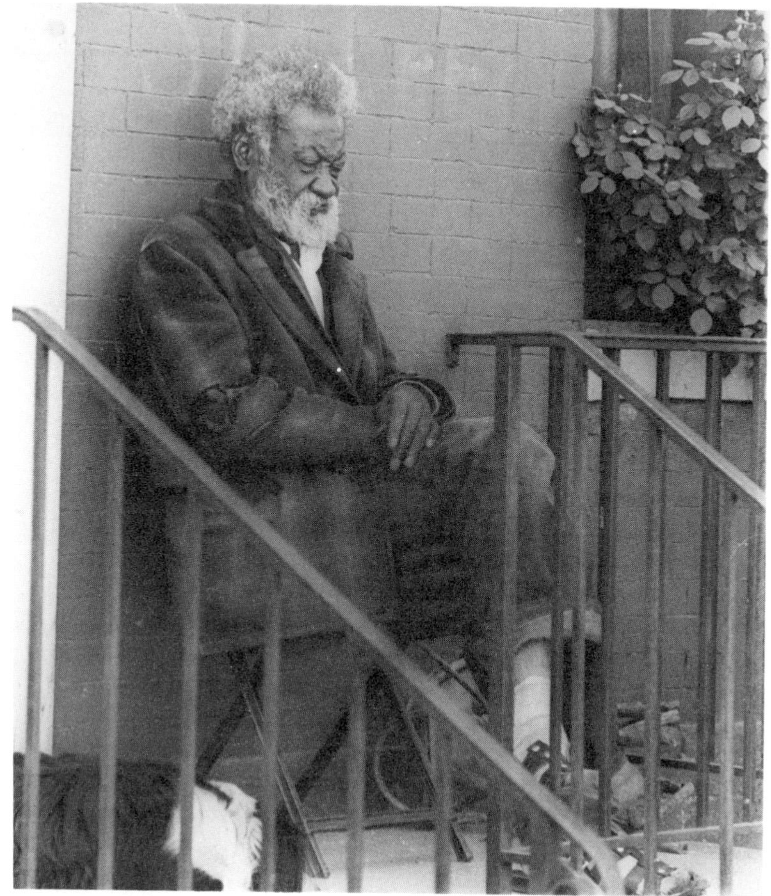

Black old age.

Photo by Harold Grandy of the New Thing Art and Architecture Center, Washington, D. C.

Table 1-2. Death rates by age, race, and sex, 1969 (rate per 1,000 population in specified group)*

	Male		Female	
	Black†	White	Black†	White
All ages	11.2	10.9	8.0	8.2
Under 1 year	35.3	21.2	28.7	16.4
1 to 4	1.4	0.7	1.1	0.7
5 to 14	0.7	0.5	0.4	0.3
15 to 24	3.0	1.7	1.1	0.6
25 to 34	5.0	1.7	2.4	0.9
35 to 44	9.2	3.4	5.2	2.0
45 to 54	16.4	8.9	9.9	4.6
55 to 64	32.1	22.2	20.7	10.2
65 to 74	67.0	48.8	46.2	25.2
75 to 84	83.5	98.8	58.8	67.2
85 and over	102.3	204.8	96.5	196.4

Source: Research Department, National Urban League, based on U. S. Public Health Service data.
*Estimated.
†Includes other nonwhite.

alized racism fall most heavily on black men —their life expectancy of 60.1 years is seven and one-half years less than that of white men, and in addition it has been *declining* (a drop of one full year between 1960 and 1970). The life expectancy of white men is 67.5 years and has remained stable since 1960. White and black women both have gained a year during the same time span with life expectancies of 74.9 and 67.5, respectively, but there remains a seven and one-half year difference between them. At age 75 a reversal occurs in which blacks begin to show a greater survival rate than whites. The explanation for this is unclear but it appears to be a "survival of the strongest" phenomenon in which the weak die early and only the strongest blacks survive. It is postulated that aged whites receive better care and thus more of the weak survive, to die at a greater rate later on.

Black elderly women outlive black men to an increasing degree, as do their white counterparts. The ratio of black women per 100 black men has increased from 115.0 in 1960 to 131.0 in 1970, and black females make up 56.7% of the total black aged population.

MARITAL STATUS

In looking at the marital situation of the elderly, one fact becomes strikingly clear. Most elderly men are married; most elderly women are widows. One finds at least three times as many widows as widowers. Two thirds of all older women are widows. This imbalance of women versus men, due to a combination of the greater female life expectancy and the fact that most women are younger than their husbands to begin with, represents one of the most poignant problems of the aged. Old men, if they survive, have greater options maritally. Chances are their wives are younger and will outlive them. But if not, the man can quite freely find a second wife. The odds are with him. There are many women to choose from. It is socially acceptable for a man to find a wife in either his own age group or any of the younger age groups. An older woman, however, is looked upon with disdain if she marries someone much younger. Each year some 35,000 older men marry, while for women the comparable figure is only 16,000, even though women in the age group outnumber men by 3 million. Table 1-3 details the aged population in terms of marital status.

Table 1-3. Distribution of the aged population by marital status

Marital status	Total	Men	Women
Total	**100**	**41**	**59**
Single	6	2	4
Married	36	24	12
Widowed	56	14	42
Divorced	2	1	1

Source: Herman B. Brotman, Administration on Aging, Department of Health, Education, and Welfare.

There is a larger number of older blacks than whites who do not live with their spouses. This has been attributed to the greater economic pressures on families, including public welfare laws that encourage black men to leave home early in life. The shorter life expectancy of black men also is an important factor, leaving a black woman widowed much earlier than a white woman.

HOUSING STATUS

With whom do the elderly live?

One of the more prevalent myths about old people is that large numbers of them live in institutions: chronic disease hospitals, homes for the aged, nursing homes, mental institutions, foster homes, etc. If one asks any group of ordinary citizens—or for that matter a group of medical, nursing, or social work students—what percentage of old people live in such settings, the answers will range all the way up to 50%. The reality is that at one time only 5% of all older people are in such institutions. This is, of course, a substantial number of people and rightly deserves serious attention. But it is important to remember that 95% of the aged are on their own in the community, living either

Table 1-4. Distribution of the aged population by living arrangements

Living arrangements	Total	Men	Women
Total	**100**	**42**	**58**
Living in a family	67	33	34
Head of a family household	36	30	6
Male head with wife present	29	29	0
Wife of head	19	0	19
Relative of family head	22	6	16
Living alone or with nonrelatives	28	7	21
Alone, head of household	26	6	20
With nonrelatives	2	1	1
Living in an institution	5	2	3

Source: Herman B. Brotman, Administration on Aging, Department of Health, Education, and Welfare.

by themselves or (more often) with a spouse, family, or friends. Out of every 10 older Americans, 7 live in families. Approximately one fourth live alone or with nonrelatives. Again the situation differs with regard to men and women. Men, because of their shorter life-span, usually live with a spouse and/or family. But only one third of women do so. Women are three times more likely to live alone or with nonrelatives. Table 1-4 provides data covering the distribution of the elderly according to their living arrangements.

In reference to the black elderly population, another widely held idea bears a more thoughtful look. It has been frequently stated that old black people are more likely to live in extended families than are the white elderly. Yet in 1960, 50.2% of black people 60 years of age and above lived alone or with only one other person, relative or nonrelative; 16% lived entirely alone. One study found that 11 of every 100 older blacks had no living relatives, compared to 6 out of 100 whites with no relatives. It is true that the black elderly are more likely than the white to have people other than spouses living with them: 20% of blacks, as compared to 12.5% of whites, had other persons in their households besides a husband and wife. We can surmise that this is due to economic necessity, which solidified in a cultural style of living earlier in the life cycle. Data contrasting men and women show that half of all black elderly men live with their wives but, again due to a longer life-span, only one fifth of black elderly women live with their husbands.

Geographical distribution

Old people, both black and white, live most frequently in central parts of cities and in rural locations.* The Midwest and upper New England areas have concentrations of older people because many of the young have left the farms. Florida has the highest proportion of elderly, with 13.2% of its population comprised of older residents. Iowa, Kansas, Maine, Massachusetts, Nebraska, New Hampshire, South Dakota, and Vermont all have greater than the national average of older people. New York State has almost 2 million older residents while California, Illinois, and Pennsylvania have more than 1 million each. A surprising observation is that New York City, on its own, has about 1 million elderly, or one twentieth of the country's entire elderly population. The highest growth in percentage from 1960 to 1965 has been found in Arizona, Nevada, Florida, Hawaii, and New Mexico—all being states with warm climate and low industrialization, which old people find appealing.

The black elderly again show a somewhat different configuration than old people as a whole. Three fifths still reside in the South,

*There are relatively few suburban elderly but it is projected that twenty years from now the suburbs may be predominately elderly.

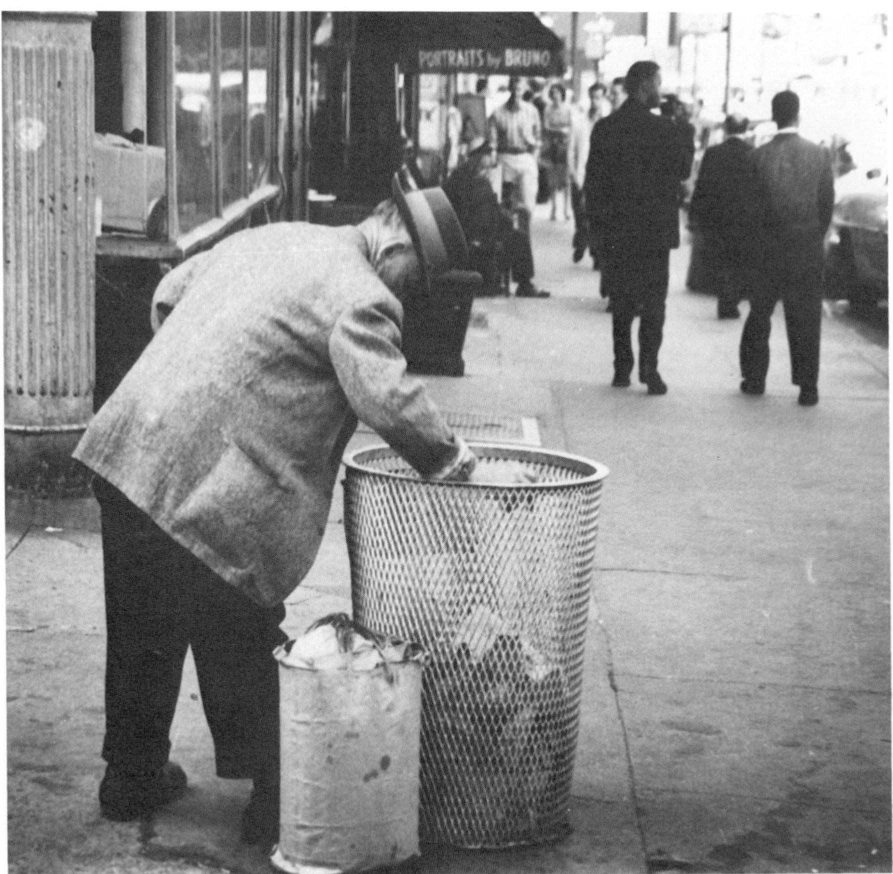

The extent of poverty in old age.

Photo by David Spilver.

many in rural areas. But because large numbers moved to urban areas in the black rural-to-urban migrations of the early 1900s, elderly blacks are now also concentrated in central cities, primarily those areas with the worst housing. Many are trapped there under the dual influence of economic hardship and a continuing racism that preserves the suburban areas for whites. One must add that the suburbs often welcome only whites with adequate finances and acceptable credentials. Public housing and housing for the elderly, the mentally ill, or addicted whites are fought with the same vehemence as black or integrated housing. The black elderly increasingly share the inner city with younger blacks and those elderly whites who cannot afford to leave. The District of Columbia is an example of this phenomenon, with a population which in 1970 was 71.8% black. Old black people accounted for 11% of this total black population. Of the approximately 70,000 elderly in the nation's capital in 1971, 57% were white and 43% black, obviously a complete reversal from the younger population, which contains proportionately many more blacks. Younger whites have tended to move to the surrounding suburbs.

Standards of housing

It has been estimated that up to 30% of the elderly in the United States live in substandard housing. This is largely a result of outright poverty or marginal income. Two thirds of all old people own their own homes. However, most of these homes were purchased in early adulthood forty to fifty years before, and many have become substandard. The cost of maintenance, utilities, and property taxes has so skyrocketed (for example, an average 30% increase between 1963 and 1969) that upkeep and needed improvements become impossible for old people on fixed incomes. The remaining one third of the elderly live, either alone or with relatives or friends, in retirement villages, rented tenements, retirement hotels, low- and middle-class government-subsidized housing, or housing sponsored by unions, churches, and benevolent associations. Some old people live in public housing, which is often seen by them as a highly desirable resource in view of the wretched alternatives available. Finally, many old people are so poor they cannot afford even public housing.

An example of this is the situation that came to light in the Washington, D. C., newspapers in 1970 when several people (one of them elderly) were found to be living in a shelter made of cardboard and scraps. They had been living there for months, in sight of the Capitol.

An essential concern for people on fixed income is the percentage that they must use for housing. Many of the 1 million elderly in New York City were surviving because of rent controls that maintained rents at a fixed rate until a tenant moved. In 1971 the state government removed rent control, leaving the elderly stranded with increasing rents.

INCOME

Extent of poverty

Poverty, like substandard housing, is typically associated with old age. People who were poor all their lives can expect to become poorer in old age. But they are joined by a multitude of people who become poor only after becoming old. Using the official 1970 poverty index of $1,852 yearly per person 65 and over (which many believe to be a stringent, unrealistic estimation of living expenses), more than one out of every four older people live below the poverty line. Thus in 1968, 4.7 million elderly lived officially in poverty. Although old people represent only 10% of the total population, they constitute 20% of the poor in America. The number of poor in the 65-plus age group increased by 200,000 from 1968 to 1969. Of the elderly poor, 85% are white.* There are clearly many more poor whites in actual numbers than blacks. However, a greater proportion of the black aged are poor and their poverty is more profound. In 1970 one half of the black aged were poor, compared to not quite one fourth of the white aged. Of all black aged females (the poorest of the poor), 47% have incomes under $1,000 yearly. We maintain that, according to a more realistic definition of poverty, 7 million of our aged live in extreme privation. In addition, in January of 1971 half of the elderly, or 10 million, lived on less than $75 a week, or *$10 per day*. The median income in 1968 for an older family was $4,592, while for an older person living alone or with nonrelatives, the figure was $1,734 yearly. Most of this money must go for food, shelter, and medical expenses—the essentials of existence. Thus the shortage of money has given rise to the old myth that the aged can live on less because they do not need as much for clothing, transportation, entertainment, recreation, or education as the young. The truth is simply that the elderly are not able to afford these items, which for younger people are considered necessary for mental health, social status, avoidance of isolation, and growth of the individual.

Middle and upper incomes

There are, of course, some middle- and upper-class elderly. Not all the old are poor. But, as we have seen, the gay rich widow is rare. In 1970 there were 7.2 million families headed by persons over 65; of these, only one fourth, or about 1.8 million, had incomes in excess of $9,000 per year.

Approximately 15% of the income of the elderly derives from accumulated assets. Those who clip coupons or collect rents are not penalized by offsetting reductions in So-

*A little-known example of poverty among whites is that found among the Jewish elderly. In Los Angeles alone a recent study found 8,000 elderly Jewish poor on public assistance and another 10,000 eligible who had not applied.

cial Security. Since 20 million older Americans are included in the population, it is extraordinary that only 179,000 families with heads of household over 65 have incomes of $25,000, even after lifetimes of work. In addition, 23,000 elderly people who are living alone or with nonrelatives have incomes over $25,000.

Sources of income

The elderly earn 29% of their aggregate income from continuing employment, while 52% comes from retirement and welfare programs, and the remainder from investments and contributions from relatives. It is commonly believed that the old are adequately provided for by Social Security and Medicare. But both of these have not met the needs of the elderly. In early 1971 the average Social Security benefits amounted to $118 per month.* Many unskilled jobs, held primarily by blacks and women, were not covered until recently. Even now, some employees (for example many domestic workers) are not covered. Medicare too needs improvements. Only 45% of the health expenses of elderly persons are met; the rest must be paid for out of their incomes. Hearing aids, glasses, dental care, podiatry, and various drugstore supplies are among items of obvious importance to old people, which are not covered under Medicare.

EMPLOYMENT

Employment should ideally be a matter of choice after age 65. Indeed old people do earn 29% of their income. But their ability to work is hampered by two major factors: the Social Security ceiling on earnings (which says in effect that an old person is allowed only a small amount of earnings, for if he earns more his Social Security check is reduced) and age discrimination in employment (both arbitrary retirement and bias against hiring older people). In addition, educational and technological obsolescence and the possible physical limitations of the elderly combine to squeeze them out of the job market. Since 1900 the number of older men in the labor force has dropped from two thirds to one fourth. On the other hand, women workers have increased from 8% in 1900 to 10% in 1970 because of the increased inclination of women to seek work outside the home.

Black aged men participate in the labor force in the same proportions as whites; but they earn less, do harder physical work, and are in poorer health (again remember that they die an average of seven and a half years sooner than white males). Black elderly women are more likely to work than white women, indicating their greater need to support themselves or supplement their husband's earnings. They, like black men, earn less, usually doing domestic and service work. Retirement by choice is less of an option because blacks' retirement benefits are often meager, in line with their previous low earnings. Indeed there may be no benefits at all. When they can no longer work, the black elderly are simply mustered out of the labor market. They frequently must turn to Old Age Assistance (OAA) as the only income source available. Thus OAA programs have a disproportionate number of aged blacks on their rolls, compared to whites, and it is important to understand why.

HEALTH

It is obvious that old people get sick more frequently than the young. Yet 81% move about on their own legs, and only 5% are confined to institutions for physical or emotional care. In 86% there are chronic health problems of one kind or another that require more frequent doctors' visits, more and longer hospital stays (an average of fourteen days per year), as well as more periods of illness at home, and result in more physical and emotional disability. In 1968 the per capita expenditure by the elderly for health care was $590, considerably greater than that required by the average person in the United States.

The mental health needs of the elderly are substantial. Emotional and mental illnesses

*Figures here predate the late 1972 Social Security Amendments, which included a 20% rise in benefits.

escalate over the course of the life cycle. Depression in particular rises with age, and suicide attains its peak in white men in their eighties. The suicide curves of white women and black men and women rise in the middle years and then decline. Depression and hypochondriasis commonly accompany the many physical ailments of old age, which range from cardiovascular disease to arthritis and hearing loss.

Organic brain disorders show increased incidence in old age. The elderly used to make up as much as 25% of all public mental hospital admissions, prior to recent efforts—at times precipitous and unfortunate—to reduce admissions.

EDUCATION

In a society where formal schooling is the key to power and status, most old people cannot compete with the young. Only 6% are college graduates, while one seventh (3 million) are functionally illiterate, with either no schooling or less than five years. No more than one half have completed elementary school. Blacks have greater illiteracy than whites but the problem of little formal education is a shared one. Our society pays little heed to experience, the "school of hard knocks," or informal education. Thus the elderly are left with their accrued body of knowledge and understanding locked within themselves, unsought and unavailable to others.

POLITICAL POTENTIAL

The potential political strength of the elderly is likely to prove to be one of the "sleeper" surprises of future politics. Almost 90% are registered to vote and two thirds vote regularly, many more than in any other age group. It remains for old people to organize themselves for political action and influence. There is even now a growing restlessness and militancy among the old for "senior power." Along with political strength can come a new sense of self-respect and a respect from others that will not be dependent on solicitude but will be a sober recognition of power at the ballot box on public issues.

MEXICAN-AMERICAN (CHICANO) ELDERLY

Little is really known about our second-largest minority. Statistical estimates of 1960 suggest that the total Mexican-American population numbers anywhere from 3.5 to 6 million people. About 80% live in urban areas, primarily in five southwestern states—Arizona, California, Colorado, New Mexico, and Texas. The elderly make up an estimated 4% of the Mexican-American population. Life expectancy is low. For example, in Colorado the life-span of the Mexican-American is 56.7 years in comparison to 67.5 for other Colorado residents. This is much lower than that for whites and even substantially lower than the blacks'. In addition to poverty, poor housing, and lack of medical care and education, which have become our historical gift to racial minority citizens, the elderly Mexican-Americans face the turmoil of drastic changes in their traditional life styles: the young are breaking rapidly with their past, the extended family is decreasing into nuclear families, and the old are cut adrift with a rich culture and tradition that is not welcomed by anyone. A sense of personal privacy and their pride make it difficult for the elderly to ask for and accept financial or medical aid. The government's Old Age Assistance is not popular and often is unused. In addition, the elderly face a language barrier and are too frequently expected to adapt to English with no instruction rather than receiving the courtesy of translations or Spanish-speaking and Spanish-oriented services.

AMERICAN INDIAN ELDERLY

As with the Chicanos, no one really knows how many American Indians there are—an ironic comment in a nation preoccupied with statistics. In 1960 the Bureau of Indian Affairs estimated the Indian population to be about a half million.* The 1970 census counted 792,730. There are no reliable estimates as to the number of el-

*Criteria include at least one-fourth Indian blood and registration on a recognized and approved tribal roll.

derly. But with an average life expectancy of 44 years,* one third shorter than the national average, it seems a wonder that any Indians survive to be 65.

Indians are the poorest people in the land. In 1964 one half of the families had incomes of less than $2,000 per year. Three fourths had less than $3,000. Unemployment in 1967 on reservations reached 37.3%, compared with 2.3% for non-Indians. Hunger and malnutrition are constant problems. If such poverty is the rule, we can be certain the elderly are even poorer. The traditional kinship support of the family is unfeasible when the family itself has no resources. The elderly are left impoverished—particularly if their children leave the reservation.

The medical care provided by the United States Public Health Service is considered totally inadequate to care for the Indian population. It is said that service for the most part is provided only for those who manage to make it to a hospital alive. The Public Health Service has no outreach program or preventive care. Thus the elderly, along with the poor, the young, and the very sick, are at a terrible disadvantage in terms of survival on the desperate trek to the nearest medical facility.

Through all of this, some Indians do manage to survive to old age, imbued with a fierce sense of reverence for their land. To elderly Indians the physical aspect of land is an essential element in their identity and sense of belonging—this in spite of the deprivation they experience in tenaciously holding on to that land.

EAST ASIAN–AMERICAN ELDERLY†

The majority of East Asian–Americans (primarily Japanese, Chinese, Filipino, Korean, and Samoan) live in California and Hawaii as a result of immigration directly to those areas. Immigration policies have profoundly affected the lives of elderly Asian-Americans, particularly with regard to family life and male-female sex ratios. In 1960 there were 12,415 elderly Chinese over 65 years of age, about 7% of the total Chinese-American population. The figure increased to 15,000 in 1970. Males outnumbered females three to one, reflecting pre–World War II immigration laws that prohibited women and children from accompanying men to the United States. Only 27% of the elderly live with a spouse, compared to 43% for the general population of elderly. Of this particular group, 95% live in cities and two thirds have settled in San Francisco alone. The median annual income in 1959 for the elderly was $1,281, with 21.6% reporting no income at all (U. S. Census); yet only one in ten in San Francisco receives Old Age Assistance. Traditional patterns of kinship and community responsibility seem to have been damaged by the experiences of immigration and forced disruption of normal family life. Many of the elderly speak little English, thus increasing their difficulties in an alien culture.

Japanese-Americans appear to have provided their elderly with greater family support and economic security, since they were not so severely restricted from bringing their families with them upon immigrating. In 1960, 29,235 Japanese-Americans, or 6% of the total Japanese-American population, were over 65 years of age. With four men for every three women, the proportion of elderly living with a spouse was 38%. Median annual income amounted to $1,163 in 1959, with 21% reporting no income. Yet it appears that most of the elderly are adequately provided for by relatives or their own savings. Elderly Japanese men usually speak at least broken English although elderly women tend to speak only Japanese. Health surveys have found that many of the elderly of this group are physically healthy and long-lived.

The Filipino-American elderly are a small group, with 6,546 persons over 65, repre-

---

*From the National Council on the Aging. (Interestingly, the Indian Health Service placed life expectancy at 64 years in 1967, but this included only those Indians on or near a reservation.)

†Data from Kalish, R. A., and Yuen, S.: Americans of East Asian Ancestry: aging and the aged, The Gerontologist **2**:36-47, 1971; and Asian-American elderly. In White House Conference on Aging, 1971. Report on Special Concerns.

senting 3% of the total Filipino-American population. Eighty-five percent are male; however, 30% of these men live with a spouse as a result of interracial marriages. Two thirds reside in urban areas. (See Chapter 6 for further discussion.)

RURAL ELDERLY

Although 40% of the elderly live in nonmetropolitan areas, only 5% actually live on farms. The remaining 35% reside in small towns. The benefits of rural and semirural life are many: fresh air and sunshine, opportunity to play and work out of doors, a leisurely life style, lack of congestion, and friends and neighbors of long acquaintance. But there are also unfavorable features: transportation for old people can be especially difficult because of poor roads, lack of public transport, and the need to maintain private cars or rely on someone else. Medical facilities are generally inadequate, since most health care and medical services are urban-based. Many communities are without a doctor or nurse. Income levels are low; few rural people are covered by private pension plans. Social Security, employment, savings, and welfare are the usual income sources but Social Security benefits are lower in rural areas because agricultural workers and the self-employed have only recently been covered. There is a shrinking tax base, and increasing scarcity of services and loss of family members are caused by the migration of young people to cities in search of work. The rural elderly are left with rising property taxes and sales taxes to maintain communities and services. A shortage of paid jobs hampers older people in their attempts to supplement their income, and present federal programs do little to help— one third of the country's poverty is found in rural areas, but only 11% of federal Manpower funds are allocated to these areas.

• • •

We have tried to acquaint you with a general profile of America's elderly as well as to detail some specifics about the more disadvantaged minorities. Successful intervention in meeting the mental health needs of old people depends on preserving a basic awareness of the general facets of their lives while focusing attention on the unique individual and his social, economic, and familial context.

REFERENCES

Birren, James E.: Handbook of aging and the individual, Chicago, 1959, University of Chicago Press.

Brotman, Herman B.: Who are the aged: a demographic view, Institute of Gerontology, Ann Arbor, 1968, The University of Michigan–Wayne State University.

Brotman, Herman B.: Facts and figures on older Americans, Washington, D. C., 1971, U. S. Department of Health, Education, and Welfare.

Butler, Robert N.: Toward a psychiatry of the life cycle: implications of socio-psychologic studies of the aging process for the psychotherapeutic situation. In Simon, A., and Epstein, L. J., editors: Aging in modern society, Washington, D. C., 1968, American Psychiatric Association.

Comfort, Alex: The process of aging, New York, 1961, The New American Library.

Doherty, Roger P.: Growing old in Indian country. In Employment prospects of aged blacks, Chicanos, and Indians, Washington, D. C., 1971, National Council on the Aging.

Doherty, Roger P.: Mexican-Americans. . . growing old in the barrio. In Employment prospects of aged blacks, Chicanos, and Indians, Washington, D. C., 1971, National Council on the Aging.

Group for the Advancement of Psychiatry: Toward a public policy on mental health care of the elderly, Report No. 79, 1970.

Hill, Robert: The plight of aged minorities in America, paper delivered at the Symposium on Triple Jeopardy, Detroit, April, 1971, The Institute of Gerontology, The University of Michigan–Wayne State University.

Hill, Robert: A profile of the black aged, Occasional papers in gerontology series, Ann Arbor, The University of Michigan–Wayne State University. To be published.

Jackson, Jacqueline J.: Some useful information about black aged, preliminary draft prepared for the National Caucus on the Black Aged, 1971.

Neugarten, Bernice L., editor: Middle age and aging: a reader in social psychology, Chicago, 1968, University of Chicago Press.

Shanas, Ethel, and Streib, Gordon F.: Social structure and the family. Generational relations, Englewood Cliffs, N. J., 1965, Prentice-Hall, Inc.

Taskforce, Special Committee on Aging, U. S. Senate, Economics of Aging: Toward a full share in abundance, Washington, D. C., 1969, U. S. Government Printing Office.

U. S. Senate Committee on Aging: The multiple hazards of age and race: the situation of aged blacks in the United States, working paper prepared by Inabel B. Lindsay, DSW, Consultant, Washington, D. C., Sept., 1971.

Yarrow, Marian, Blank, Paul, Quinn, Olive W., Youmans, E. Grant, and Stein, Johanna: Social psychological characteristics of old age. In human aging: a biological and behavioral study, Public Health Service Pub. No. 986, 1963 (paperback reprint, 1971).

Youmans, E. Grant: Aging patterns in a rural and an urban area of Kentucky, Bull. No. 681, Agriculture Experiment Station, University of Kentucky, March, 1963.

2
HEALTHY, SUCCESSFUL OLD AGE

Old age can be an emotionally healthy and satisfying time of life with a minimum of physical and mental impairment.

Mr. S, a 76-year-old retired businessman, was spontaneous, talkative, and relevant. He had appropriate and varied affect and no sign of psychomotor retardation. When interviewed, he spoke in a frank and integrated manner about his achievements. Although some general forgetfulness was noted on his history, there was no sign of a marked intellectual decline and no memory impairments were found on the mental status examination.

He was born on a farm in central Europe, the oldest of ten children. He was already employed at age 9 and left home at age 13. He described his parents as having some problems, and stated that he felt closer to his mother but attained a greater understanding of his father as years went by. At age 23 he married and emigrated to the United States. His marriage was viewed by him as an excellent one, and his wife is in good health. After a prostatectomy at age 60, Mr. S experienced a decrease in sexual desire but continues sex relations on a less frequent basis. His relationship with children and grandchildren is satisfying, with moderate interaction. He remembers that his children's adolescent rebellions gave him a chance to look anew at his own early years.

Mr. S had made plans for his older years and continues to plan optimistically for the future. He feels concerned about death and hopes he will have a sudden death or die in his sleep. He feels some interest in religion but denies any marked change since youth. He has made out a will and arranged for a burial site.

In viewing his aging condition he shows a reasonable recognition of his capacities and limitations, with no obvious denial. He appears to have accepted his physical changes. He is no longer very active but takes walks and moves about the house and yard with regularity. He shows no history of lifelong psychopathology, and there is no evidence of new psychopathology as he ages. There is no psychological isolation, and it is deemed unlikely that he will in the future have a functional breakdown.

Mr. S is an example of an elderly person who has adapted to old age with minimal stress and a high level of morale. With old age, just as with any other age, one can learn much about pathological conditions by understanding healthy developmental processes. Unfortunately Mr. S and other healthy old people are rarely the subjects of research investigation or theoretical constructs. The study of "normal" development has seldom gone beyond early adult years, and the greatest emphasis has been on childhood. The healthy aged tend to be invisible in the psychology of human development, and this is in accord with the general public avoidance of the issues of human aging.

NEGATIVE STEREOTYPE OF OLD AGE

Few people in the United States can think of old age as a time of potential health and growth. This is partly a realistic reflection, considering the lot of many old people who have been cast aside, becoming lonely, bitter, poor, and emotionally or physically ill. American society has not been generous or supportive of the unproductive—in this case old people who have reached retirement age. But in a larger sense the negative view of old age is a problem of Western civilization. The Western concept of the life cycle is decidedly different from that of the Orient, since they derive from two opposing views of what "self" means and what life is all about. Oriental philosophy places the individual self, his life-span, and his death *within* the process of the human experience.

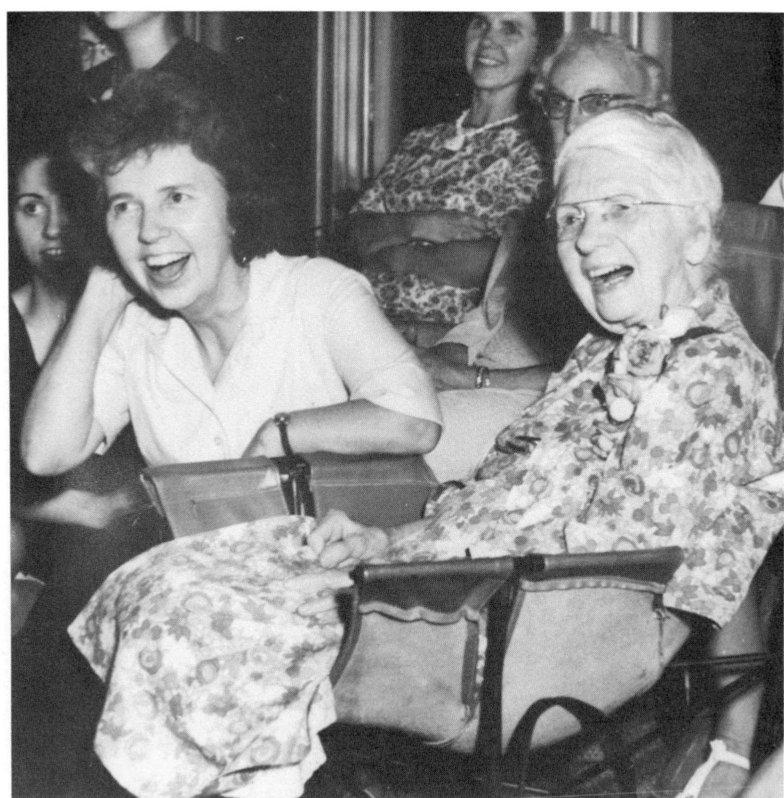

Triumphant old age.
Photo by Russell Lewis.

Life and death are familiar and equally acceptable parts of what self means. In the West, death is considered as *outside* of the self. To be a self (a person) one must be alive, in control, and aware of what is happening. The greater and more narcissistic Western emphasis on individuality and control makes death an outrage, a tremendous affront to man, rather than the logical and necessary process of old life making way for new. The opposite cultural views of East and West evolved to support two very different ways of life, each with its own merits; but the Western predilection for "progress," conquest over nature, and personal self-realization has produced difficult problems for the elderly and for those preparing for old age. This is particularly so when the national spirit of the country and the spirit of this period in time have emphasized and expanded the notion of measuring human worth in terms of individual productivity and power. Old people are led to see themselves as "beginning to fail" as they age, a phrase that refers as much to self-worth as it does to physical strength. Religion has been the traditional solace by promising another world wherein the self again springs to life, never to be further threatened by loss of its own integrity. Thus the consummate dream of immortality for Western man is fulfilled by religion while the integration of the aging experience into his life process remains incomplete. Increasing secularization produces a frightening void, which frequently is met by avoiding and denying the thought of one's own decline and death and by forming self-protective prejudices against the old.

Medicine and the behavioral sciences have mirrored societal attitudes by presenting old age as a grim litany of physical and emotional ills. *Decline* of the individual has been the key concept and *neglect* the major treatment technique. Until 1960 most of the medical, psychological, psychiatric, and social work literature on the aged was based on experience with the sick and the institutionalized even though only 5% of the elderly were confined to institutions. A few research studies that have concentrated on the healthy aged give indications of positive potential for the entire age group. But the general almost phobic dislike of aging remains the norm, with healthy old people being ignored and the chronically ill receiving half-hearted custodial care. Only those elderly who happen to have exotic or "interesting" diseases or emotional problems or substantial financial resources ordinarily receive the research and treatment attentions of the medical and psychotherapeutic professions.

WHAT IS A HEALTHY OLD AGE?

In thinking about health, one is led to the understanding that, in addition to the general lack of interest in the elderly, science and medicine have historically been more concerned with treating "what went wrong" than with clarifying the complex, interwoven elements necessary to produce and support health. Typical of this is the treating of coronary attacks after the fact rather than prescribing a preventive program of diet, exercise, protection from stress, and absence of smoking. Most of the major diseases of the elderly could be cited as examples of this same phenomenon. The tedious and less dramatic process of prevention requires an understanding of what supports or what interferes with healthy development throughout the course of the life cycle.

The World Health Organization has defined health as "a state of complete physical, mental and social well-being and not merely the absence of disease or infirmity" (WHO, 1946). This, of course, represents an ideal with many possible interpretations. But the broad elements of health—physical, emotional, and social—are the framework in which one can begin to analyze what is going well in addition to what is going wrong. The attempt must be made to locate those conditions which enable humans to thrive and not merely survive.

Old age does have unique developmental work to do. Childhood might be defined as a period of gathering and enlarging strength and experience, whereas a major developmental task in old age is to clarify, deepen, and find use for what one has already attained in a lifetime of learning and adapting. The elderly must teach themselves to conserve their strength and resources where this is necessary and to adjust in the best sense to those changes and losses that occur as part of the aging experience. The ability of the elderly person to adapt and thrive is contingent on his physical health, his personality, and his earlier life experiences and on the societal supports he receives: adequate finances, shelter, medical care, social roles, recreation, and the like. An important point to emphasize is that, as true for children, adolescents, and the middle-aged, it is imperative that old people continue to develop and change in a flexible manner if health is to be promoted and maintained. Failure of adaptation at any age or under any circumstance can result in physical or emotional illness. Optimal growth and adaptation can occur all along the life cycle when the individual's strengths and potentials are recognized, reinforced, and encouraged by the environment in which he lives.

Popular ideas of human development need revision to encompass the experience of the elderly. An old person should not have to view himself as "failing" or "finished" because one or another element of his life is changing or declining. For example, a loss in physical health or the loss of a loved one is indeed a serious blow, but the potential for continuing adjustment and growth needs therefore to be even more carefully exploited than under less critical circumstances. In our too-quick assumption that old age is a relentless downhill course we ignore the lifetime-gathered potential of the elderly for strength as well as for a richer emotional, spiritual, and even intellectual and social life than may be possible for the young. Youth must concentrate on the piece-by-piece accumulation of personality and experience. Old age, in its best sense, can mean enjoyment of the finished product—a completed human being.

BECOMING "OLD"

To attempt to clarify and disentangle what "old" means, we must emphasize that the concern here is not with those characteristics of old people which are the result of preexistent personality factors. The kind of personality one carries into old age is a crucial factor in how one will respond to the experience of being elderly; personality traits produce individual ways of being old. However, we wish to deal with the more general characteristics of old age and the changes that are fairly uniformly common to the aging population in the United States.

Physical changes

Some of the outward alterations experienced by elderly persons are graying of hair, loss of hair and teeth, elongation of ears and nose, subcutaneous fat losses, particularly around the face, skin wrinkles, fading of eyesight and hearing, postural changes, and a progressive structural decline that may result in a shortened trunk with comparatively long arms and legs. Not all of these changes happen to everyone—nor at the same rate. A person can be a "young" 90-year-old in a physical sense or an "old" 60-year-old. Little is known about the onset and progress of many of these changes, since they were long thought to be simply the inescapable and universal consequences of growing old. But recent research has revealed that some, or perhaps many, are results of disease states that occur with greater frequency in late life and may be treatable—possibly preventable and probably retardable. Atherosclerosis and osteoporosis are cases in point. Even heart disease and cancer may someday be conquered, although not many years ago someone dying of cancer was said to be dying of "old age." Other reasons for bodily changes have been identified as results of unusual amounts of exposure to some pathogenic element—too much sun (causing skin wrinkles), cigarette smoke, and air pollution, to name a few. Genetic traits can be responsible for changes like graying hair and loss of hair. Yet in the best of all future worlds, with acute and chronic disease states identified and eliminated, undesirable genetic traits nullified, and pathogenic environmental conditions removed, a process called aging will still occur. The potential for life can be lengthened and enhanced, but the mysterious flow of human existence from birth through death will prevail. As many old people realize more calmly than the young, aging and death must be accepted as part of human experience.

The overall physical health of the body plays a critical role in determining the energies and adaptive capacities available to the elderly. Old people experience a good deal more acute and chronic disease than the younger population. Specific physical disabilities and diseases such as cardiovascular and locomotor afflictions are particularly debilitating, especially when they affect the integrative systems of the body—the endocrine, vascular, and central nervous systems. Severe or even mild organic brain disease can interfere markedly with functioning. Perceptual losses of eyesight and hearing can deplete energy and cause social isolation. However, although 86% of the elderly have one or more chronic health problems, 95% are able to live in the community. Their conditions are mild enough to enable 81% of the elderly to get around with no outside assistance. If significant breakthroughs occur in research and treatment of diseases of the elderly (heart disease, cancer, arthritis, arteriosclerosis, and acute and chronic brain syndromes), one can envision a very different kind of old age. Assuming adequate environmental supports, including proper nutrition, old age could become a time of lengthy good health with a more gentle and predictable decline. The elderly would not have to battle the ravages of disease, and a fuller measure of their physical strength could be available for other uses. Already today one can see the possibilities in those elderly people who are disease-free. They can more vigorously cope with the emotional and social changes specific to their age group and in so doing have the opportunity for a successful and satisfying later life.

Emotional changes

As with physical changes, much that is associated with the more negative emotional aspects of aging is the result of disease states. Old people are often described as slow thinkers, forgetful, rigid, mean-tempered, irritable, dependent, and querulous. They may suffer from anxiety, grief, depression, and paranoid states. Yet if one were to separate out the personality traits demonstrated in earlier life, realistic responses to actual loss of friends and loved ones, and personal reactions to the idea of one's own aging and death, much of the remainder would be the predictable emotional responses of human beings at any age to physical illness or social loss. The emotional aspects of aging will be more fully discussed in Chapter 3.

Social changes

It is in the social realm of an old person's life that the most clearly age-specific patterns can presently be seen. The nature of families and societies in the course of the life cycle decrees certain conditions that can be described as "natural" for the elderly. They find themselves the eldest group in the population with two, three, or even four generations below them. Many have grown children and grandchildren with whom they are involved. Grandparentage becomes a new social role. The elderly husband and wife each face prospects of widowhood and membership in a peer group with a large proportion of widowed contemporaries. There are increasing numbers of women compared to men as they age. Many of the elderly are less involved than previously in work and income-related activities and thus have more time available for their own use.

Beyond these certain basic social conditions, the elderly experience wide variations from culture to culture.* They may be venerated or scorned, treated oversentimentally or rejected, protected or abandoned. At times they are arbitrarily respected for great wisdom and counsel or at other times, paradoxically, seen as burdens that waste their society's strength and resources. In the United States the overwhelming majority of old people face a prevailing sense of being put on the shelf and forgotten after age 65. A split and contradictory set of roles exists for elderly men, since some of them remain active in government, political parties, religious affairs, and business life. They may have strong executive and administrative responsibilities. In the United States Supreme Court, 85% of all service has been supplied by men over 65. Such opportunities exist for relatively few older men, however; and old women, because of their cultural roles as homemakers, have almost no positions of public power and status.

The feelings of social loss among the aged are tremendous. Mandatory retirement and Social Security regulations put them out of the work force when many would prefer employment. Income becomes drastically reduced, in many cases to outright poverty. The mobile nuclear family system may leave an isolated situation for households of the elderly—of whom 26% live alone and 32% with just a spouse. Children and grandchildren may live miles away and maintain infrequent contacts.† Elderly men find themselves unprepared for finding life meaningful after retirement. Elderly women, after a lifetime of being wives and mothers, can be emotionally traumatized in widowhood. Society provides few supports and little encouragement; individual old people must

*Cross-cultural studies in the psychology of later life give insights concerning universal features of aging and offer opportunities for borrowing new social and cultural arrangements.

†It must be added, however, that outright neglect or isolation from families is *not* the norm, except when geographical distances are a factor. Many families are supportive of their elderly even though they may live in separate households, which both generations may prefer.

forge their own roles—when and where they can.

Old age, then, is a multiply-determined experience that depends on an intricate balance of physical, emotional, and social forces, any one of which can upset or involve the others. An old person who is socially lonely may not eat well and therefore may develop physical symptoms of malnourishment, which in turn cloud intellectual functioning. Hearing loss can lead to a suspiciousness that irritates people and causes them to shun the person's company, leaving him isolated. A widower, grieving the loss of his wife, may develop psychosomatic symptoms and lose his job. It is evident that much suffering could be eliminated by application of knowledge and skills already available. People need to be fed and sheltered decently; they must have medical and psychiatric care; they need loving and supportive personal contacts; and finally they require meaningful social roles. Health is not really an elusive concept, but it does require that we make commitments *as* human beings *to* human beings.

HISTORICAL FACTORS IN ADAPTATION

People are shaped not only by their own personal history, family environment, and inherent personality characteristics but also by the larger world around them. So in understanding the aged it is useful to consider those factors in local, national, and world history which may have influenced them as they grew from infancy to old age.* The present 65-plus population was born around the turn of the century at a time when Herbert Spencer's social Darwinism or "survival of the fittest" was the popular social theory. Huge fortunes were amassed by families with names like Gould, Morgan, Rockefeller, and Carnegie while poorly paid immigrant workers provided labor. The Protestant ethic, inspired by Calvin's philosophy of success through hard work and self-sacrifice, was the dominant religious influence. The Labor movement and Women's Suffrage and Child Labor laws were evolving as protection against exploitation. Thus the nation had reached a crossroads between accepting the notion of survival of the strongest and attempting the protection of all, including the weak. This raw dichotomy was the earliest societal experience of the now-elderly population. Many of them still feel the tug of these forces in their personal lives and insist upon being independent in the face of real personal limitations. They often berate themselves for not being allowed or able to work, since they were taught as children that leisure and idleness are sinful. They may accept their difficult economic and social conditions as evidence that they are not among the elite, or "fittest," and thus do not deserve better. They are not as sure as their children and grandchildren are that government and social policies must be designed to serve them rather than merely those with more income, and they tend to be somewhat ambivalent about Social Security and Medicare. The massive depression of the 1930s served to propel scores of "rugged individualists" into reluctant acceptance of governmental intervention in their lives, but many emotionally felt such intervention to be evidence of personal failure rather than overwhelming social forces. Two world wars, a Korean war, and the war in Southeast Asia have made the lives of the elderly a time of frequent preparation for, participation in, or recovery from war. Many have lost children and grandchildren. They have contended with the tumultuous concept of progress through industrialization and automation and with the technological notion of human obsolescence. This has served to increase their sense of uselessness as their own skills are performed by machines and they themselves are seen as burdens.

POPULAR MYTHS ABOUT AGING

The dominance of *chronological aging* is a myth, and a more apt measure of actual age might be that old maxim "You're as old

*For an overview of the experience of today's elderly it is useful to read Barbara Tuchman's *The Proud Tower* and Frederick Lewis Allen's *The Big Change*.

as you feel." Young 80-year-olds can look very different from old 80-year-olds. It is well established that large disparities often exist between physiological, psychological, chronological, and social ages. People age at such different rates that physiological indicators show a greater range from the mean in old age than in any other age group, and people may become more diverse rather than similar as they age. Of course certain diseases have a leveling effect that causes a look-alike appearance from person to person. Massive organic brain damage and the major illnesses can so damage body and brain that their victims may react and behave very much like each other, as do invalids of all age groups. Poverty and illiteracy also tend to obscure individual uniqueness and variation.

Another widespread myth surrounding aging is the conviction that all old people are "senile." *Senility,* although not an actual medical term, is excessively used by doctors and laymen alike to explain the behavior and condition of the elderly. Many of the reactive emotional responses of old people, such as depression, grief, and anxiety, are labeled senile and thus considered chronic, untreatable states. Senility is an especially convenient tag put on old women by doctors who do not wish to spend the time and effort necessary to diagnose and treat their complaints. The popular medical school term for old people is "crocks"; thus attitudes are formed that affect future practice. To be sure, brain damage from cerebral arteriosclerosis and senile brain disease is a realistic problem, probably causing 50% of cases of mental disorder in old age. But even with brain disease there can be overlays of depression, anxiety, and psychosomatic disorders that are responsive to medical and psychotherapeutic intervention.

A third myth, the *tranquility myth,* presents a strange and contradictory position, considering the general public disdain and neglect of the elderly. This myth sets forth the sugar-coated "Grandma-with-her-goodies" vision of old age as a time of idyllic serenity and tranquility when old persons enjoy the fruits of their labors. It reminds one a little of the old cliché that poor black people really are rather happy in their discriminated-against condition and probably would not want it any other way. A combination of wishful thinking about their own future old age and denial of the realities that presently exist is evident in the younger generation's image of happy-go-lucky old people.

Mrs. G and her husband retired with an estate of a quarter of a million dollars. He had been a successful doctor in a midwestern city. Dr. G was 69 when he chose to retire and his wife was four years younger. Only two years later he was dead. Their son, age 44, died of a coronary a year afterward. Mrs. G paid many of the expenses of her son's terminal illness and also helped her daughter-in-law meet the college expenses of her grandchildren. Ten years later at 77 years of age Mrs. G, the respected and wealthy physician's wife, was herself impoverished and enfeebled. Her money had run out.

We cite this example to illustrate how people who may have entered old age in the most favorable circumstances can nonetheless be subject to major and continuing emotional and financial crises.

There is the *myth of unproductivity* associated with old age. It is assumed that older people can no longer produce on a job or be active socially and creatively. The elderly are presumed to be disengaged from life, declining and disinterested. But in the absence of disease and social adversity, this does not happen. Old people tend to remain actively concerned about their personal and community relationships. Many are still employed. The 1971 Bureau of Labor statistics show 1,780,000 people over 65 years of age employed full time and 1,257,000 employed part time. Numbers of others do "bootleg work" to avoid reporting their earnings, because of Social Security income ceilings.

The *myth of resistance to change* is equally as suspect as all the others. It is true that adult character structure is remarkably stable, but ability to change depends more on previous and lifelong personality traits than on anything inherent in old age. Often when conservatism occurs it derives not from aging, but from socioeconomic pressures. An example might be the decision of older people to vote against school loans because of the increase those loans would mean in their personal property taxes.

NEW INTERPRETATIONS OF AGING FROM RESEARCH

In attempting to gain a more realistic picture of aging, a few investigators responding to the paucity of information in this area began studying healthy old people. Community-resident and socially autonomous elderly people were examined from a wide range of research perspectives in studies beginning in the late 1950s and early 1960s. Busse was responsible for some of the first work and Shock has studied some 600 men longitudinally every eighteen months.* The National Institute of Mental Health undertook collaborative studies involving separate academic disciplines and medical specialties over a period of eleven years. The NIMH findings were surprisingly optimistic and in general reinforced the hypothesis that much of what has been called aging is really disease.

Decreased cerebral (brain) blood flow and oxygen consumption were found to be probable results of arteriosclerosis rather than an inevitable companion of aging. Healthy elderly men with an average age of 71 presented brain physiological and intellectual functions that compared favorably with those in a younger control group with an average age of 21. Some evidence of slowing in speed and response was found, but this correlated with environmental deprivation and depression as well as physical decline.

The elderly were found to have the same psychiatric disorders as the young with similar genesis and structure. Adaptation and survival appeared to be associated with the individual's self-view and sense of ongoing usefulness, as well as his continuing good physical health. Current environmental satisfaction and support were found to be of critical import to psychological stability. Individuals who were "self-starters" and could structure and carry out new contacts, activities, and involvements were found to have the least disease and the longest survival rates. The interrelating between sound health and adaptability was validated by the sensitivity of psychometric test results to even minimal disease. In general the healthy aged were characterized by flexibility, resourcefulness, and optimism, whereas manifestations of mental illness were attributed to medical illness, personality factors, and social cultural effects rather than the aging process.

SOME SPECIAL CHARACTERISTICS OF OLDER PEOPLE

A number of characteristics that one sees quite frequently in older people are connected with the unique sense of having lived a long time and having accepted the concept of life as a cycle from birth through death.

Desire to leave a legacy

Human beings have a need to leave something of themselves behind when they die. This legacy may be children and grandchildren, work or art, personal possessions, memories in the minds of others, even bodies or parts of them for use in medical training and research. Motivations for the tendency toward legacy are generally a combination of not wanting to be forgotten, of wanting to give of one's self magnanimously to those who survive, of wishing to remain in control in some way even after death (for example, through wills), of desiring to tidy up responsibly before death. Legacy provides a sense of continuity, giving the older person a feeling of being able to participate even after death.

*Longitudinal research in aging presents difficulties in methodology. When a sample is studied over a span of time, it becomes complicated to differentiate intrinsic changes from those due to environment. Greenhouse and Morrison (1971) and Schaie (1965), among others, have considered these problems.

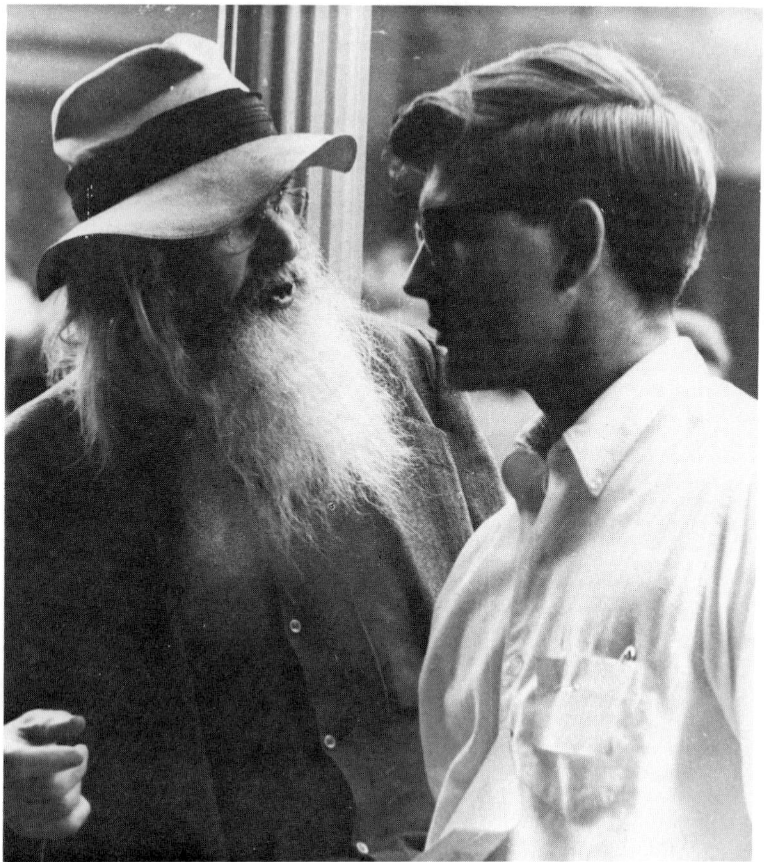

The "elder" function of old people.

Photo courtesy Jerome Lewis.

The "elder" function

Closely connected with legacy, the "elder" function refers to the natural propensity of the old to share with the young the accumulated knowledge and experience they have collected. If unhampered and indeed encouraged, this "elder" function takes the form of counseling, guiding, and sponsoring those who are younger. It is tied to the development of an interconnectedness between the generations. It is important to a sense of self-esteem to be acknowledged by the young as an elder, to have one's life experience seen as interesting and valuable; on the other hand, it can be devastating to be shrugged off by seemingly uninterested younger people as old-fashioned and irrelevant. Not all older people, however, have a nurturant feeling toward the young. Some, because of their life experience, look upon the young with envy and distrust. Mental health personnel can learn much about how to help older people by respecting and benefiting from what the elderly have to teach. This occurs through listening to them with an open mind, reading the writings of older people, viewing their arts, and hearing their music.

Attachment to familiar objects

An increasing emotional investment in the things surrounding their daily lives—home, pets, familiar objects, heirlooms, keepsakes, photo albums, scrapbooks, old letters—may be noticed. Such objects provide a sense of continuity, aid the memory, and provide comfort, security, and satisfaction. Fear of loss of possessions at death is a frequent preoccupation. Older people gen-

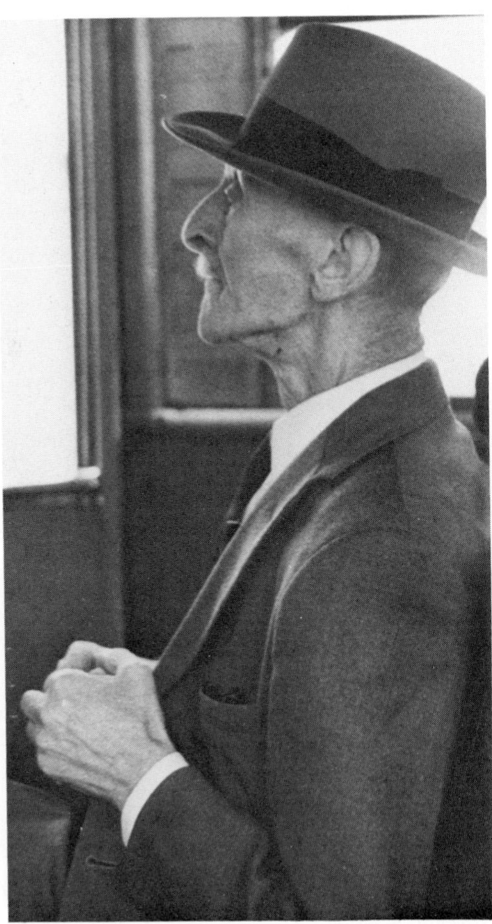

A sense of the life cycle.
Photo by David Spilver.

erally feel better if they can decide in an orderly manner how their belongings will be distributed and cared for. Younger family members or friends should take such concerns seriously, offering their help rather than denying that the older person will someday die. Possessions may have to be painfully given up before death as a result of moves from a house to an apartment, an institution, etc. Some institutions are now recognizing the value of encouraging people to bring some of their own familiar possessions with them.

Change in the sense of time

There may be a resolution of fears about time running out, with an end to time panics and to boredom, and the development of a more appropriate valuation of time. While the middle-aged begin to be concerned with the number of years they have left to live, the elderly tend to experience a sense of immediacy, of here and now, of living in the moment. This could be called a sense of "presentness." The elemental things of life —children, plants, nature, human touching, physically and emotionally, color, shape— assume greater significance as people sort out the more important from the less important. Old age, because of its natural tendencies, can be a time of emotional and sensory awareness and enjoyment.

Sense of the life cycle

Older people experience something that younger people cannot: a personal sense of the entire life cycle. We shall discuss this further in Chapter 8. There may be a greater interest in philosophy and religion, in enduring art or literature. In Japan it is common for old men to write poetry, thus giving another expression of life and its meaning. A sense of historical perspective and a capacity to summarize and comment upon one's time as well as one's life sometimes develop.

Creativity, curiosity, and surprise

Creativity does not invariably decline with age. Many persons recognized as creative have continued their work far into old age —Cervantes, Voltaire, Goethe, Tolstoi, Picasso, and Casals—to name a few. It is of course easy to name the persons of such achievement who continue to be productive in late life. But less well known is the fact that *most* old people remain productive and active in the absence of disease and social problems. Many become creative for the first time in old age, and the list does not begin and end with Grandma Moses. Factors that impede or support creativity and activity must be studied.

Curiosity and an ability to be surprised are other qualities that have a strikingly adaptive quality. Such qualities are especially attractive to younger people, who take heart and hope in them for their own old age. This type of enthusiasm probably reflects lifelong personality traits and serves the individual well in old age. Such older people are described as lively, full of life, spry, bright-eyed, and zestful.

Sense of consummation or fulfillment in life

A feeling of satisfaction with one's life is more common than recognized but not as common as possible. It is a quality of "serenity" and "wisdom," which derives from resolution of personal conflicts, reviewing one's life and finding it acceptable and gratifying, and viewing death with equanimity. One's life does not have to be a "success" in the general sense of that word in order to result in serenity. The latter can come from a feeling of having done one's best, from having met challenge and difficulty, and sometimes from simply having survived against terrible odds.

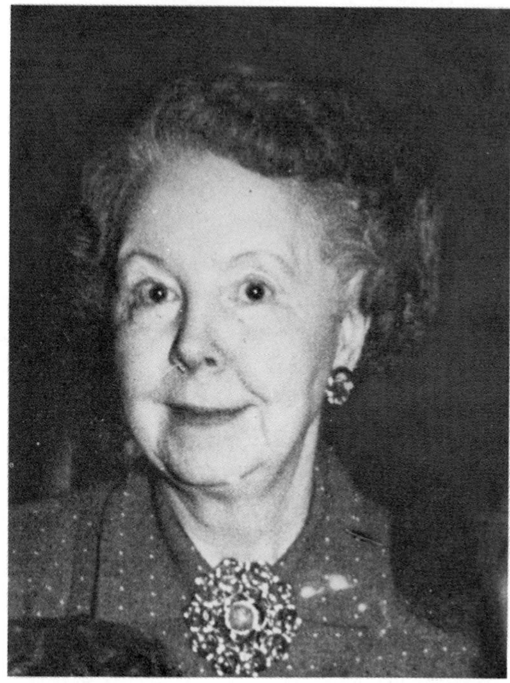

A sense of fullfillment.

MIDDLE AGE AND THE TRANSITION TO OLD AGE

An understanding of old age requires consideration of the transition from the middle years. Neugarten and Lowenthal have contributed much to the study of mid-life. Middle age is usually regarded as the period from age 40 to 65, during which most people are engaged in providing the livelihood for a family and finishing the rearing of children. The middle-aged are the people in command in society in terms of power, influence, norms, and decisions. They make up 40% of the population and carry much responsibility for the 10% who are over 65 years of age and the 50% under 25.

Two themes that predominate in mid-life are the growing awareness of personal aging (eventual death) and the changes in life patterns that occur as the middle-aged person's children grow up, his own parents grow old, and he assumes new roles personally and socially. People become aware of a different sense of time; they begin to think about how long they have left to live rather than about how long they have lived. Men are aware of the possibility of their own imminent death whereas women, who have a longer life-span and often are married to an older spouse, worry about the death of the husband. They may consciously or unconsciously prepare for widowhood.

A personal sense of death can no longer be easily denied and avoided. The death of parents leaves the middle-aged next in line. Friends and peers begin to die, unmistakable physical changes occur, one's own children reach adulthood. But the perception of death may be a matter-of-fact acceptance rather than negative fears and worries. It can lead to greater respect for and attention to one's physical health; Neugarten has called this "body monitoring": the activities undertaken to keep the body in physical condition and to care for any physical illnesses or chronic conditions that have developed. It also leads to a reassessment of one's life, a stock-taking in terms of marriage, career, personal relationships, values, and other commitments made earlier in youth. Career changes and divorces are not infrequent, and sometimes the whole way of life may be changed. Mid-life has been compared to a second adolescence—one in which people reassess, change, strike out in new directions. (A third such period may occur after retirement, when again one sees reevaluation, with new identities and directions emerging.) A conception of personal death must become consciously realized. At first this can be frightening and painful but if favorably resolved, a mature resignation frees the person from fear. Mid-life and eventually old age can then be enjoyed but with a full awareness of death, which lies beyond. Appreciations of some of the elemental things that people tend to value more highly as they age—human love and affection, insight, pleasures of the senses, nature, children—are probably a result of the restructuring and reformulation of concepts of time, self, and death.

Studies thus far seem to indicate that the majority of people adjust and adapt remarkably well to the demands and problems of middle life. But difficulties do occur and are sometimes called "mid-life crises." Middle-aged people may panic and attempt to recapture youth by adopting inappropriate dress, manners, and behavior. They may envy the young and feel inferior to them or, on the other hand, hate and disparage them. There can be an overexaggeration of body monitoring, which becomes hypochondriacal. There can be such a fear of change that people will remain in pressured or boring jobs and marriages or will leap into almost identical situations if they do decide to take action. There may be preoccupations with age and appearance and self-consciousness about how to act and relate. Depression and alcoholism tend to increase. Although the "empty nest" (when children have left home) and the menopause do not ordinarily cause serious problems for women (and indeed may bring a sense of freedom and spontaneity), both of these may become overemphasized. Sexual promiscuity in order to prove youth and attractiveness may develop, as well as increased religiosity that has a hollow and desperate ring to it. Men may be haunted by a need to "succeed." All of these represent unresolved fears of aging and attempts to deny it by trying to turn back the clock. One can see fixation, rigidity, fatalism, pessimism, or overexpansiveness.

Middle age can be and is for most people the prime of life. But it can be complicated by periods of genuine crises, ranging from the superficial and reversible to the profound and more pathological. The middle-aged person who truly wants to be young again is rare, but most would like to preserve the good health and energy that mark youth. In its best sense mid-life can become a time of increasing sensitivity, self-awareness, use of capacities and skills to the fullest, and separation of that which is valuable from the less valuable in order to use time wisely and enjoyably. It can in this sense become a healthy preparation for the transition to old age.

THE CHANGING AWARENESS OF OLD AGE

A large aged population is a new phenomenon, with the aged moving from a position of rarity to one of commonality. Old people have become more highly visible since the nineteenth century as greater life expectancy and various social and economic conditions have unfolded the life cycle, making its stages stand out in bolder relief. An example of the fast-changing nature of this age group is the fact that 70% of the present 65-plus population have joined that group since 1959. Each day there are 1,000 more older Americans; each year 365,000 more. By the year 2000, older people could make up one fourth of the total population. As their numbers grow, old people have slowly begun to be of interest to American sociologists and psychologists. G. Stanley Hall was a pioneer, writing the first major American book on the psychology of old age in 1922. Politicians have begun to grasp the value of supporting programs to benefit the elderly since they have become a major voting bloc. But the medical and psychotherapeutic professions, which come most closely in contact with old people, still have not made an active commitment to their special concerns and problems. The elderly may soon challenge this by dint of their growing self-awareness and sophisticated use of public opinion and public policy. Their increasing good health and survival rates may at last bring the elderly hope for a vital participation in a better future for themselves and all of us.

REFERENCES

Beard, Belle Boone: Social competence of centenarians, Athens, Ga., 1967, University of Georgia Printing Department.

Berezin, M. A.: Some intrapsychic aspects of aging. In Zinberg, N. E., and Kaufman, I., editors: Normal psychology of the aging process, New York, 1963, International Universities Press.

Birren, J. E.: Handbook of aging and the individual: psychological and biological aspects, Chicago, 1959, University of Chicago Press.

Birren, James E., Butler, Robert N., Greenhouse, Samuel W., Sokoloff, Louis, and Yarrow, Marian R.: Human aging, National Institute of Mental Health Pub. No. (HSM) 71-9051, 1971. (This is the paperback reprint of the work originally published in 1963.)

Bromley, D. B.: The psychology of human aging, Baltimore, 1966, Penguin Books, Inc.

Busse, Ewald W.: Therapeutic implication of basic research with the aged, Strecker Monograph Series No. 4, The Institute of Pennsylvania Hospital, 1967.

Butler, R. N.: Myths and realities of clinical geriatrics, Image and Commentary **12**:26-29, 1970.

Carp, Frances M.: Senility or garden-variety maladjustment? Journal of Gerontology **24**:203-209, 1969.

Granick, S., and Patterson, R.: Human aging, II. An eleven-year follow-up biomedical and behavioral study, National Institute of Mental Health Pub. No. (HSM) 71-9037, 1971.

Greenhouse, S. W., and Morrison, D. F.: Statistical methodology. In Human aging: a biological and behavioral study. 1963. Reprinted as Pub. No. (HSM) 71-9051, 1971.

Greenleigh, Lawrence: Timelessness and restitution in relation to creativity and the aging process, Journal of the American Geriatrics Society **8**:353-358, 1960.

Group for the Advancement of Psychiatry: Toward a public policy on mental health care of the elderly, Report No. 79, 1970.

Growing old in America: the unwanted generation, Time Magazine, Aug. 3, 1970.

Guttman, David L.: The country of old men: cross-cultural studies of the psychology of later life. In Occasional papers in gerontology, vol. 5, Institute of Gerontology, Ann Arbor, 1969, University of Michigan–Wayne State University Press.

Hall, G. S.: Senescence: the last half of life, New York, 1922, D. Appleton & Co.

Jacque, E.: Death and the midlife crisis, International Journal of Psychoanalysis **46**:502-514, 1965.

Lowenthal, Marjorie F., and Chiriboga, David: Transition to the empty nest: crisis, challenge, or relief? Archives of General Psychiatry **26**:8-15, 1972.

Neugarten, Bernice L.: Awareness of middle age. In Neugarten, B. L., editor: Middle age and aging, Chicago, 1968, University of Chicago Press.

Palmore, Erdman: Normal aging: reports from the Duke longitudinal study, 1955-1969, Durham, N. C., 1970, Duke University Press.

Schaie, K. W.: A general model for the study of developmental problems, Psychological Bulletin **64**:92-107, 1965.

Shanas, Ethel: The health of older people: a social survey, Cambridge, Mass., 1962, Harvard University Press.

Spence, D. C., Feigenbaum, E. M., Fitzgerald, Faith, and Roth, Janet: Medical student attitudes toward the geriatric patient, Journal of the American Geriatrics Society **16**:976-983, 1968.

Strehler, B. L.: Time, cells and aging, New York, 1962, Academic Press, Inc.

World Health Organization: Constitution of the World Health Organization, Public Health Report **61**:1268-1277, 1946.

3

COMMON EMOTIONAL PROBLEMS

Loss is a predominant theme in characterizing the emotional experiences of elderly people. The psychological treatment goal is obtaining insight and restitution possibilities within the limits of the life situation and individual personalty. Losses in every aspect of late life compel the elderly to expend enormous amounts of physical and emotional energy in grieving and resolving grief, adapting to the changes that result from loss, and recovering from the stresses inherent in these processes. The elderly are confronted by multiple losses, which may occur simultaneously: death of marital partner, older friends, colleagues, relatives; decline of physical health and coming to personal terms with death; loss of status, prestige, and participation in society; and, for large numbers of the older population, additional burdens of marginal living standards. Inevitable losses of aging and death are compounded by potentially ameliorable cultural devaluation and neglect.

In the complex of factors affecting subjective experience, overt behavior, and level of adaptation of the elderly, any or all of the following may be significant.

- Environmental or extrinsic factors
  - Personal losses or gains
    - Marital partners; other loved and significant figures (friends, children)
  - Social forces (losses or gains)
    - Status losses, prestige loss: in social groups other than family and as paterfamilias
    - Socioeconomic adversities: income drop, inflation
    - Unwanted retirement: arbitrary retirement policies
    - Cultural devaluation of the elderly: sense of uselessness, therapeutic pessimism, forced isolation, forced segregation
- Intrinsic factors
  - Nature of personality: character structure (defensive and integrative mechanisms), life history, survival characteristics
  - Physical diseases: disease of any organ system; perceptual decrements; sexual losses; disease of integrative systems (hormonal, vascular, and central nervous systems); brain damage; arteriosclerosis, senile dementia, etc.; physical limitations; arthritis
  - Age-specific changes (largely obscure and mysterious, but inexorable with objective passage of time)—losses of speed of processes and response; involutionary processes; others (heredity, survival qualities); changes in body size and appearance ("slipping" and "shrinkage")
  - Experience of bodily dissolution and approaching death (subjective passage of time)

Old people often are handicapped by their own bodies, which respond to challenge with less energy and strength than were formerly available, particularly if major illnesses have taken their toll. Emotionally, a rapid succession of losses can leave individuals with accumulated layers of unresolved grief along with fatigue and a sense of emptiness.* There may be little societal support for grief and mourning as the rituals of religion and custom are increasingly questioned and discarded.

---

*Goldfarb and his co-workers have reported that the dreams of older people deal with concern over diminishing resources and leave them feeling weak and vulnerable. The studies showed similar results whether the subjects were in or out of institutions: Barad, M., Altschuler, K. Z., and Goldfarb, A. I.: A survey of dreams in aged persons, Archives of General Psychiatry **4**:419-424, 1961. Altschuler, K. Z., Barad, M., and Goldfarb, A. I.: A survey of dreams in the aged. II. Noninstitutionalized subjects, Archives of General Psychiatry **8**:33-37, 1963.

It is an odd distortion of reality when the elderly are popularly depicted as weak, unassuming, gently tranquil people who passively wait out their last days. Becoming old, being old, and dying are active physical and emotional processes that test the mettle of each person. Reluctance to accord the elderly appropriate recognition for their strengths and capacities indicates a failure to understand what is required in being old. We have lost our naiveté about the carefree nature of childhood as we have developed our understanding of the difficult and frightening developmental work each child must do to grow up. But simplistic illusions about old age continue, with little conceptualization of the normative stages one must pass through in late life.* Certain dramatic events (for example, widowhood) have been more widely studied than others, but there is as yet no cohesive, reliable body of information against which one can measure adjustment patterns.

EMOTIONAL REACTIONS TO AGE-RELATED LIFE CRISES

Certain life crises occur in old age regardless of socioeconomic and cultural circumstances, as part of the current aging experience in the United States.

Widowhood

With 56 out of every 100 of the elderly now becoming widowed (three times as many women as men), the loss of spouse represents a major psychological issue. The mourning process itself occurs at the same time as the need to make practical though emotion-laden decisions about where to live, what do about the family home and possessions, how to dispose of the spouse's personal effects, what kind of contact to maintain with the spouse's relatives, and what to do about new social roles. Although research data are not available on the progress of couples (or of individuals, for that matter) through the entire life-span, one can observe the interdependence that results from years of living together. Yarrow, Butler, et al. (1963) found that losses of significant persons were important factors where there were any evidences of deteriorated functioning in healthy aged men. Other investigations point toward associations between bereavement and increased medical and psychiatric morbidity.* The widowed and their children may be ambivalent about the more involved roles that many grown children feel compelled to accept in relation to the remaining parent. Friends and associates tend to socially ostracize the widowed individual for varieties of reasons: pain over the reminder of the loss of a friend; anxieties and denial of their own aging; awkwardness in knowing how to comfort a grieving person; and uneasiness about accepting a single man or woman into a cultural pattern of couples. Thus widows and widowers may be forced to seek out each other's companionship or fall back on their own resources.

Marital problems†

Couples who enter old age together find new situations awaiting them. There is a greater amount of close contact and free time for each other. With retirement, the elderly man spends most of his day at home for the first time in his adult life. Wives may complain of husbands being underfoot all day with nothing to do as the wives continue their accustomed routines of housework. Some men actively pursue new interests but many encounter difficulties in finding a meaningful substitute for work. As one or the other becomes ill and requires

*"Senescence" is a term that has been used to describe the developmental stages of later life. It is an analogue to pubescence and adolescence; no similar term has been formulated for middle age.

*The interdependence or mutual support of *some* elderly couples can become symbiotic to the extent that the remaining member may die shortly after the death of the other, even though he has been seemingly healthy. In other cases severe depression may ensue.

†Very little data is available on old-age marital relationships. There have been no studies of husband and wife through the life-span; therefore, we must largely theorize from clinical experience.

nursing care, the healthy spouse is torn between the desire to provide such care for the sick person and a need to have a life of his own outside the sickroom. Typically, because of a shorter life expectancy and a tendency to be older than their wives at time of marriage, it is the husband who becomes ill, often chronically so, and the wife nurses him until his death. If the illness is a long and draining one, the wife can be expected to feel some bitterness and sense of exploitation. This becomes a more serious problem when the wife denies her feelings and insists upon the pretense that her husband is no burden. The husband, sensing his wife's frustrations, may react with hurt and anger, and a troubled marital relationship ensues wherein both need guidance and reassurance.

Sexual problems

Sex relations, although tending to be diminished in frequency, are practiced by many old people; however, problems can arise physically and emotionally in relationship to aging and illness. Surgery requiring a colostomy, for example, can seriously deter sexual expression for aesthetic and physical reasons. Physiological changes in females (for example, untreated "senile" vaginitis) and prostatic problems in males are some of the possible organic impediments to sexual intercourse. Old people, like young, tend to react with anxiety and depression over threats to potency and sexual fulfillment. In addition, new fears can present themselves. One of the more common worries is fear of the effects of sexual exertion on the heart or circulatory system. Studies remain inconclusive in clarifying the validity of concern in this area, but it does appear that more fear is present than is warranted. Other problems result from spending a long life together: one partner may begin to find the other less and less sexually attractive as they age or be simply bored by the routine of the same partner over a period of years. During widowhood the surviving spouse has an especially difficult situation, particularly the woman, since chances for remarriage are so slight. The elderly are inclined to follow the strict sexual customs of their youth—no sex outside of marriage—and are therefore forced into celibacy regardless of personal inclination.

Iatrogenicity (a physician's induction of pathological reactions) is pertinent to our considerations. By means that range from the injunction to "take it easy," given to the active man now suffering from a cardiac disorder, to the failure to prepare the patient who is about to have a prostatectomy and orchidectomy, the physician may contribute to depressive reactions so common in old people. (We shall be discussing sex more fully in Chapters 6 and 14.)

A 76-year-old retired political scientist who was still active sexually required a prostatectomy and orchidectomy for malignancy. He was not psychologically prepared, developed extreme anxiety at the time of operation, and had a profound suicidal depression following the procedure. He put himself to bed, ate poorly, talked little, discouraged visitors, and died eight months later. Autopsy revealed that metastases did not fully account for his death.

Discrepant rates of change, narcissism, fear of death, and the relationship to the children are among the critical variables that seem pertinent to marital problems in late life and require study.

A daughter of a 78-year-old patient wrote concerning the present relationship of her parents: "I might note here that when I was growing up my father objected to even the words darned or damned. He now swears freely and will mutter Jesus Christ under his breath the minute he hears mother call. He seems to feel that both her present philosophical outlook and her physical inabilities could be improved if she 'had the guts.' He bitterly resents her balkings and her standard 'I can't answer. . .' His answer to her frequent plea 'love me' is 'give me something to love'. . . He is crushed by her condition. She is crushed by his cruelty and intolerance."

• • •

The wife of a 75-year-old patient bitterly complained of her husband's glum, depressed nature. He denied being as depressed as she insisted. He had the typical "ironed-out" facies of parkinsonism, although no other manifestations of this disorder were present. If people were better informed about some of the physical changes commonly seen in late life, anxieties and misperceptions might be alleviated.

Retirement

Women enjoy a mixed blessing in relation to retirement. Many never work outside the home and therefore are not as subject as men to the generally arbitrary retirement policies of employers. The traditional housewife's job identity is threatened in mid-life as her children leave home but as she adjusts to caring for only herself and her husband, she has a definite pattern of work—at least until her husband dies. Even in her widowhood a women continues to have the routines of homemaking available to her. One of the negative aspects of the traditional female homebound role is that, as a widow or even earlier, a woman may have insufficient financial resources and be forced to go to work, although frequently untrained and inexperienced for the job world. However financially handicapping eventual retirement may be, the emotional trauma of retirement would not seem to be a serious problem for most women until in the future women, earlier in life, begin to identify with a professional or work life outside the home.

For men, retirement is a concern that can affect the very essence of their lives. A large number of men derive an almost single-minded identity from their work (some even becoming "workaholics"—addicted to work). Many develop no diversified interests outside their employment and are caught up in a narrow definition of who they are and what they are worth as people. Work and life become so interconnected that the loss of a job can demolish the reason for living.

Mr. J, a retired legal adjudicator, was diagnosed as having an adjustment reaction to old age—in this case, to retirement. He was irritable, sad, anxious, fearful, and perplexed. He described himself as always having been fidgety, but this trait had increased since his retirement. Time dragged heavily, and he missed feeling useful. He had voluntarily retired four years ago (at 66), having done little planning for his old age or the future. He tended to deny his aging state and felt frightened and depressed about the future. He had shown no previous adjustment or personality problems.

The syndrome of the restless and depressed retired man is common indeed, with little hope for wide-ranging solutions in the near future. There is both commonsense and research evidence that men adjust better if they can choose when and how completely they wish to retire, but such evidence is of little import in a youth- and production-oriented economic system. Eventually a redefinition of work itself as well as the role of men may bring a more satisfying retirement picture. Perhaps work, leisure, and study could be alternated throughout the life cycle instead of being parceled out according to age group. Men should also be encouraged to take a more active part in other aspects of life—with more involvement in the care of children and home, a sharing of responsibility for financial support with the wife, more leisure time throughout life for rest and study, and active involvement in cultural and social activities. A call for male as well as female liberation is in order if men are to escape the crushing burden of overidentification with work and the problems of stress, coronary disease, retirement shock, and shortened life expectancy that are associated with it.

Sensory loss

Significant hearing loss, which affects men* more often than women, occurs in some 30% of all older people and is potentially the most problematical of the perceptual impairments. It can reduce reality testing and lead to marked suspiciousness, even paranoia.

From clinical observations it has long been thought that a relationship exists between hearing loss and depression. The National Institute of Mental Health's study of elderly men provides evidence of such a relationship and its connection with reaction time. An analysis of variance (a statistical procedure) based on the data tabulated showed an interaction between depression

---

*Brearley, C. W.: The general problem of deafness in the population, Laryngoscope **50:**856-905, 1940.

Table 3-1. The relation of auditory acuity and depression to reaction time*

Diagnostic category	Very healthy older men		Healthy older men	
	Number of subjects	Mean reaction time	Number of subjects	Mean reaction time
No decrease in auditory acuity; no depression	11	0.21	12	0.22
Decrease in auditory acuity; no depression	7	0.21	3	0.26
No decrease in auditory acuity; depression	8	0.24	2	0.30
Decrease in auditory acuity; depression	0	—	2	0.33
Total	26		19	

*From Butler, Robert N., and Perlin, Seymour: Human aging, Washington, D. C., 1963, Government Printing Office, p. 300.

and decreased auditory acuity, which was statistically highly significant.

Hearing loss causes greater social isolation than blindness, since it reduces or complicates verbal communication with other people. Onlookers may mistake the hard-of-hearing as mentally abnormal or "senile." There is little social sympathy, and deaf old people are often excluded from activities to become less and less well oriented. The loud or badly articulated speech associated with hearing loss can have a negative effect on others and the hard-of-hearing are given less consideration than the elderly blind, probably because verbal communication with them is so difficult.

Although most old people need glasses, poor vision is not as widespread as is usually thought. About 80% have fair to adequate visual acuity to age 90 and even beyond. Often one eye may continue to function, even if the other does not. The elderly find the possibility of cataracts, glaucoma, and other disorders frightening because of the isolating and immobilizing effects. Visual loss can cause decreasing mobility, poor orientation, and frightening visual impressions that resemble hallucinations. Reading, television, and other pastimes are reduced or eliminated. Further, old people feel more vulnerable to danger and crime when handicapped by sensory loss.

Smell also declines with age, and up to 30% of people who are over 80 years have difficulty identifying common substances by smell. Taste too is affected, since two thirds of taste sensations are dependent on the ability to smell; in addition, taste buds decrease sharply in number with age.* There is also a falloff of tactile response as both perception and motor expression decline in reaction to stimuli. However, the slowing of speed and response, which at first appears to be a characteristic of old age, was found in the NIMH studies to be also related to environmental deprivation and depression.

On a more positive note, Beard in 1967 studied 270 male and female centenarians (100 years old or more) and found only 5.2% blind and only 1.9% completely deaf. However, 58.5% had only fair to poor vision. Hearing disappeared more slowly than sight. Women lost more vision than the men, and men lost more hearing than did women.†

Aging, disease, and pain

The chronic and acute illnesses and diseases in old age provide the fulcrum determining the physical functioning and energy levels that are available to elderly people. Just as loss and grief define the critical emotional variable for the old, so illness presents the prime physical variable. The Roman adage "mens sana in corpore sano," a sound mind in a sound body, recognizes

*In Shakespeare's *As You Like It,* old age is described as "sans teeth, sans eyes, sans taste, sans everything."

†Beard, Belle Boone: Social competence of centenarians, Athens, 1967, University of Georgia Printing Department.

the interrelationships between the two. Psychometric tests have proved to be unusually sensitive to even minimal disease. Physical illness frequently generates both appropriate and distorted emotional reactions, since it represents so much that is inherently frightening to human beings. Latent fear and anxiety about death grow real with illness. Feelings of helplessness and vulnerability buried deep within the individual are resurrected in the face of implacable illness and the aging process. Hope for cures from medicines, luck, or a supreme being diminishes in the light of the general knowledge most people now possess about aging and the current irreversibility of many chronic diseases. Old people's sense of pride in their own body's reliability is shaken when they experience greater susceptibility to communicable diseases, air pollution, dampness, cold weather, and exertion. Moreover, aging and disease threaten people's sense of who they are—their identities—as their bodies change "in front of their eyes." People report feelings of shock and disbelief at their mirror images, in reaction both to aging (is that old person me?) and to illnesses, which even more rapidly change the size, shape, and appearance of the body.

A common feature of old age, which begins in the middle years, is "body monitoring"—the need to concern oneself with the care of one's body and its functions in a more concerted way than before. Bodily processes that formerly took care of themselves or required minimal attention begin to demand more and more time as people age. Among the elderly, 86% have some kind of chronic health problem requiring more visits to the doctor, added stays in the hospital, special diets, exercises, drugs, rehabilitative therapy, or additional provisions for daily life at home. With 81% of the elderly ambulatory and to a substantial degree responsible for their own self-care (only 5% are in institutions and, even there, many have some degree of self-care), it is apparent that body monitoring is a compelling preoccupation. Some old people welcome the relief from other anxieties, which occurs as they absorb themselves in their own care. But others are annoyed, wearied, or bored by the routines imposed upon them by ill health and the decline of their bodies. The composer Stravinsky in his eighties wrote of his irritation at having to spend so much time on his body when he wanted to write music. One can assume that his complaint is echoed by many who wish to continue active, interesting lives.

Pain is another frequent preoccupation for the old. The periodic aches and pains of rheumatism, the throbbing relentless pains of arthritis, the sharp distress of angina pectoris—these are examples of pain in some of its shapes and forms. The elderly deal with pain according to their life style, personality, and cultural background, as well as the nature and extent of the pain. (Individual pain thresholds vary from person to person and vary also in intensity at different times in the same individual.) For many persons, the use of drugs offers the most consistent relief, yet drugs sometimes produce side effects that can be particularly devitalizing or disorganizing to old people—dizziness, loss of appetite, weakness, nausea, or dulling of consciousness. Twelve of the twenty-two most frequently prescribed drugs have a sedating effect. Old people often fear drugs on the basis of frightening past experiences, and at times clarity of consciousness and preservation of strength may be more important than absolute freedom from pain.

Hospitalization and surgery

Heart and circulatory diseases, digestive conditions, and disturbances of the nervous system are the primary causes of hospitalization after age 65. Hospitalization is drastic and dramatic proof that something is wrong or may be wrong. Fears become heightened and, since so many of the elderly now die in hospitals and nursing homes rather than at home, such institutions come to be viewed as places to die as well as places to regain health. There is still far too little attention paid to the emotional feelings of sick people and this is especially the case with the elderly. The emphasis on treating physical disease, the often cold and cheerless environment of hospitals, the generally efficient but overworked and impersonal medical staff, and too rigid visiting regulations combine to make the elderly person feel isolated, unprotected, lonely, and bored. There is little to do except watch television, a pastime that becomes limited if hearing or sight is impaired. Occupational and recreational therapies are usually minimal. Removal from the home environment (with consequent deprivation of adequate contact with family and friends, lack of responsibility, and restriction of mental and somatic activity) encourages anxiety, irritability, disorientation, and eventual regression.

Insufficient thought has been given to the side effects of various surgical procedures. An example is the "black patch" syndrome, which until relatively recently puzzled the medical profession. Following bilateral cataract surgery when patches were placed over both eyes, some old people became delirious and disoriented. It was observed that the syndrome did not occur when one eye was operated on at a time, leaving the sight in the other available to the patient. Finally, the conclusion was correctly drawn that the black patch reaction was simply the result of loss of contact with people and environment. Therefore, operating on one eye at a time and providing additional sensory stimuli will allow patients to maintain orientation. It seems logical that other undesirable side effects of surgery might be alleviated through just such careful thinking through of the problems.

Dying and death

Preparation for death involves a condition unknown in past or present experience, for one cannot truly imagine one's own nonexistence. Yet, strangely, although fear of death is part of human experience, old people tend to fear it less than the young do and often are more concerned about the death of those whom they love than about their own. Many can accept personal death with equanimity. In terminal illness it may even be welcomed as a release from pain and struggle. Reactions to death are closely related to a resolution of life's experiences and problems as well as a sense of one's contributions to others.* Profound religious and philosophical convictions facilitate acceptance. The process of working through one's feelings about death begin with a growing personal awareness of the eventual end of life and the implications of this for one's remaining time alive. For some people the process begins early; for others the physical signs of aging occur before awareness is allowed to surface. Some few attempt to deny death to the very end. A resolution of feelings about death may be responsible for those elusive qualities, seen in various old people, known as "wisdom" and "serenity." The German philosopher Feurbach has written that "anticipation of death is seen as the instrument of being—of authentic existence." There are of course varying degrees and levels of acceptance; perhaps the most satisfying is that described by another philosopher, Spinoza: "The adult who sees death as completion of a pattern and who has spent life unfettered by fears, living richly and productively, can integrate and accept the thought that life will stop."

In the NIMH study, 55% of old people in good health seemed to have resolved the problem of their death, 30% manifested denial, and 15% candidly expressed fear.

Few elderly persons today have the opportunity to die at home as their parents and grandparents did. More than 50% of all deaths take place in hospitals, and many in nursing homes. The process of dying is made more difficult by this shift from home to institutions, where the emphasis is on physical rather than emotional concerns. Short and inflexible visiting hours and lack of accommodations for intimate family contact encourage families and friends to withdraw from dying persons, in anticipatory grief (working out feelings of grief as though the

*The psychoanalytically influenced explanation of fear of death as "castration anxiety" suggests a denial of the reality of death on the part of psychoanalysts themselves.

person were already dead). Thus the old person, who may have resolved many of his own difficult feelings about death itself, is left without human comfort and warmth as death approaches. Old people often remark that their greatest fear is of "dying alone."

There is an increasing interest in the subject of death and dying, as evidenced by a growing body of research and literature. One of the best-known reports is the Kübler-Ross work (1970) on the stages of dying, in which she suggests five more or less distinct stages or levels of experience during the actual course of dying. The first stage is denial of death, in which the person simply refuses to believe the evidence of his own approaching demise. In the second stage, denial is replaced by anger and rage at the injustice and unfairness of life's ending. Thirdly, the person moves into a bargaining stage during which he tries to make a deal with God or fate in return for his life (promises of being a better person, showing more concern for others, etc.). When this is seen to be futile, the person moves into a period of depression and preparatory grief over the loss of life and loved ones. Finally, in the last stages, a level of acceptance is reached—a quiet expectation of death and a lessening of interest in the outer world, including loved ones.

COMMON EMOTIONAL REACTIONS AS EXPRESSED IN OLD AGE

The elderly experience human feelings that are similar for people of every age, but as with each age, there is a uniqueness in the character of such feelings as they reflect the life events of old people. Both the uniqueness and the similarities bear examination if one is to clarify the distinctive nature of old age.

Grief (mourning)

As has been previously discussed, grief as a result of loss is a predominate factor in aging. Loss of the marital partner or other significant and loved people can be profound, particularly since it is difficult in later life to find any kind of substitute for such losses. This is illustrated in the tender and grief-stricken passage by St. Augustine in his *Confessions:*

> I pressed her eyes closed, and a hugh wave of sorrow flooded my heart and flowed outward in tears. . . What, then, was it which caused grevious pain within me, if not the fresh wound arising from the sudden breaking of a very sweet and cherished habit of living together? Since I was thus bereft of such great comfort from her, my soul was wounded and it was as if life which had been made one from hers and mine was torn to shreds. . . It was a relief to weep in Thy sight about her and for her, about myself and for myself.

The primary adaptive purpose of grief and mourning is to accept the reality of the loss and to begin to find ways of filling up the emptiness caused by the loss, through identifying with a new style of life and new people. Parkes (1970), in his studies of London widows, describes the futile search for the lost love object in which the mourner is torn between the desire to recover or resurrect the dead person and the knowledge that this is irrational.* A cultural adaptation is found in the practice of ancestor worship in Shintoism and Buddhism—where the mourner believes the presence of a departed loved one remains (to be fed, prayed to, etc.) yet in a new spirit form that does not allow direct physical contact. Thus both the reality of death and the wishful recovery of the person are provided for, in a religious belief that gives structure to the grief process.

A typical grief reaction has an almost predictable pattern of onset, regardless of age—numbness and inability to accept the loss, followed by the shock of reality as it begins to penetrate. There are physical feelings of emptiness in the pit of the stomach, weak knees, perhaps a feeling of suffocation, short-

*Studies indicate that some widowed people have hallucinations and delusions of contact with the lost spouse. These may last for years and are more likely to occur in individuals who had been happily married. The most common hallucination reported was feeling the dead spouse's presence; others thought they saw, heard, were touched by or spoken to by the spouse.

ness of breath, and a tendency to deep sighing. Emotionally the person experiences great distress. There may be a sense of unreality, including delusions and obsessive preoccupations with the image of the lost person and acting as though the deceased were still present. Generally feelings of guilt are present as well as anger and irritability, even toward friends and relatives. There is usually a disorganization of normal patterns of response, with the bereaved person wandering about aimlessly, unable to work or take social initiative. Anxiety and longing alternate with depression and despair. Insomnia, digestive disturbances, and anorexia are common. Acute grief ordinarily lasts a month or two and then begins to lessen; on the average, grief may be largely over in six to twelve months although further loss, stress, or some reminder can reactivate it.

Exaggerated grief reactions may occur:

> A 66-year-old woman was as angry and depressed over the death of her husband sixteen months after his death as she was in the immediate weeks. She had passed through the "markers" of a year—the anniversary of their marriage, Thanksgiving, Christmas, Valentine's Day, Easter, and summer vacation reminiscence. But she could not shake her oppressive depression. She was furious at her brother-in-law, who she felt would find ways to cheat her of her inheritance. She chastised her two sons for their neglect. It was only through open exploration of her anger, first with her sophisticated clergyman and then with a psychiatrist, that her depression began to lift.

"Morbid" grief reactions are distortions or prolongations of typical grief. Such reactions may take the form of delay, in which the grief is delayed for days, months, or even years, and in its extreme form is generally bound up with conscious or unconscious antagonism or ambivalence toward the deceased. Inhibited grief, according to Parkes, produces minimal mourning but other symptoms develop such as somatic illnesses, overactivity, or disturbed social interaction. Chronic grief, yet another of the morbid grief reactions, is the prolongation and intensification of normal grief over an extended or limited period of time.

Anticipatory grief is the process of mourning in advance, before an actual loss is sustained. This form of mourning can occur during long illnesses; for example, a wife caring for a sick husband may go through a grief reaction and may have reached some degree of acceptance before his death occurs. Such grief is seen as a protective device that prepares the bereaved for their loss, but it can lead to problems if it causes loved ones to disengage themselves prematurely from the dying person, leaving him isolated and alone.

Interrelationships between grief and vulnerability to both physical and emotional illness have been the subject of a number of investigations. Bereavement as a loss is hypothesized to be the single most crucial factor in predicting decline or breakdown in functioning on a physical or emotional level. In addition, losses of health, money, possessions, employment, or social status or changes in appearance seem to be possible factors in precipitating decline or lowering resistance.

Guilt

Old age is a time of reflection and reminiscence that can evoke a resurgence of past conflicts and regrets. Guilt feelings may play a significant role as the old person reviews his life, attempting to consolidate a meaningful judgment as to the manner in which life has been lived and to prepare for death and cope with any fears of death. The sins of omission and commission for which an individual blames himself weigh even more heavily in the light of approaching death and dissolution. If expiation and atonement are to occur, they must occur now; time for procrastination begins to run out. Individuals who have held grudges for a lifetime may decide to resolve their differences. Some may undertake a variety of reparations for the past. Others become more religiously active, in the hope of forgiveness. Such feelings should be dealt with seriously and not simply treated with facile reassurance. For many the resolution of guilt feelings is an essential part of final acceptance of their lives as worthwhile.

Other forms of guilt are the "death survival's guilt"* from outliving others and "retirement guilt" from no longer being employed and working. The latter is especially hard on Horatio Alger types.

Loneliness

In infancy being alone is a condition that provokes terror, anger, and disconsolation. A baby's early cries communicate the primitive drive for physical survival. But very early a new element is introduced. As the child alternately experiences the gratifying warmth and comfort of his mother and the aloneness of his crib, he learns a new fear, the fear of not being able to get back to mother—of being left alone. Thus there appear to be two elements in the early sense of loneliness: *aloneness,* or the fear for physical survival in a threatening uncertain world, and *loneliness,* the fear of emotional isolation, of being locked inside oneself and unable to obtain the warmth and comfort that one has learned is available from others if one can gain it. Growth and a refinement occur as children move outside of themselves and their isolation, not only toward other people but also toward an absorption in play, learning, work, and other creative efforts. That moment is significant when the child first learns to escape his own aloneness or consciousness of himself and becomes totally involved in a task—a moment described as an escape from loneliness, which is not dependent on the presence of another person. (Paul Tillich describes this as a distinction between loneliness and solitude.)

The etiology of loneliness developmentally is significant in regard to old people, not in a simplistic sense of comparing them to children but in attempting to comprehend the special character of loneliness in old age. The primitive fears concerning physical survival and emotional isolation recede as human beings grow to adulthood and learn to successfully provide for their own physical sustenance and achieve emotional satisfactions through family, friends, and work. But with old age, the combination of harsh external forces and a diminishing self-mastery revives once again the latent threats. The old adage that we are born alone and we die alone reflects the experience that each of us encounters in the course of the life cycle. But, unlike the usual experience of children, the elderly person does not suffer so much from a fear of being unable to relate as from the reality of having no one to relate to. With the death of loved ones, there is a diminishing circle of significant people who are not readily replaceable. Former compensations of work may be gone. Children and grandchildren, if they exist, may live far away. The all too limited outlets of religion, hobbies, television, pets, and a few acquaintances, which form the daily existence of so many of the elderly are not enough to satisfy emotional needs.

The American dream of self-reliance and independence can further isolate the old person within himself. At a time when increased human contact could be supportive, old people hold on to cultural notions that living alone and "doing for oneself" must be maintained. Familiarity with and determination to continue such patterns make communal living in hospitals, nursing homes, or group homes difficult in sheerly social terms. It has been observed that old people in more group-oriented societies such as the rural kibbutzim in Israel can enjoy the companship and involvement inherent in a close living situation with others without the same loss of self-esteem and sense of dependency felt by "rugged individualists." Cultures that advocate societal and group responsibility for the individual are perhaps more in sympathy with the natural needs of older people.

---

*Chodoff especially has emphasized "survival guilt" as a result of concentration camp experiences. We have observed this also in old people who have outlived their peers and spouses, although of course many take pride in survival as well. See Chodoff, P. C.: Late effects of the concentration camp syndrome, Archives of General Psychiatry 9:323-333, 1963.

Depression

Depressive reactions increase in degree and frequency with old age as a corollary to the increased loss of much that is emotionally valued by the elderly person. Unresolved grief, guilt, loneliness, and anger are expressed in mild to severe depressions with symptomatology including insomnia, despair, lethargy, anorexia, loss of interest, and somatic complaints. (See Chapter 4.)

Anxiety

The sense of free-floating anxiety intensifies in elderly people as illness and imminent death undermine illusions of invulnerability built up as protection during a lifetime. (A very powerful anxiety is the fear of becoming a pauper.) In addition, new modes of adaptation become necessary, creating additional anxieties in the face of constant change. Notice is seldom taken of the amount of new learning an old person must undergo to adapt to the accelerating changes in body, feelings, and environment. As with any new learning, anxiety develops in proportion to the task at hand, the resources available to master it, and the chances for and consequences of failure. Anxiety manifests itself in many forms: rigid thinking to protectively exclude external stimuli (a person may "hear" what he wants to hear), fear of being alone, and suspiciousness to the point of paranoid states. It may also become somatized into physical illness. Frequently anxiety and its expressions are incorrectly diagnosed as "senility" and wrongly considered untreatable.

One type of anxiety derives from life history, the observations of old people during one's childhood. Fear that they will have the diseases of old age that as children they observed in their grandparents or in other older people is another ingredient in denial or projection in the aged.

A 70-year-old retired chemist who had been born when his mother was 40 years old had seen her develop severe parkinsonism and become increasingly helpless when he was 20 years old. He carried this image with him all his life but after he retired it became obsessional. He gradually convinced himself and his doctors that he did have the disease. If he did, it was clinically negligible.

Sense of impotence and helplessness

A significant reaction for older men, particularly those white men who as a group can be postulated to have once held the power and influence of the society, is a sense of their present impotence and helplessness. The highest suicide rates occur among older white men in their eighties. The elderly black male and all women, black or white, are affected by loss of esteem and cultural status as they age but do not experience quite the same degree of loss of power and privilege. In fact, an interesting reversal can occur for older women within the traditional marital relationship. As their husbands decline, wives may assume more of the initiative, taking over financial management, nursing care, and household repairs; they may, therefore, feel more status and influence than at any previous point in their lives.

Rage

Another of the emotional manifestations of old age is a sense of rage at the seemingly uncontrollable forces that confront the elderly, as well as the indignities and neglect of the society that once valued their productive capacities. The description of some old people as cantankerous, ornery, irritable, or querulous would be more realistically interpreted if one became sensitive to the degree of outrage the elderly feel, consciously or unconsciously, at viewing their situation. Much of the rage is an appropriate response to inhumane treatment. Some old people, of course, rage against the inevitable nature of aging and death, at least at some point in their coming to terms with these forces, but this too would seem to be a legitimate reaction. Dylan Thomas's words, "Do not go gently into that good night," express the desire of many to be alive to the end and to die with a sense of worth and purpose, if not righteous indignation at being obliged to leave life.

COMMON ADAPTIVE TECHNIQUES

Defense mechanisms*

The elderly have throughout their lifetimes acquired individual and characteristic methods of handling anxiety, aggressive impulses, resentments, and frustration. Such methods, known as defense mechanisms, are internal, automatic, unconscious processes whereby the personality protects itself by attempting to provide psychological stability in the midst of conflicting or overwhelming needs and stresses that are part of human existence. As people mature, some new defenses may be added and old ones discarded, but others persist throughout life, taking on different tones and colorations at different stages in the life cycle. Emphasis here will be on the defense mechanisms that most often appear in old age and on nuances that are characteristic of older people.

Denial

The denial of old age and death found in the young person's attitude of "This won't happen to me" may also occur in old age in the form of "This isn't happening to me." In one of its extreme forms denial can manifest itself in a "Peter Pan" syndrome, with the old person pretending to be young and refusing to deal with the realities of aging. There may be a self-attribution of strength—claiming that one is still capable of everything. Not all denial is pathological. It is, in fact, a necessary and useful component for maintaining a sense of stability and equilibrium. But the usefulness of denial is eroded when it begins to seriously interfere with the developmental work of any particular age. In old age, an individual who denies that he is sick and refuses to take medicine or see a doctor is showing an example of denial that no longer accomplishes a life-protective purpose.

Denial, like other defenses, often responds to psychotherapy:

Chief complaint: "I can't catch my breath." This is the case of a man who was always in a hurry and had eventually to stop to catch his breath.

A 68-year-old, highly intelligent and intellectual sociologist developed a severe cough upon his return from an extended and exciting journey abroad. An X-ray shadow increased the medical suspicion of malignancy. Without prior discussion and preparation the patient was inadvertently but directly told this by a secretary arranging his admission for surgery. The operation revealed a lung abscess and the patient responded well physically both to the operative procedure and in the recovery period, with one exception: he could not catch his breath. His internist suggested an extended vacation, and later tranquilizers, and offered reassurance. After some months the doctor strongly recommended psychotherapy, as he realized the patient was becoming increasingly agitated and depressed without adequate medical explanation. The patient was extremely tense and restless. He appeared somewhat slovenly. His pants hung loose from his suspenders and his fly was partly open. In short, he gave the impression of having some organic mental disorder but he spoke clearly and well. Despite his obvious gloom, he managed some humor and clarity in giving his present and past history.

His situation was socially and personally favorable. He had a good relationship with a devoted wife. He had many good friends and professional colleagues. He was well regarded professionally. He was under no pressure to retire, and consultancies were open to him. He had a wide range of interests in addition to his professional field. His relationships with his brothers and sisters were good. With the exception of the chief complaint, his physical status was excellent. He believed his physician's report that there was no major organic disease; in other words, he was not suffering from a fear that he was being misled. But despite all of this he was tense and depressed. Recurrent dreams included one in which "a paper was due" and another in which he was "behind in an exam." He had never taken out any life insurance. He had made no conscious admission to himself that he might age. He had made nothing of birthdays. Nor did he have a very clear concept of the natural evolution of the life cycle. He did not have a sense of stages and development of middle and later life. He had an enormous capacity for work and had kept busy all his life as though unaware of the

*"Nowhere in the literature is there a complete, dynamically meaningful analysis of defenses. Most writers have utilized lists which are incomplete, not logically ordered or mutually exclusive," according to Cohen, R. A., and Cohen, Mabel B.: Research in psychotherapy: A preliminary report, Psychiatry **24**:46-61, 1961. We would recommend the glossary of defenses in Bibring, Grete, et al.: The Psychoanalytic Study of the Child **16**:62-71, 1961.

passage of time. He had never been bored. He had great capacity for self-discipline and was not given to marked expression of either grief or anger but only to a narrow spectrum of affects, including fearfulness and pleasure. He was a kind of Peter Pan and he and his wife eventually concluded in the course of his psychotherapeutic work that he, and in some measure she, had imagined themselves as remaining in their twenties instead of in their late sixties. As he reviewed his life and the realities of aging and death, he became freer in his expression of more negative affects. His depression and tension improved and he remained well in a follow-up of some six months. He was no longer short of breath.

Projection

Some elderly persons attempt to allay anxieties by projecting feelings outward onto someone or something else. They may appear suspicious and fearful, with characteristic complaints of merchants cheating them, doctors ignoring them, their children neglecting them. They often become concerned about physical safety on the streets. Much of what is named projection may indeed be legitimate complaints and fears about situations that exist, either potentially or in actuality, and others may be denying reality by labeling them projection. Of course actual projection itself does occur, signifying internal stress (people with hearing losses are prime victims) and can reach paranoid proportions unless the stress is alleviated.

Fixation

Fixation is most often associated with old age as a carryover defense from earlier life, implying that the fixation point occurred somewhere in childhood. But if one views old age as having developmental work of its own, fixation is a useful concept in describing the elderly person who may reach a particular level of development and be unable to go further. An example might be the person who has adapted well to living alone, without a spouse, but cannot accept in an insightful manner the need for outside help as physical strength wanes. Such a person may unconsciously want to stop the action and refuse to accept a new change.

Regression*

Regression, or a return to an earlier level of adaptation, is an overused and catchall explanation for much behavior in old age. Familiar descriptions of old people as "childlike," "childish," or "in second childhood" imply a reverse slide back to earlier developmental stages with no cognizance of a lifetime of experience that unalterably separates them from their childhood patterns of coping. A pejorative connotation is given, with the notion that old people lose their "adultness" under stress of illness and age and begin to act like children. Regression implies a disruptive, deteriorative, nonadaptive retreat in which the personality is not up to facing the stress it must overcome; the weakness is internal. But in old age much of the stress is from external sources that strain the resources of even the most healthy personalities. The use of the concept of regression to describe the attempts of old people to adapt in such situations is similar to the popular use of "paranoid" to describe the reactions of black people to racism. What appears to be something pathological may indeed be the normal and necessary patterns of behavior.

Displacement

A person whose life is drastically undergoing change may displace his feelings by declaring that the world is going to ruin or that things are not the way they were when he was young. Others openly criticize young people, blame doctors and nurses for neglect, and berate family members for slights and lack of concern. The function of displacement is to reassure the person that he is all right and that any problems to be found can be explained by unfortunate circumstances around him.

Counterphobia

Counterphobia is the compelling and sometimes risky tendency to look danger

*Originally a neurological rather than a psychological concept, constructed by English neurologist Hughlings Jackson.

in the face in an attempt to convince oneself that it can be overcome. An old man with dizzy spells may insist on climbing a ladder to fix his own roof. Another, with a history of visual blackouts, may demand that he drive the family car just as before. A woman with heart trouble ignores her racing pulse as she continues to carry tubs of laundry from her basement. In each case the individual ignores a realistic appraisal of his limitations and relies upon sheer force of will to undo the danger.

Idealization

One type of defense is the idealization of the lost object, be it person, place, life style, or status. A person may, for instance, idolize a deceased mate, glorifying the past and the good old days. The purpose is to make one's life seem meaningful and not wasted.

Rigidity

There is little evidence that older people become rigid in personality as they age. Rather, when rigidity is seen, it is a defense against a general sense of threat or actual crises.

Other defensive behavior

Selective memory

The dulling of memory and the propensity to remember distant past events with greater clarity than events of the recent past have generally been attributed to arteriosclerotic and senile brain changes in old age. However, it appears that such memory characteristics can at times have a psychological base, in that the older person may be turning away from or tuning out the painfulness of the present to dwell on a more satisfying past.

Selective sensory reception

A process of "exclusion of stimuli" described by Weinberg (1956) has been observed in elderly people, by which they block off the sensorium that they feel unprepared to deal with. This is more often observed in people with hearing problems, who at times seem to hear what they want to hear. This may be the only way an old person can control the amount of input impinging upon him.

Exploitation of age and disability

Elderly people can use changes occurring in their lives to obtain secondary gains —that is, benefits which in and of themselves may be satisfying or desired. An example is shown by the old person who insists he must remain in a hospital or other care facility, even though he no longer needs medical care, because he enjoys the extra attention and sense of importance accruing from the illness. Or an individual with a proclivity to control others can use illness or impending death to manipulate those around him. Examples are the tyrant on the sick bed who terrorizes family and friends through guilt and the invalid who commandeers personal services from everyone through appearing totally helpless and passive. Exploitation of age and disability can also result in freedom from social expectation; with the elderly person not feeling bound by the social amenities and established patterns. In this sense the defensive behavior may allow the person to try on a new identity or a new way of relating. Behavior that in youth might have been considered unacceptable or even bizarre can be viewed in old age as pleasantly idiosyncratic or at least harmless.

Restitution, replacement, or compensatory behavior

Numerous activities may be adopted to make up for a loss. These may include practical measures such as memory pads and reminders of all sorts to compensate for poor memory. Or they can take the form of finding new persons to replace lost ones. Attempted restitution is frequently seen, in which a person tries to give back or get back that which has been lost or taken away.

Use of activity or busyness

General busyness, known as "working off the blues," is a defense against depression, anxiety, and other conditions that are painful or unacceptable. It involves concentrating on activity of some kind, whether productive or nonproductive, with the purpose of warding off the unwanted feelings.

Insight as an adaptive technique

Successful adjustments to real life conditions are not optimally possible if feelings and behavior are unconsciously motivated and therefore not subject to conscious control. Similarly, it can prove nonadaptive to be unaware of the natural course of life: what to expect, what can be changed, and what cannot. Thus insight requires not only an inner sense of one's self and motivations but also an inner knowledge of the human life cycle—a realization of life and how it changes. The elderly individual who has a steady comprehension of the life process from birth to death is thereby assisted in his efforts to decide what to oppose and what to accept, when to struggle and when to acquiesce and, ultimately, to understand the limits of what is possible. Insight includes the willingness and ability to substitute available satisfactions for losses incurred. It is the most widely used and successful adaptation found in healthy older people.

Related to adaptation is the changing adaptiveness found with psychopathology, which will be discussed in Chapter 9. Paranoid personality structures appear to become even less adaptive with age as the few persons in the paranoid's circle die, isolation hardens, and crises occur. On the other hand, the schizoid personality structure seems to insulate against loss. The obsessional and compulsive personality whose fussbudget behavior may have impaired his effectiveness earlier in life may adjust well to the void of retirement or losses, through meticulous and ritualistic activities.

THE LIFE REVIEW

The tendency of the elderly toward self-reflection and reminiscence used to be thought of as indicating a loss of recent memory and therefore a sign of aging. However, in 1961 one of us (RNB) postulated that reminiscence in the aged was part of a normal life review process brought about by realization of approaching dissolution and death. It is characterized by the progressive return to consciousness of past experiences and particularly the resurgence of unresolved conflicts which can be looked at again and reintegrated. If the reintegration is successful, it can give new significance and meaning to one's life and prepare one for death, by mitigating fear and anxiety.

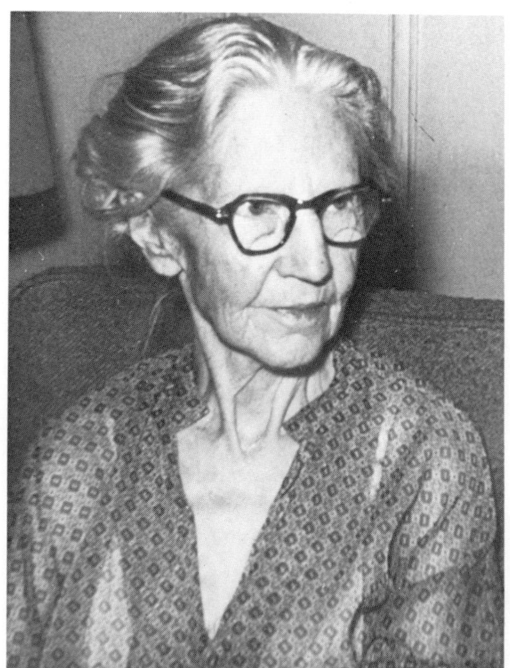

The life review.

Photo by Robert N. Butler, M.D.

This is a process that is believed to occur universally in all persons in the final years of their lives, although they may not be totally aware of it and may in part defend themselves from realizing its presence. It is spontaneous, unselective, and seen in other age groups as well (adolescence, middle age); but the intensity and emphasis on putting one's life in order are most striking in old age. In late life people have a particularly vivid imagination and memory for the past and can recall with sudden and remarkable clarity early life events. There is renewed ability to free-associate and bring up material from the unconscious. Individuals realize that their own personal myth of invulnerability and immortality can no longer be maintained. All of this results in reassessment of life, which brings depression, acceptance, or satisfaction.

The life review can occur in a mild form through mild nostalgia, mild regret, a tendency to reminisce, story-telling, and the like. Often the person will give his life story to anyone who will listen. At other times it is conducted in monologue without another person hearing it. It is in many ways similar to the psychotherapeutic situation in which a person is reviewing his life in order to understand his present situation.

As part of the life review one may experience a sense of regret that is increasingly painful. In severe forms it can yield anxiety, guilt, despair, and depression. And in extreme cases if a person is unable to resolve problems or accept them, terror, panic, and suicide can result. The most tragic life review is that in which a person decides life was a total waste.

Some of the positive results of reviewing one's life can be a righting of old wrongs, making up with enemies, coming to acceptance of mortal life, a sense of serenity, pride in accomplishment, and a feeling of having done one's best. It gives people an opportunity to decide what to do with the time left to them and work out emotional and material legacies. People become ready but in no hurry to die. Possibly the qualities of serenity, philosophical development, and wisdom observable in some older people reflect a state of resolution of their life conflicts. A lively capacity to live in the present is usually associated, including the direct enjoyment of elemental pleasures such as nature, children, forms, colors, warmth, love and humor. One may become more capable of mutuality with a comfortable acceptance of the life cycle, the universe, and the generations. Creative works may result such as memoirs, art, music. People may put together family albums, scrapbooks and study their genealogies.

One of the greatest difficulties for younger persons (including mental health personnel) is to listen thoughtfully to the reminiscences of older people. We have been taught that this nostalgia represents living in the past and a preoccupation with self and that it is generally boring, meaningless, and time-consuming. Yet as a natural healing process it represents one of the underlying human capacities upon which all psychotherapy depends. The life review as a necessary and healthy process should be recognized in daily life as well as used in the mental health care of older people.

REFERENCES

Altschuler, K. Z., Barad, M., and Goldfarb, A. I.: A survey of dreams in the aged. II. Noninstitutionalized subjects, Archives of General Psychiatry **8**:33-37, 1963.

Barad, M., Altschuler, K. Z., and Goldfarb, A. I.: A survey of dreams in aged persons, Archives of General Psychiatry **4**:419-424, 1961.

Birren, James E., Butler, Robert N., Greenhouse, Samuel W., Sokoloff, Louis, and Yarrow, Marian R.: Summary and interpretations. In Human aging, Washington, D. C., 1963, U. S. Government Printing Office.

Butler, Robert N.: The life review: an interpretation of reminiscence in the aged, Psychiatry **26**: 65-76, 1963.

Butler, Robert N.: Re-awakening interest, Nursing Homes **10**:8-19, 1961.

Butler, Robert N., and Perlin, Seymour: Physiological-psychological-psychiatric interrelationships. In Human aging, Washington, D. C., 1963, U. S. Government Printing Office.

Gitelson, Maxwell: The emotional problems of elderly people, Geriatrics **3**:135-150, 1948.

Glaser, B. G., and Strauss, A. C.: Awareness of dying, Chicago, 1965, Aldine Publishing Co.

Gorer, Geoffrey: Death, grief, and mourning, New York, 1965, Doubleday & Co., Inc.

Hinton, J.: Dying, Baltimore, 1967, Penguin Books, Inc.

Hollingshead, August B., and Redlich, Fredrick: Social class and mental illness, New York, 1958, John Wiley & Sons, Inc.

Kübler-Ross, Elisabeth: Five stages a dying patient goes through, Medical Economics, pp. 272-292, Sept. 14, 1970.

Lindemann, Erich: Symptomatology and management of acute grief. In Parad, Howard J., editor: Crisis intervention: selected readings, New York, 1965, Family Service Association of America.

Marris, Peter: Widows and their families, London, 1958, Routledge & Kegan Paul, Ltd.

Neugarten, Bernice L.: The awareness of middle age. In Owen, Roger, editor: Middle age, London, 1967, British Broadcasting Corp.

Parkes, C. Murray: The first year of bereavement, Psychiatry 33:444-467, 1970.

Parkes, C. Murray: Seeking and finding a lost object, Social Science and Medicine 4:187-201, 1970.

Perlin, Seymour, and Butler, Robert N.: Psychiatric aspects of adaptation to the aging experience. In Human aging, Washington, D. C., 1963, U. S. Government Printing Office.

Rossman, Isadore, editor: Clinical geriatrics, Philadelphia, 1971, J. B. Lippincott Co.

Tolstoi, Leo: The death of Ivan Ilych (1886), New York, 1960, Signet Classic Paperback.

Weinberg, Jack: Personal and social adjustment, In Anderson, J. E., editor: Psychological aspects of aging, Washington, D. C., 1956, American Psychological Association.

Weisman, A. D., and Kastenbaum, R.: The psychological autopsy: a study of the terminal phase of life, Community Mental Health Journal, Monograph No. 4, New York, 1968, Behavioral Publications, Inc.

4

FUNCTIONAL DISORDERS

OVERVIEW OF PSYCHOPATHOLOGY IN LATE LIFE

The mental disorders of old age are of two kinds: the *organic disorders,* which have a physical cause (Chapter 5), and the *functional disorders,* for which at present no physical cause has been found and for which the origins appear to be emotional—related to the personality and life experiences of people. The extent of mental disorders in old age is considerable. It has been estimated by the American Psychological Association in 1971 that at least 3 million, 15%, of the older population need mental health services. We would consider this to be a conservative estimate. A million older people are at this moment in institutional settings, for a variety of reasons. The effects of institutionalization itself ensure further emotional problems on top of those already existing. At least 2 million people living in the community have serious chronic disorders, predominantly physical but also mental. It is evident that the majority of people having chronic physical illness also have associated emotional reactions requiring attention. In addition are those persons who need treatment for primarily mental illnesses. Added to this list are the 7 million who live in poverty in conditions that are known to contribute to emotional breakdown or decline. Finally, the effects of lowered social status and self-esteem take a toll on mental health. The true proportion of psychiatric need among older people has not been fully documented.

Institutional care

In 1963, of the 292,000 older persons with mental disorders who were institutionalized in a variety of settings, 43% were in nursing homes and related facilities and 57% were in state, county, city, or private hospitals. In 1968 there were almost 400,000 resident patients (of all ages) in state and county mental hospitals. Of that 400,000, 30% were elderly (two thirds of the elderly were women). Figures for residence of the elderly in hospitals included these 120,000 persons of age 65 and over in state and county mental hospitals, an additional 15,000 in private hospitals, and 3,000 in Veterans Administration hospitals. It is estimated that about one third to one half of elderly patients were admitted to hospitals as younger patients and the remainder were admitted at age 65 or older.

About 29,000 elderly people entered state and county mental hospitals in 1968 for the first time, representing 17% of all first admissions. In private mental hospitals, nearly 11,600 elderly people were similarly admitted, or 12% of first admissions. Undoubtedly the lower percentage of private versus public admissions reflects the lower incomes of many of the elderly, which preclude private care. In any case, it is clear that older people make up a substantial number of the first admissions as well as the total residents. However, they have received little attention other than custodial care.

Furthermore, older patients are being increasingly pushed from inadequate mental institutions into other inadequate custodial facilities, known euphemistically as "the community." Since 1940, even before introduction of the tranquilizing drugs, the resident hospital populations began a downward slope as attempts were made to shorten hospital stays. In the 1950s and 1960s, lower rates of admission began to be encouraged along with the shorter hospitalizations. From 1960 on, the emphasis was on transferring the older patients out of hospitals, wholesale. The rhetorical reason given was that it was "better" for people; actually the reason was a fiscal policy in which the states could save money by obtaining federal financial support for use of community facilities. The various nursing homes, personal care homes, and foster care facilities to which old people are being transferred, often indiscriminately, are frequently of dubious quality. Many are firetraps, offer poor nursing and medical care, give little or no psychiatric care, are unsafe in supervision, etc. Regulations and controls are inadequate and unenforced. Since 1965 and the enactment of Medicare and Medicaid amendments to the Social Security Act, there has been a proliferation of such facilities as the care of the aged has become profitable business. The controversial 1972 legislation regarding "intermediate care facilities" will lead to further transferring of older mental patients out of mental hospitals. As has been said, "The patient goes where the money flows." We certainly support the growing trend toward *appropriate* care outside of hospitals when it is in the interest of patients. But the present transfer policy is unsound, medically and psychiatrically. Data show that transfer of the very old increases morbidity and mortality. Many people have lived in hospitals for twenty, thirty, or more years and have made some sort of adjustment. Many have developed such a "hospitalitis" or "institutionalitis" that it is difficult for them to survive in a new and strange environment. Now suddenly—when they are 70, 80, or even 90 years old—they are being transferred, often without their consent, into largely underregulated and inadequate community facilities. Such transfers are obviously not for the patients' benefit. Instead, they represent political and financial arrangements between states, the federal government, and private enterprise.

Outpatient care

Old people are not seen as outpatients in psychiatric clinics, in community mental health centers, and in the offices of private psychiatrists or other therapists in proportion to their emotional and psychiatric needs. Only about 2% of persons seen in psychiatric clinics are over 60. About 4% to 5% of the people seen in community mental health centers are over 65. And only about 2% of private psychiatric time involves older persons. In all of these settings the elderly are often not seen for treatment but, rather, for routine diagnostic work-ups and rapid disposition.

Two major groups of older mental patients

It is important to bear in mind that older people in mental hospitals or in nursing homes and related facilities form two large groups. In the first are people who were admitted to mental hospitals early in life and who grew old there or have been transferred to community settings. This tragic group reflects society's failure to provide adequate care so that their lives could be salvaged. Many of course became ill before the development of "modern" treatments such as electroshock therapy, various forms of individual and group therapy, and the tranquilizers and antidepressant drugs. But this cannot explain why so many have been neglected for so long. They are the victims of prejudicial attitudes toward the mentally ill and of inadequate and fluctuating state hospital budgets that have made sound diagnosis and good treatment impossible.

The second group of people are those who developed mental illness for the first time in late life. Many have chronic, organic brain syndromes; but a surprising number have reversible brain disorders as well as functional illnesses like depression and paranoid tendencies. The long-term and the recently admitted patients differ from each other in diagnosis and prognosis; therefore, their treatment should reflect these differences. At present they are often all misleadingly identified as geriatric patients, with not even those who have reversible brain syndromes being singled out for treatment.

Drug problems

The oft-heralded "tranquilizer revolution" has lead to abuses and misuses that make one suspect that these drugs are employed more for the benefit of the therapist or the quiet serenity of institutions than in the best interest of patients. Patients may be kept on high dosages for years at a time, with minimal medical monitoring. Drug treatment is often the *only* treatment given. Between 1956 and 1972 the state and county mental hospital population declined from 559,000 to 308,000. As a result, there are increased numbers of people in the community whose fundamental problems in living have not been solved but who are simply pacified. The side effects of prolonged tranquilizer use are tolerated more easily by physicians than by their patients. For example, tardive dyskinesia is a serious and irreversible syndrome that appears to be a side effect of phenothiazine therapy. It seems to be more common in the brain-damaged, such as elderly people with brain syndromes. Yet many doctors discount the potential long-term effects of drugs, feeling that the problems of the elderly and the mentally ill are so incomprehensible that massive experimental drug usage is warranted.

Research on mental illness in community-resident aged

The Langley Porter Institute's Studies of Aging, under the general direction of Alexander Simon and Marjorie Fiske Lowenthal, represents one of the first major attempts in the United States to explore the associated characteristics of mental illness among community-resident older people.* These studies examined 600 San Francisco residents over age 60 and 500 who were hospitalized for mental illness. Physical illness was found to be unequivocally related to psychiatric complaint. In contrast, widowhood and retirement were demoralizing but not clearly causative of hospitalizable mental illness, according to their findings.

A study in Syracuse (Gruenberg, 1961) was concerned with the more limited problem of "certifiability" for mental hospitalization, and the work *Five Hundred Over Sixty* (Kutner et al., 1957) dealt with life problems and measures of psychological adjustment rather than mental illness. Three gerontological research programs—the Kansas City Study of Adult Life (Williams and Wirths, 1965), the National Institute of Mental Health work, and studies by the Center for the Study of Aging at Duke University—were based on volunteer samples, within the range of "normal" patterns of personality and adjustment.

It is difficult to compare the results of these studies because of the different methodologies and notions of what constitutes mental illness. But all of them add valuable insights and information to this growing field.

Diagnostic nomenclature

We are including an abbreviated outline of the American Psychiatric Association's *Diagnostic and Statistical Manual of Mental Disorders* (DSM II) at the end of this chapter. The outline presented there includes psychotic and nonpsychotic organic brain syndromes, functional psychotic conditions, neuroses, personality disorders, psychophysiological disorders, and transient situational disturbances of late life. We have omitted any items that are not specifically pertinent to older people.

This nomenclature leaves much to be desired in diagnosing conditions of older persons, particularly in the case of acute and chronic brain syndromes. However, for hospital charts, insurance forms, and various other administrative purposes it is necessary to be familiar with the latest nomenclature (1968), as well as the earlier terms used in DSM I (1952). The literature of the aging field reflects the changing terminology,

---

*Lowenthal, Majorie Fiske, Berkman, Paul L., and associates: Aging and mental disorder in San Francisco—a social psychiatric study, San Francisco, 1967, Jossey-Bass, Inc.

which might be quite confusing to the reader without these references.

It is well to remember that to base treatment on a medical, disease-oriented diagnosis from the statistical manual can be misleading and limiting.* For example, an old person who is diagnosed as having severe brain damage (by sophisticated psychiatric examination and psychological test scores) may function quite well in a supportive milieu. Another person may have minimal brain damage but have no economic, personal, and social supports and thus have more trouble functioning—not because of any inherently serious mental condition but because he has no environmental supports. Thus diagnosis and treatment, as well as prevention, must go beyond the traditional psychiatric diagnostic evaluation to include the context in which symptoms develop and the healthy assets and resources of the personality.

We might add here that the use of insurance forms that require a therapist to state the diagnosis on a patient creates a sticky, ethical problem. The patient's interest may be compromised if a diagnosis is given that can be later used irresponsibly. We have no assurances about the confidentiality of insurance records; and they do get lost, misplaced, and confused with other patients' records. On the other hand, a vague, general diagnosis can make the whole matter of insurance information irrelevant, especially when statistics are collected from these sources on the "mental illness" of policyholders. But when it comes down to cases, most practitioners choose to protect their patients when possible. One rarely sees diagnoses such as schizophrenia, homosexuality, or antisocial personality. The nomenclature more commonly used includes such designations as anxiety neurosis, depressive neurosis, marital maladjustment, and other terms that are not as revealing.

*In *The Vital Balance* (1963), Karl Menninger wrote: "Psychiatry should provide a better understanding of human beings in trouble. . . without pejoratively labeling them."

FUNCTIONAL DISORDERS

For a long time mental illness in old age was thought to be related to brain damage. There were some nonpsychiatric writers such as Goethe who recognized and described depression in old age, as he did in his novel, *Wilhelm Meister's Lehrjahre*. By 1930 more and more investigators were cautioning clinicians not to misdiagnose as arteriosclerotic or senile psychosis when in fact depression was the problem. Studies in England by Post, Roth, and their colleagues emphasized the significant incidence of affective (referring to people's emotions or feelings) illnesses in old age. These workers developed methods for differentiating depression from organic illness through studies of outcome (for example, discharge from hospitals, death) and psychological tests. Tests of orientation and memory such as the Mental Status Questionnaire (MSQ) of Goldfarb became helpful in establishing the organic diagnosis.

The incidence of mental illness increases as people age. Table 4-1 shows the average annual incidence rates per 100,000 population of total psychoses (functional and organic) for the state of Texas, 1951-1952. This table demonstrates also the markedly increasing incidence of psychopathology, decade by decade, with advancing age. The Na-

Table 4-1. Average annual incidence rates of psychoses (per 100,000 population of total psychoses, functional and organic, Texas, 1951-1952)*

Age-group	Males	Females	Total
To 15 years	1	1	1
15 to 24 years	42	48	45
25 to 34 years	90	117	103
35 to 44 years	98	127	112
45 to 54 years	106	135	120
55 to 64 years	133	127	130
65 to 74 years	155	122	137
75 and over	274	183	228
Total rates	68	78	73

*From Jaco, E. Gartly: The social epidemiology of mental disorders, New York, 1960, Russell Sage Foundation.

tional Institute of Mental Health has presented data confirming the same generalizations (WHO, 1959).

Further knowledge shows that the increasing mental illness in old age is explained in large measure by the rising occurrence of depression and organic brain disorders. In the 1950s and 1960s in England and America, independent researchers simultaneously highlighted the importance of recognizing depressions. Estimates vary, but probably about 30% to 40% of major illness (that is, illness likely to lead to hospitalization) is composed of functional disorders.* However, the remaining 70% that are organic cases may contain as many as 50% reversible (acute) organic states due to such varied causes as malnutrition, congestive heart failure, drug reactions, and infections. Depression can be and often is an accompanying part of the organic conditions, and it too can be treated and possibly reversed along with the acute brain syndromes.

Psychotic disorders

Psychosis implies varying degrees of personality disintegration and of difficulty in testing and correctly evaluating external reality. Delusions and hallucinations are characteristic, as well as inappropriate behavior and attitudes and a diminished control of impulses.

Late-life schizophrenia (also called late paraphrenia or senile schizophrenia)

Schizophrenia is a severe emotional disorder marked by disturbances of thinking, mood, and behavior; but thought disorder is the primary feature. Hallucinations, delusions, and poor reality testing are characteristic.

In our experience it has been rare to see a newly developed schizophrenic disorder in an older person. "Paraphrenia," as it is called in England and the Continent, may be equivalent to the diagnosis of so-called paranoid states in America. Kay and Roth state "The relationship between paraphenic, paranoid and schizophrenic illness has long been disputed, and no view at present commands general acceptance." Late paraphrenia is used by European authors for cases with a paranoid symptom complex in which signs of organic dementia or sustained confusion are absent and the delusional and hallucinatory symptoms do not appear to be due to major affective disorder or to paranoia, in which delusions would be better systematized. However, in the course of time the illness changes features, which makes diagnosis uncertain. Social factors often include little human contact. Deafness is a common physical factor.

Many older people have developed types of schizophrenia in earlier years and carried them into old age. These persons are often called "chronic schizophrenics." The classic age of onset is adolescence. One sees schizophrenic patients who have been hospitalized as long as fifty or sixty years; many never received treatment and were simply "stored" out of sight in hospitals, beyond the mainstream of medicine and psychiatry. (Privately paying patients usually fared better: they were likely to be hospitalized on occasions of decompensation and then released to their homes where further care could be given as needed.) The following is an example of a chronic schizophrenic patient hospitalized for forty years:

Mr. M is 67 years of age. The diagnosis in his case was schizophrenic reaction, chronic undifferentiated type, of moderate severity, with onset at approximately 21 years of age. He was also diagnosed as showing a moderate depressive reaction for the past two years.

Mr. M was hospitalized about forty years ago and in the last six months has been moved to a foster care home. He has only minimal impairment of his recent memory and his level of intellectual functioning has not declined. His impairments of judgment and abstraction are interpreted as psychogenic and not organic. Psychiatric symptoms include hypochondriacal ideas, suspiciousness, depressive trend, illusions, obsessions, compulsions, phobias, nightmares, sexual maladaptation (he claims he never had sexual intercourse), and

*Kay, D. W. K., Beamish, P., and Roth, M.: Old age mental disorders in Newcastle-upon-Tyne: a study of prevalence, British Journal of Psychiatry 465:146-158, 1964.

psychosomatic symptoms. There is a history of auditory hallucinations.

Since age 21, when he began feeling "hot, dizzy, unable to breathe and I've been no good since," he has been treated with tonics, sedatives, and electroconvulsive therapy. He began work at 12 and had a good work history until he became ill.

Developmental history included the death of a father at age 15; immigration to the United States from Germany at that time, with a mother, brother, and two sisters; financial difficulties; language problems and stuttering that impeded his school work. Neither he nor any of his siblings married. He was apparently inordinately close to his sisters and hated his brother. He wanted to spend his later years traveling with his sisters but they died.

Mr. M was moved to the foster care home where his blind brother had been placed earlier. He has become increasingly nervous and depressed ever since the transfer. His defense is to continue to be future-oriented. Although he sees himself as trapped in a home with a despised brother and deserted by the death of sisters, he holds out the hope that he "may find the answer" to a better life for himself.

In addition to his personality characteristics it seems clear that there was little basic understanding of the environmental stresses on Mr. M at the time of his breakdown and little treatment given, beyond minimal care. But forty years later he is still "hoping" for a cure and a better future. One could say either that he is denying reality or that in spite of everything he has refused to give up.

In the later years schizophrenia may coexist with a chronic brain syndrome as illustrated in the next summary:

Mrs. W was diagnosed as showing schizophrenic reaction, paranoid type, and chronic brain syndrome associated with arteriosclerosis and senile brain disease (mixed). The schizophrenia was regarded as chronic, severe, and of many years' duration whereas the chronic brain syndrome is of recent origin.

She is 74 years old, her husband is dead, and she has been intermittently hospitalized since her early twenties. Her appearance is one of sadness, suspiciousness, and distance. Major psychiatric symptoms include depressive trend, grandiose ideas, auditory and visual hallucinations and illusions. The chronic brain syndrome is evidenced by difficulty in maintaining attention and set, irrelevance, fabrication, perseveration of ideas, shifts of mood, and inappropriate and shallow affect. It is difficult to differentiate between the two disorders. At first the brain syndrome is most evident, but as one talks with Mrs. W she seems to have less and less ability to integrate and suppress her delusional systems. At this point the schizophrenia becomes clearly obvious.

Major affective disorders (affective psychoses)

The affective disorders are distinguished from schizophrenia because they are primarily *mood* rather than thought disorders. A single mood, either extreme depression or elation, is characteristic and accounts for whatever loss of contact with the environment exists. There is no apparent connection with an event in real life, although this may be debatable.

Involutional melancholia (involutional psychotic reaction). This is a psychotic reaction that takes place during the involutional period, originally referred to as the end of ovarian functions (menopause)* but now used in connection with aging in general. Depressive and occasionally paranoid types are seen. Onset occurs from age 40 to 55 in women and 50 to 65 in men, thus suggesting a relationship to certain emotion-laden life events.† For example, a woman in her forties may find her children leaving home and her life changing. The man in his fifties may begin to recognize the limits on whatever achievements he may have hoped for and realize that retirement is not far off. As women identify more and more with careers, one would expect similar reactions at this time for them. The impact of these life events depends on the individual's personality, previous life experience, and contemporary circumstances. Anger is usually a distinctive element in these, as in all depressions. Some writers liken depression to an internal temper tantrum.

---

*Whether there is any connection with the physiological aspects of menopause at all is questionable. Millions of women go through menopause without major depressive reactions.

†Exogenous depressions are explained by outside events in one's life. Endogenous depressions are internal and apparently not caused by immediate outside occurrences. They may be related to early developmental deprivations and losses. They also may be caused by the inner process known as the life review in older persons. It is often not possible to differentiate clearly between the two types of depression.

The course of involutional melancholia tends to be a prolonged one, manifested through feelings of guilt, anxiety, agitation, delusional ideas, insomnia, and somatic preoccupation. There is no previous history of manic-depressive illness. Differentiation from other psychotic reactions is difficult.

Manic-depressive illnesses (manic-depressive psychoses). These illnesses are marked by severe mood swings from depression to elation and may show either both extremes or cyclic episodes of one mood alone with recurrence and remission. They occur most frequently in women, in higher social classes, and among professional people.

Psychotic depressive reaction

The diagnosis of psychotic depressive reaction is used to refer to severe depressions that are related to some definable life experience (the less severe are called depressive neuroses or reactive depressions). Ordinarily the person has no history of repeated depression or cyclothymic moodiness. People who in middle or somewhat later life develop these or any other depressions often have been high-striving, ambitious, overly conscientious, or obsessive compulsive. Reality testing and ability to function are impaired. The precipitating factor is usually a serious loss or disappointment.

It is often difficult to differentiate between depressive and organic states (Chapter 9). There are even some investigators (Gillespie, Kassel, etc.) who feel that organic senile psychosis is itself a functional state brought about by the accumulated stresses of aging.

Paranoid states

Paranoid states are psychotic disorders presenting a delusion, usually persecutory or grandiose, as the main abnormality. From this delusion follow disturbances in mood, behavior, and thinking. Paranoid states are therefore different from the affective psychoses and schizophrenias, in which mood and thought disorders are the essential problem. Intellectual functions are not impaired. Paranoid states are usually of short duration but are sometimes chronic as in classic paranoia. They tend to occur under adverse conditions—imprisonment, deafness, isolation, disfigurement, infections, drunkenness, involution, or blindness. Isolation from human contact and a hearing loss that results in misinterpretation of incoming stimuli are perhaps primary precipitating factors. Women are affected more than men, although paranoid states are quite common in the elderly of both sexes.

Actual classic paranoia itself is extremely rare, marked by an elaborate, well-organized paranoid system in which the person may consider himself remarkably endowed with superior ability and powers. Allen and Clow describe four types of paranoid reactions generally seen in older people: "1) a type which may be called 'consistent' since it reveals the inevitable but overreactionary annoyances at real physical and environmental limitations, characteristic to some extent of all over 60; 2) a type characterized by episodic paranoid conditions with generally favorable prognosis; 3) the paranoid type of involutional psychosis in which the prognosis is frequently poor; and 4) a type displaying a paranoid trend associated with organic brain disease where the prognosis precludes complete recovery."*

Sometimes the paranoid symptoms may be very discrete or circumscribed. An older woman in her late seventies may seem free of major psychopathological symptoms, but at nighttime she thinks that the neighbor above is purposely taking a cane and pounding the ceiling or that fumes are being sent out from the radiators in the bathroom. However, study may uncover the fact that this is a discrete, circumscribed delusion related to fears, say, of being alone at night or lacking visual orientation in the dark. Such symptoms are, characteristically, isolated and may not influence everyday activities.

Folie à deux is a mental disorder in which two persons who are intimately associated with each other develop the same delusions. One person is dominant. The submissive

---

*From Allen, E. B., and Clow, H. E.: Paranoid reaction in the aging, Geriatrics 5:66-73, 1950.

partner may be more shaky in his or her beliefs and when separated from the stronger personality may give up the delusional system. It is more frequent among people with similar backgrounds such as siblings, parents, and children; but it can develop among unrelated (nonconsanguineous) persons, including man and wife. Misperception may attain paranoid proportions:

The frightened voice of a woman begged me (RNB) on the phone to see her and her mother because (and she lowered her voice) mother wants to move again. Otherwise "they" will get her.

At the appointed hour a woman of 42 and of faded attractiveness arrived, with a frail, sharp-faced woman of 70. In the office they insist on my seeing them together, not separately. They describe the harassment they have received from two men living below. They mention the possibility that some wires are used to listen to them, perhaps in connection with their TV set or toaster. The older woman reveals excellent intellectual functioning, but she states that a man in the apartment above is shooting rays at her body, including "indecent places." He wants to kill her and she is powerless. He brings pains to her hands and knees, scorches parts of her body, and "stuns my consciousness." She refuses to see doctors, considers medications "harmful," and denies any illnesses (despite obvious malnutrition, manifestation of probable hypovitaminosis, arthritic changes, and a Meniére-like syndrome). She also insists that she has aged very little. Her unmarried daughter, deeply conflicted, nearly "believes" there are men responsible. Such quasi folie à deux is not rare.

See Chapter 13, treatment of paranoid reactions, for further information on folie à deux.

Several theories have been offered to explain the genesis of paranoid personalities and states. Freud believed unconscious homosexuality was the basis and thus analyzed the famous Schreber case (Schreber was a German jurist). Others dispute this single-factor approach and instead conceptualize that paranoid behavior is the result of family and interpersonal forces of distortion and a basic, profound insecurity. The personality of the paranoid patient grown older is one that may have been marked by sullen quietness, sensitivity, disdain, and fearfulness about a frightening, inimical world. Some move through life with certain uncertainty or uncertain certainty, eccentric and the object of public attention.

The slim bronzed white-haired man stalked the resort boardwalk during all the seasons. He often carried flowers in one hand and a transistor radio in the other. He would seem totally inattentive of others, muttering unintelligible sounds at various decibel levels.

• • •

Many, perhaps most, paranoid people go through life outside hospitals. They may be relatively harmless to others but are, of course, harmful to themselves for they are unable to experience intimacy and full psychological growth. They are seen as cranks, eccentrics, hard to get along with, touchy, angry. They are avoided, and what few human and other attachments they may have in life inevitably disappear with advancing age. Following is an example of the increasing late-life isolation of the paranoid personality:

Dr. J, a 72-year-old man, was diagnosed as having paranoid personality with obsessive features, chronic, severe, and of lifelong duration. His second diagnosis is depressive reaction, moderate, and of two or three years' duration. He compensates well in a suitable, supportive, and structured environment.

Dr. J is a dentist in semiretirement who is irritable, suspicious, depressed, and anxious. He is extremely intelligent and integrated very well during interviews. He was paranoid, belligerent, and self-centered; yet it was remarkable how he could put aside his belligerence and tell of his delusions.

He was in semiretirement because of a failing practice and not of his own choice. He applied for room in an old age home because he felt he was at the end of his rope. He sees his situation as resulting from the imperfections of the world and other people but at other times describes his life adjustment as poor and says he hates himself.

He was born in Poland, came to the United States at 20, was unusually attached to his mother, and had "nothing in common" with his siblings. His father died when Dr. J was 12. He rebelled against education and did not enter dental school until he was 32. He married at 37 against his own desires, out of fear of an implied breach of promise suit, and was divorced four years later. He never considered remarriage. Marriage was his first and only sexual experience. He practiced dentistry in a poor neighborhood and had no close, personal relationships. He distrusted others and felt that only his alertness saved him from being exploited by others.

As Dr. J grew older, his isolation became more complete and he developed an angry depression through which he despised himself and the world. He seems unable to experience pleasure.

As Dr. J illustrates, the paranoid person may paradoxically get along in the community by being isolated. No one bothers with him and he bothers no one. But eventually a problem will emerge in which the person no longer can care for himself and must obtain help in some way. This is frequently the paranoid person's path to the mental hospital or, as in Dr. J's case, to an old age home.

The elderly paranoid person can be dangerous. Paranoid rage and murderousness do occur:

A slight, 89-year-old man who needed a cane to walk killed his daughter, a librarian, with a hatchet. "I wanted to see her die before I do," he said.

The body of the daughter, 57, was found in her bed with deep wounds in her head and body. Her father, who notified police by telephone that he had slain his daughter, was booked on a murder charge.

"The devil prompted me to do this," he told police.

However, such extreme behavior is the exception. In general, the following rule of thumb can be followed in evaluating paranoid states: "Show me one truly paranoid person and I will show you ten who are truly persecuted." Much of what appears to be paranoid behavior is a reaction to extraordinary and unbearable stress—physical, emotional, and environmental.

Neuroses

In spite of their clinical significance, neuroses in old age are largely ignored in the literature. With neurosis there is neither gross distortion of reality nor profound personality disorganization, although thinking and judgment may be impaired. Neurosis represents attempts at resolving unconscious emotional conflicts and is characterized by anxiety. Probably most older people who develop neurotic symptoms had similar difficulties earlier in life. Neuroses are not inevitable in old age but are extremely common.

Anxiety neurosis

Anxiety neurosis can either appear for the first time in old age or represent an increase in a previous history of neurosis. It may take the form of a nameless dread and sense of threat when no obvious danger is present or it may be an exaggerated response to real trouble and danger. Also, like people of all ages, old people may be struggling to curb unconscious and unacceptable impulses, aggressive or sexual. Finally, anxiety symptoms may portend some oncoming physical disease or condition that is beginning to unfold.

Hysterical neurosis—dissociative and conversion types

The dissociative type is seen when an older person becomes anxious to the point of personality disorganization, resulting in fugue states, stupor, amnesia, confusion, and sleepwalking. It may merge into a psychosis. Conversion neurosis occurs when emotional conflict changes into physical symptoms. An example is seen in the person who cannot move an arm or leg, although there is no physical reason for not doing so. Only the special senses or the voluntary nervous system are involved. The mechanism for causing this is unconscious as opposed to the conscious manipulations of the malingerer. The autonomic nervous system is not involved and thus provides diagnostic differentiation from psychophysiological (psychosomatic) disorders. In older people with this tendency, symptoms or illnesses may be exaggerated and in this way a "secondary gain" be achieved, in the form of extra attention and help.

Obsessive compulsive and phobic neuroses

Obsessive compulsive and phobic neuroses may also be found. The former type is seen when unacceptable thoughts or actions occur, which the person cannot stop (excessive handwashing, touching something repeatedly, etc.); the latter represents an intense fear of something that is no real danger in itself but represents a displacement of something fearful. An example might be a fear of death, which can be expressed symptomatically as a fear of closed spaces. Both of these neuroses tend to have developed prior to the aging period, but they may appear for the first time in old age.

Depressive neuroses (reactive depressions or depressive reactions)

Depression is the most common of the neuroses found in older people.* Usual indicators of the presence of depression are feelings of helplessness, sadness, lack of vitality, frequent feelings of guilt, loneliness, boredom, constipation, sexual disinterest and impotence. In severe depressions insomnia, early morning fatigue, and marked loss of appetite may be seen. Hypochondriasis and somatic symptoms are common. A depressive neurosis can be triggered by loss of love or a loved one, disappointments, criticism or other threats, both real and imagined.

Mr. P is a 69-year-old insurance salesman who was diagnosed as having depressive neurosis, moderate, with an estimated duration of fifteen years.

In 1941 he was in serious financial difficulties of his own making, and legal proceedings followed. He became depressed and made a serious suicidal attempt (opened his veins in the bathtub). He recovered and was then tried, convicted, and imprisoned for six months. He tells this with a stir of matyrdom and denies guilt or regret over it. He was able to recover his insurance license but thereafter suffered a declining career. He and his wife had basic disagreements, which were exacerbated by his semiretirement. He became more and more depressed and felt misunderstood and victimized. He evidenced considerable anger toward his wife and gave a history of many extramarital affairs. He denied depression but obliquely indicated he *may* get depressed over not having done enough for others, such as children, but he would not be depressed *for himself*. He slept poorly and was afraid of death.

His early life was one of deprivation and poverty. He was puny and sickly and was diagnosed as malnourished. At 11 he left his home, fanatically religious father, and "charitable" mother and developed his own moral code of independence ("don't like to be helped"). In truth he is extremely dependent on women (wife and mistresses) but scoffs at them as pitiful figures: ("It is a curse to be a woman"). He handles his inadequate and depressed feelings by a kind of compensating grandiosity—a fantasy life in which he would make the world all right. When one thinks of his early losses and his more recent ones, it becomes apparent that his current depression is a reactivation of earlier depressed feelings.

Busse has emphasized decreased self-regard as much more important than guilt in the causation of depression in older people, and this has been repeatedly stressed in the psychiatric literature. However, we feel it is simply not so. Old people are still capable of actions that produce guilt, even when they are on a death bed. Old age does not wipe out vindictiveness, anger, greed, or similar characteristics that are hurtful to others. The elderly also must deal with their guilt from the past, particularly during the life review process through which they examine past actions. As one elderly woman said, "That's the story of my life, doctor. I wish I were dead." And even recognizing that reduced self-regard is an important ingredient in depression does not gainsay the fact that the more guilty are more vulnerable. A prolonged depressive reaction following the death of someone close is often related to problems with the deceased person earlier in life. Thus the grief is burdened by guilt.

Mrs. Allen P is an 85-year-old Southern gentlewoman of charm as well as so-called helplessness. She was admitted as a voluntary mental patient

*Müller and Ciompi, at the University of Lausanne, have major studies in progress on the late-life outcomes of patients hospitalized with a variety of psychiatric disorders before 65. The material on 555 cases of depression, for example, shows a lessening intensity with age, greater tendency to somatization, etc. These studies on the natural history of psychiatric disorders inescapably provide insights concerning the life cycle. These particular studies, of course, do not concern the development and evolution of psychiatric disorders that occur for the first time in late life. More studies of both categories, along with longitudinal psychodynamic, life cycle investigations of the lives of people who have not suffered psychiatric disorders before or after 65, are indicated. The "control group" of the natural courses of life events is the least examined.

eight years ago, just after the death of her husband. Following the retirement of her wealthy husband, she was said to have developed delusions of poverty, and she showed increasing bitterness toward him. After he had sustained a cerebral vascular accident, she pushed him in his wheelchair down a flight of stairs because he would not speak. Upon admission, she was described as having delusions of poverty, being confused, and being extremely controlling and complaining. The psychological studies showed little or no intellectural deterioration but, rather, many superior intellectual capacities. She was tense and paranoid. Psychotherapy was strongly recommended but was refused by the patient.

She remains lively, cantankerous, and bitter. She expresses her anger with great determination and notable effect. To illustrate, she once urinated in church in the company of her one surviving son. She did not acknowledge any awareness of her anger toward her son and dismissed the episode by noting, "The young man next to me seemed embarrassed by the smell." She also coerced the staff to provide a commode in her room because "I can't get to the bathroom at night on time." And she fights the nurses by utilizing it unnecessarily during the day.

She is a voluntary patient. She is not overtly psychotic. She is in good physical health. She is monied. She is obviously full of life. She has *chosen* to live out her remaining years in comparative oblivion in a mental hospital rather than live in the outside world closer to her surviving family. She discourages visitors, including her favorite granddaughter. On the other hand, it is equally clear at times that she strains to be related. One might speculate that this self-imprisonment offers her the opportunity for expiation for past wrongs, a way of readying herself for Judgment Day.

Severe depressive reactions are often found associated with physical disease, especially with diseases that leave people incapacitated or in pain.* Dovenmuehle and Verwoerdt† (1963) and others have demonstrated correlations between the two. Unfortunately the presence of physical or organic disorders tends to discourage practitioners from treating the depressions that accompany or are added to them. Family members may agree with nontreatment, feeling it would be too much for the person to handle. The following is an example (from case notes of RNB) of a depressed man with an organic brain syndrome who was "protected" from treatment, even though it was felt he could have benefited:

I was asked to see a 76-year-old man who lived alone in a large apartment. His son had arranged for around-the-clock nursing because his father was confused, disoriented, and not able to take care of himself. I learned that his wife had been placed in a nursing home eight months before because of increasing confusion and depression further complicated by serious heart disease. The husband became increasingly upset upon his visits to see her. The wife had died four months before, and the son had decided to spare his father that "dreadful news." Therefore, he was not taken to the funeral. The father had given up reading newspapers and so had not seen the obituary. Despite the father's worsening condition, a psychiatrist had not been called because "It is too late. He is simply senile. There is nothing that can be done." In the two visits that I made I did not succeed in making very profound contact with him. It was apparent that he was severely depressed as well as suffering from organic damage. Among a number of suggestions I made to the family was that he be told of his wife's death. But the son did not agree to this.

The man's depressive illness had dated from his separation from his wife. It seemed likely that he was preoccupied by her situation and imagined her to be deeply suffering, both from her physical disease and their separation. Not knowing she was dead, he was in no position to make even the initial movements toward the resolution of grief. He may even have imagined her suffering to have been worse than it really was, especially since he may have seen through his son's efforts at deception and may have misinterpreted these efforts to mean that the son was covering up her suffering. He may have felt guilty over his own apparent inability to visit with his wife, and regarded himself as a deserter who deserves punishment.

One might understandably say "you're drawing an awful lot of conclusions from very little contact, only two hours." Perhaps his central nervous system was so diseased that he could not have understood the news of his wife's death anyway.

*There is also evidence of physiological concomitants of depression in the aged (Birren, Butler, Greenhouse, Sokoloff, and Yarrow: Human aging: a biological and behavioral study, Washington, D. C., 1963, reprint 1971, U. S. Government Printing Office). Hormonal changes have been demonstrated in depression at younger ages by Bunney and others.

†Dovenmuehle, R. H., and Verwoerdt, A.: Physical illness and depression symptomatology. II. Factors of length and severity of illness and frequency of hospitalization, Journal of Gerontology 18:260-266, 1963.

Table 4-2. Differential diagnosis of depressions*

		Criteria for evaluation		
		Loss of love object	**Self-esteem**	**Relationship to others**
Psychic states	Mourning	Real	Not impaired	Not disturbed
	Neurosis	May be real or fancied	May be impaired	May be disturbed
	Psychosis	May be real or fancied	Shattered, with end point at suicidal stage	Chaotically disrupted

*From Hall, Bernard: Medical World News, March 22, 1968, p. 53.

And, if he was sufficiently able to grasp the message, why should he be subjected to grief under the circumstances?

I strongly suspect that the son was quite correct when he concluded that his father would understand and would suffer. Where the son and I parted company was that he could not visualize that grief can be resolved and that some (but not all) of his father's symptomatology might have lifted as a consequence.

A differential diagnosis of depression is often difficult because many of the typical symptoms are similar whether the depression be classified as "normal," neurotic, or psychotic. Table 4-2 gives some useful clues to diagnosis. Depression varies all the way from the transient "blues," which everyone experiences, to the extremes of psychotic withdrawal or suicide. Depressive symptoms may be obvious and apparent or occult and hidden. The origins can be external (reactive) or internal (endogenous) or both. Drugs like the tranquilizers and hypotensive medication (for example, the Rauwolfia series) can cause the whole range of depressions. Sleep is often disturbed in depression, but there are no distinctive patterns as between reactive and endogenous forms. In general, the more depressed individuals, especially the agitated, sleep less in the latter half of the night.

One of the treatment problems with depressed people is that they tend toward negativism and withdrawal—making it difficult to locate and stay in contact with them. A Greek biographer, Plutarch, wrote of such a man:

The physician, the consoling friend, are driven away. "Leave me," says the wretched man, "me the impious, the accursed, hated of the gods, to suffer my punishment."

Hypochondriacal neurosis

Hypochondriasis is an overconcern with one's physical and emotional health, accompanied by various bodily complaints for which there is no physical basis. Hypochondriasis is commonly associated with depressive feelings but it may stand alone. It has many meanings, one of which may be a symbolization of the older person's sense of defectiveness and deterioration (Chapter 9, self-drawings). It may be a means of communication and interaction with others—family members, doctors, nurses, social workers. It can be used to displace anxiety from areas of greater concern. And it can include identification with a deceased loved one who had similar symptoms. Finally, it can serve as punishment for guilt, as an inhibition of impulses, and as an aid in the desire to control others. The following list summarizes the psychic functions of hypochondriasis in persons of all ages.

1. To symbolize and make concrete one's sense of defectiveness or deterioration
2. To serve as a ticket to interaction with caretakers (or punishers), doctors, nurses, etc.
3. To displace anxiety from areas of greater concern
4. To serve as part of identification with a deceased loved one through similar symptoms
5. To serve as punishment for guilt
6. To avoid or inhibit unwanted behavior or interactions

7. To punish others
8. To regulate (usually reduce) interpersonal intimacy*

Meyersberg's unpublished work on "crocks" is an excellent study of hypochondriasis. He speaks of the typical withdrawal of the physician in the face of treatment defeat, the voluminous clinic and hospital records for these patients, the magical expectation of patients that treatment personnel will alleviate their suffering. There is much overlap between depression and hypochondriasis. Most depressive individuals show some hypochondriacal preoccupations, and hypochondriasis has a gloomy and depressive mood associated with it. But whereas a basically depressed person will withdraw and not seek help, the hypochondriac sees his problems as physical and goes to the doctor, thus at least relieving the isolation. Meyersberg sees hypochondriasis as a prophylactic measure, in that the person may be taking steps that ward off more incapacitating mental illness. Thus medical help, although not curing the problem, may be a preventive measure, particularly if it can lead the patient to examine the real reasons he is seeking help. Even if it cannot, a service is being provided, perhaps to everyone's dismay. Anxiety should be listened to and accepted. Hypochondriasis causes special difficulties if it is connected with a real organic condition. Then, diagnosis and treatment may be difficult.†

Personality disorders

In this broad group of disorders we see defects in personality development that are of lifelong nature. There is little sense of anxiety or distress associated with them. Maladaptive patterns of behavior are deeply ingrained.

Certain personality disorders serve different adaptive functions, depending on the stage in the life cycle. This phenomenon, the changing adaptive nature of psychopathology, was observed in the NIMH studies by Perlin and Butler. For example, a so-called schizoid or introspective personality may function somewhat better in old age. Such an individual tends to be insulated against the experiences of life and therefore may feel relatively more comfortable in the loneliness and difficulties of old age. On the other hand, he may become even more of a recluse with almost no human contact. The man or woman with a paranoid personality has perhaps the most problems in later life as he loses his few friends and relationships and becomes increasingly isolated.* The inadequate, dependent person may welcome and enjoy the opportunity for greater dependence in old age and the freedom from work responsibilities. Obsessive compulsiveness can become useful in taking care of oneself and keeping busy with many details; in fact this type of individual can create a whole life for himself by "taking care" of things—possessions, spouse, grandchildren, bodily ailments, etc. (as Mr. H has done).

Mr. H has been retired three years. His obsessions and compulsions are useful mechanisms in filling the vacuum of a forced retirement. "My home is always in order," says Mr. H, as he putters around the house, arranging everything according to strict schedule in a careful, meticulous manner. He is thrifty and even hoarding of his possessions, not to mention his feelings.

*From Patterson, R. D., Freeman, L. C., and Butler, R. N.: Psychiatric Aspects of adaptation, survival and death. In Granick, S., and Patterson, R. D., editors: Human aging. II. HSM 71-9037, Washington, D. C., 1971, U. S. Government Printing Office.

†Unpublished work of Dr. Herman Arnold Meyersberg and colleagues (George Washington University Medical School, Washington, D. C.), 1966.

*Occasionally a folie à deux may result, involving the older person and someone close to him. One kind of "eccentricity" is observed when a mother and daughter, two brothers, or two sisters become recluses, living in a house that ages as they do—or, more precisely, deteriorates. It is usually the health department that becomes alerted for purposes of cleanup or eviction. Electricity may be off, plumbing and toilets may not function, there may have been small fires, human feces may be found on the bathroom floor, cat litter may be evident, window screens may be rusting, the house may need painting and repairs, the garden may be overgrown.

He takes care of his health with religious fervor and follows the doctor's orders precisely. He has arranged for two grave sites (one in St. Louis and one in Florida) so he can be well taken care of in case he dies, whether at home or on vacation. He has checked actuarial tables to predict his death at age 88, leaving no stone unturned.

The cyclothymic personality may also be helpful by activating the individual periodically. From a therapeutic perspective it is important to realize the possible adaptive qualities of personalities. Obsessional persons may be encouraged to make constructive use of ritualism. The therapist can help hysterical persons keep alive their dramatic qualities and, at times, their childlike expectations.

Sexual deviations in older people are overestimated and overstated. Most sexual pathology is related to young adulthood.* Sensationalism in court cases concerning children who have been "molested" has been misleading in many instances. The sexual element may have been less significant than the loneliness of the older person, who may have no children or grandchildren. Some elderly men have fantasies of rejuvenation in contact with young children,† rather than any direct sexual preoccupation. Children of course must be protected from any exploitation that may occur. But the older person needs sympathetic understanding rather than punishment, and efforts should be made to provide that which is lacking in their lives. In some cases, total misinterpretation occurs. We have known of old people who were supposedly molesting younger children and have been arrested for exhibitionism; actually they were confused, needed to urinate, and found the most convenient spot.

Criminal activities are rare in late life. Violent crimes are seldom committed, although embezzlement and other less violent crimes do occur. Old "sociopaths" do fade away, it seems. We seldom have seen aged "con artists." Thus geriatric delinquency is not a problem to rouse one's keen interest.

*Gebhard, P. H., Pomeroy, W. B., Christenson, Cornelia, and Gagnon, J. H.: Sex offenders: an analysis of types, New York, 1965, Harper & Row, Publishers.

†This idea is of a standard biblical conception. The elderly King David, for example, was advised to "lay" with young girls.

Psychophysiological disorders (also called psychosomatic disorders or "organ neuroses")

The psychophysiological disorders are physical symptoms caused by emotional factors and involving an organ system under control of the autonomic nervous system. Anxiety leads to these chronic and exaggerated expressions of emotions characterized by effects on secretion, mobility, and vascularity in various tissue and organ systems. Alfred Adler, Flanders Dunbar, and Franz Alexander contributed much to our understanding of the interplay between physiological and psychological events.

It is important to differentiate psychosomatic disorders from conversion reactions and hypochondriasis. The following are signs of psychosomatic disorders.

1. The autonomic nervous system is involved, and not the voluntary musculature and sensory perceptive systems.
2. The disorder does not reduce anxiety, thus contrasting with the conversion reaction, in which the phenomenon of *la belle indifférence* (beautiful indifference) occurs.
3. There is a physiological rather than symbolic origin of symptoms.
4. There is a definite somatic threat because of structural change.

In older people, some of the common psychophysiological reactions include skin reactions such as pruritus* ani and vulvae, psychogenic rheumatism, hyperventilation syndromes, irritable colon, nocturia,† and cardiac neuroses with fear of sudden death. Preoccupations with bowel habits are common, perhaps less related to age than to cultural considerations. Laxatives, certain food habits, and theories of diseases in the early 1900s were very influential in the

*Itchiness.

†Frequency of urination at night.

childhoods of contemporary older people: theories of ptomaine poisoning, focal infections, and fletcherism (the meticulous chewing of food) are all heritages of both the national and the medical culture. Constipation is a common complaint, and nocturia can be extremely disconcerting.

In our experience some psychosomatic disorders—for example, ulcers—are less common in old age; other types—especially muscular, skeletal, genitourinary, and dermatological problems—are perhaps more common. Psychotherapy is helpful.

Mr. B visited to ask our help for a pruritic scalp condition on his essentially bald pate; he "incidentally" told us of the recent death of his wife. He could not get himself to say Kaddish, the mourner's prayer in the Jewish faith. The scalp condition was similar to the rim of a skull cap, worn by men in the synogogue. We treated his already infected lesions and discussed his wife and the question of saying Kaddish. He later reported having said the prayer and of having a "clear" scalp. (He also reported newly growing hair!)

How important is diagnostic classification?

Strömgren has stated that classification of the disorders of old age is complex and that they "very often have no clear-cut borderlines. In many cases the onset is so insidious that it is impossible to state the time at which a person is passing from the 'healthy' group to the 'ill' group. In addition, the nosological entities in many cases are not sharply defined, with the result that frequently it may, in principle, be impossible to say definitely whether the case under consideration should be included in the group."*

We hold that the diagnostic task must be functional, determining what is remediable. We must not allow ourselves to fall into the time-wasting quagmire of the "how many angels can sit on the head of a pin?" type of diagnostic game-playing.

*From Strömgren, E.: Epidemiology of old-age psychiatric disorders. In Williams, R. H., Tibbitts, C., and Donahue, Wilma, editors: Process of aging, vol. 2, New York, 1963, Atherton Press.

SOME SUBJECTS PERTINENT TO MENTAL BREAKDOWN

Lack of mourning rites

The elderly in the United States today do not receive necessary cultural support for grief and mourning. Learning how to mourn productively and restoratively requires models in ritual and custom as well as in personal experiences with others who mourn. Lack of such support can prolong depression and leave grief unresolved. Patterns of mourning for the dead are in disarray as many time-honored customs become discarded (wearing black clothing, abstaining from social events for a period of time, etc.) and others are practiced piecemeal (religious rituals, the rallying around of friends and family, etc.) Still other patterns are recent and psychologically-suspect innovations (funeral directors or morticians who "console" the family, the use of barbiturates to calm nerves and deaden the feelings). Gorer (1965) remarks that, up to 1900, every society in the world had definite rules for mourners to follow.* This is no longer true, and the picture might accurately be described as "every man or woman for him/herself" as long as mourning does not bother anyone else. Our culture seems reluctant to acknowledge the pain of death and to bear the agony of experiencing it through to acceptance. Some churches and many individuals deny the existence of death, preferring to speak of it as "merely sleep" or "the beginning of life hereafter." This may reassure individuals but it does not help them resolve the pain of separation and the need to find new attachments.

In the United States people receive some support in the period of initial shock, from the time of the death to burial. But after that the church services are over, the undertaker disappears with a sizeable portion of the mourner's money, and relatives and friends go home, taking away their casserole

*Gorer, Geoffrey: Death, grief, and mourning, New York, 1965, Doubleday Anchor Press.

dishes and other gestures of help and support. But for the mourner the intense period of mourning is just beginning and it must usually be experienced alone. Onlookers will try to divert the mourner's attention to other things. Crying is considered indulgent and possibly harmful rather than a psychological necessity. Gorer compares our present attitudes toward death and mourning with the prudish attitudes toward sex in the past: death has become an obscenity—one should not discuss it in public, the feelings are "bad," and any indulgence in mourning must be done in secret.

Gorer goes on to point out the maladaptive behavior that results. Exaggerated depression, aimless busyness, deification of the dead person, or callous denial of others' grief as well as one's own may occur. People may become excessively preoccupied with death or violence. Since death is an unavoidable crisis inherent in the human life cycle, it is peculiar that a society can so determinedly avoid the provisions of cultural custom and ritual that could make it easier to bear. However, such a coming to terms with death would require a coming to terms with the value of human life. This would mean some considerable reshuffling of values in American society.

Suicide in old age

The highest rate of suicide occurs in white males in their eighties. Suicide is one of the ten leading causes of death in the United States. The elderly, about 10% of the population, account for roughly 25% of reported suicides—about 5,000 to 8,000 yearly.* The peak rate of suicide for white women occurs in middle age. However, throughout the world, suicide rates have been increasing for women, especially older women.† Rates for black men and women are lower, with a peak in middle age. Table 4-3 shows suicides per 100,000 population by age and sex.‡ The increased suicide rate with age is found in all countries which keep reliable statistics.

Table 4-3. Suicides per 100,000 population by age and sex in 1964*

Age	Male	Female
Total	16.1	5.6
5 to 14	0.4	0.1
15 to 24	9.2	2.8
25 to 34	16.9	7.0
35 to 44	21.3	10.1
45 to 54	29.9	11.6
55 to 64	36.1	10.2
65 to 74	37.0	9.8
75 to 84	47.5	6.4
85 and over	59.3	4.1

*Based on U. S. Public Health Service data.

The 75-year-old man suffocated after he tied a plastic bag over his head and pulled it tight with a pajama drawstring. He was despondent over ill health.

• • •

Police in Blaine, Minnesota, reported that an 85-year-old man, depressed over a painful illness, arranged for his own funeral, then drove to the mortuary and shot himself in his car. Police said he telephoned the Wexler Funeral Home Sunday and inquired about the cost of cremation, telling an employee he would be over later. He wrote a note to his wife. Authorities found him dead in his car with a $300 check made out to the funeral home.

• • •

Rear Admiral Fred B, 56, who retired from the Navy last year after thirty years of service was found dead in a hotel room with a .22 caliber bullet wound in his head. A pistol was found near the body. Police ruled the death a suicide.

In the German language suicide means self-murder (selbstmord). This etymology tells something of the motives of hatred of self or others which are present in many suicides. Freud in 1925 said that perhaps no one could find the psychical energy to

*Resnik, H. L., and Cantor, J. M.: Suicide and aging, Journal of the American Geriatrics Society 18:152-158, 1970.

†Weiss, J. M. A.: Suicide in the aged. In Resnik, H. C. P., editor: Suicidal behaviors, Boston, 1968, Little Brown & Co.

‡The actual rate of suicide is underreported because of shame and guilt. Some religious groups such as Catholics and Orthodox Jews have denied burial rites to suicides. It is also underestimated because of deception to protect life insurance.

kill himself unless in the first place he was thereby killing at the same time someone with whom he had identified himself. Menninger (1938) has written that the suicide victim wishes to die, to kill, and to be killed. Indeed, suicide is three times more common than homicide. Perhaps it is emotionally less threatening to consider killing oneself than others.

Other theoretical views concerning motivation for suicide include Durkheim's notion of *anomie or alienation.* Old white men commit suicide at greater rates than black men or women in general (after the different life expectancies of each group are accounted for). We surmise that the explanation lies in the severe loss of status (ageism) that affects white men, who as a group had held the greatest power and influence in society. Black men and most women have long been accustomed to a lesser status (through racism and sexism) and ironically do not have to suffer such a drastic fall in old age. In fact there are some indications that black people enjoy a rise in social status as they age.*

Control is another motivational element. Seneca said "Against all the injuries of life, I have the refuge of death"; and Nietzsche stated "The thought of suicide gets one successfully through many a bad night." Death itself is certain but its timing and its character are not. One can defy and control death by virtue of initiating the act of one's own death. Control also extends beyond the grave—survivors are deeply affected and a grim, unmistakable legacy of guilt, shame, and regret may be left for them to bear.

A *sacrificial romantic* quality can be present as in the double suicide pacts of lovers, old or young.

> In death pacts between lovers we meet the age-old belief, found in myth and history, that two people who die together are united forever beyond the grave. This belief is also encountered in the German Romantic Period. In Japan it is known as *shinju.* It is but a step from such a belief towards symbolization of the grave as a bridal bed.*

A *rational* or *philosophical* decision to kill oneself is undoubtedly more common in old age as people perceive themselves to be failing. Old men, especially, may decide to kill themselves rather than leave their widows penniless from the cost of a long illness. Married couples may commit double suicide or a combination of mercy killing of one and suicide of the other.

> Documents left by the married couples yield a typical picture of an ageing man and woman, one or both suffering from grave illness which is never absent from their thoughts. A deeply devoted pair, childless, in modest circumstances and with few interests and friends, they are deeply absorbed in their own small world. Prolonged insomnia speeds the decisive act. "We are at the end of our tether" is a phrase which repeatedly occurs. Here is a typical situation. A 56-year-old ex-miner, with impaired vision and an injured leg, underwent an operation for cancer of the bowel. The operation was not successful and he was confined to his bed with frequent, violent attacks of pain. His wife was disabled by Parkinson's disease and had been partly paralyzed for fifteen years.*

Perhaps the most preventable are the suicides related to *depression.* Albert Camus, French novelist and essayist, saw suicide as submission and stated "there is only one truly serious problem and that is suicide." Suicide in these cases is a passive, perhaps desperate, giving up. Depressive reactions are very widespread and important in old age. These include not only psychotic depression or the special depression associated with lucid moments of the cerebral arteriosclerotic patient, but also those of an everyday nature resulting from loss, grief, and despair. Depressions frequently follow physical illnesses, including viral illnesses, and are not uncommon in Parkinson's disease. Varying degrees of depression may be observed in connection with lowered self-esteem due to reduced social and personal valuation and status. Retirement may be a fac-

---

*Wylie, F. M.: Attitudes toward aging and the aged among black Americans: some historical perspectives, Aging and Human Development **2:** 66-70, Feb., 1971.

*From Cohen, J.: Forms of suicide and their significance, Triangle **6**:280-286, 1964.

tor. Finally, guilt over one's actions in either the past or the present can lead to depression. Organic brain syndromes are a serious and complicating factor in late-life depressions.

Older people use all the usual methods of killing themselves: drugs, guns, hanging, and plunging. In the United States firearms and explosives are at the top of the list because of lack of gun control. Suicide may also be accomplished "subintentionally," by the slower means of not eating, not taking medicines, drinking too much, delaying treatment, and taking risks physically. This long-term process of suicidal erosion is of course not part of suicide statistics, since suicide is seen as a single act. Most laws regarding commitment require specific evidence of danger to oneself or to others (rightfully protecting the civil liberties of people). Therefore, such long, drawn-out self-destructive behavior often presents a touchy legal problem: does one try to intervene or not?

A 72-year-old woman insisted on living by herself and not with her daughter and the latter's family. She did not want to be a burden. Nonetheless, she had diabetes and congestive heart failure. By living alone she reduced the "threat" of effective prompt care in any emergency. Moreover, she lived in a cheap inner-city boarding house. It was unsanitary, the heat was not always adequate, and she had to walk up three flights of stairs.

It seems clear to us, in the above situation, that the woman's right to make her own choices is paramount, regardless of concern for her health. Indeed, it may be far more beneficial for her to have such choices than to be in a "safe" environment. The decision to take away choice must always be made very conservatively, seeking out every possible alternative. However, the concept of "danger to oneself or others" needs to be rethought with the long-term suicide in mind.

Mental health personnel should take suicide threats of older persons seriously. Persons attempting suicide are more likely to fail if below age 35 and to succeed if over 50. It is most rare for an attempt by anyone over 65 to fail. Men are more successful than women. (For suicidal clues, see Chapter 9.)

Reducing the frequency of depression and providing for its effective treatment when present are the major ways of reducing suicide in old age. One must be especially alert with people whose depressions seem to have lifted. They may be gathering enough energy to commit the suicide they had contemplated earlier. When there is evidence of suicidal preoccupations, one must schedule extra time and additional sessions. It is important to openly discuss the subject rather than, ostrichlike, hope it will go away. Rescue fantasies—that the therapist will always be on call or will rush to save them—must be dealt with and clarified. Grueling as it may seem, a "psychological autopsy" following a committed suicide is mandatory to try to understand what happened and whether anything could have been done. The Weisman-Kastenbaum procedure is useful. Outreach services are imperative to reach depressed people who may have withdrawn and become isolated. Old age must offer the older person something to live for. Bartko, Patterson and Butler reported that the degree of organization (activities, friendships, family relationships, interests, usefulness) in the daily life of old men was a good predictor of survival in originally healthy subjects.* Jung was correct when he said that man cannot stand a meaningless life. Suicide is evidence of that.

Physical effects of "giving up" psychologically

Suicide is not the only consequence of giving up. A team of researchers headed by George Engel (Schmale and Engel) at the University of Rochester Medical Center explored the relationship between psychological attitudes and the onset of physical disease. They found that between 70% and 80% of patients had felt like "giving up" at the time their illness developed. The study

---

*Bartko, John, Patterson, Robert, and Butler, Robert N.: Biomedical and behavioral predictors of survival among normal aged men: a multivariate analysis. In Palmore, E., and Jeffers, Francis C., editors: Prediction of life span, Lexington, Mass., 1971, Heath Lexington Books.

suggests that if a person responds to his life with hopelessness, depression, and submission, he may trigger a biological change that encourages the development of an already present disease potential. Their work included patients with infections, cancer, cardiovascular diseases, rheumatoid arthritis, diabetes, and diseases of the nervous system. Predictions of physical illness were able to be made on the basis of psychiatric interviews. Engel emphasized that it was not the magnitude of an event but the way in which a person reacted to it that determined whether one "gave up." Again, the treatment of despair and depression must be emphasized.

DIAGNOSTIC NOMENCLATURE OF THE AMERICAN PSYCHIATRIC ASSOCIATION (SELECTED SECTIONS)*

II. ORGANIC BRAIN SYNDROMES (OBS)

A. Psychoses

Senile and presenile dementia

290.0 Senile dementia
290.1 Presenile dementia

Alcoholic psychosis

291.0 Delirium tremens
291.1 Korsakov's psychosis
291.2 Other alcoholic hallucinosis
291.3 Alcohol paranoid state
291.4 Acute alcohol intoxication
291.5 Alcoholic deterioration
291.6 Pathological intoxication
291.9 Other alcoholic psychosis

Psychosis associated with intracranial infection

292.0 General paralysis
292.1 Syphilis of central nervous system
292.2 Epidemic encephalitis
292.3 Other and unspecified encephalitis
292.9 Other intracranial infection

Psychosis associated with other cerebral condition

293.0 Cerebral arteriosclerosis
293.1 Other cerebrovascular disturbance
293.2 Epilepsy
293.3 Intracranial neoplasm
293.4 Degenerative disease of the CNS

*From Diagnostic and statistical manual of mental disorders (DSMII), Washington, D. C., 1968, American Psychiatric Association.

Psychosis associated with other cerebral condition—cont'd

293.5 Brain trauma
293.9 Other cerebral condition

Psychosis associated with other physical condition

294.0 Endocrine disorder
294.1 Metabolic and nutritional disorder
294.2 Systemic infection
294.3 Drug or poison intoxication (other than alcohol)

B. Nonpsychotic OBS

309.0 Intracranial infection
309.13 Alcohol (simple drunkenness)
309.14 Other drug, poison, or systemic intoxication
309.2 Brain trauma
309.3 Circulatory disturbance
309.4 Epilepsy
309.5 Disturbance of metabolism, growth, or nutrition
309.6 Senile or presenile brain disease
309.7 Intracranial neoplasm
309.8 Degenerative disease of the CNS
309.9 Other physical condition

III. PSYCHOSES NOT ATTRIBUTED TO PHYSICAL CONDITIONS LISTED PREVIOUSLY

Schizophrenia

295.0 Simple
295.1 Hebephrenic
295.2 Catatonic
295.23 Catatonic type, excited
295.24 Catatonic type, withdrawn
295.3 Paranoid
295.4 Acute schizophrenic episode
295.5 Latent
295.6 Residual
295.7 Schizo-affective
295.73 Schizo-affective, excited
295.74 Schizo-affective, depressed
295.90 Chronic undifferentiated
295.99 Other schizophrenia

Major affective disorders

296.0 Involutional melancholia
296.1 Manic-depressive illness, manic
296.2 Manic-depressive illness, depressed
296.3 Manic-depressive illness, circular
296.33 Manic-depressive, circular, manic
296.34 Manic-depressive, circular, depressed
296.8 Other major affective disorder

Paranoid states
- 297.0 Paranoia
- 297.1 Involutional paraphrenia
- 297.9 Other paranoid state

Other psychoses
- 298.0 Psychotic depressive reaction

IV. NEUROSES
- 300.0 Anxiety
- 300.1 Hysterical
- 300.13 Hysterical, conversion type
- 300.14 Hysterical, dissociative type
- 300.2 Phobic
- 300.3 Obsessive compulsive
- 300.4 Depressive
- 300.5 Neurasthenic
- 300.6 Depersonalization
- 300.7 Hypochondriacal
- 300.8 Other neurosis

V. PERSONALITY DISORDERS AND CERTAIN OTHER NONPSYCHOTIC MENTAL DISORDERS

Personality disorders
- 301.0 Paranoid
- 301.1 Cyclothymic
- 301.2 Schizoid
- 301.3 Explosive
- 301.4 Obsessive compulsive
- 301.5 Hysterical
- 301.6 Asthenic
- 301.7 Antisocial
- 301.81 Passive-aggressive
- 301.82 Inadequate
- 301.89 Other specified types

Sexual deviation
- 302.0 Homosexuality
- 302.1 Fetishism
- 302.2 Pedophilia
- 302.3 Transvestitism
- 302.4 Exhibitionism
- 302.5 Voyeurism
- 302.6 Sadism
- 302.7 Masochism
- 302.8 Other sexual deviation

Alcoholism
- 303.0 Episodic excessive drinking
- 303.1 Habitual excessive drinking
- 303.2 Alcohol addiction
- 303.9 Other alcoholism

Drug dependence
- 304.0 Opium, opium alkaloids, and their derivatives
- 304.1 Synthetic analgesics with morphinelike effects
- 304.2 Barbiturates
- 304.3 Other hypnotics and sedatives or "tranquilizers"
- 304.4 Cocaine
- 304.5 Cannabis sativa (hashish, marihuana)

Drug dependence—cont'd
- 304.6 Other psychostimulants
- 304.7 Hallucinogens
- 304.8 Other drug dependence

VI. PSYCHOPHYSIOLOGICAL DISORDERS
- 305.0 Skin
- 305.1 Musculoskeletal
- 305.2 Respiratory
- 305.3 Cardiovascular
- 305.4 Hemic and lymphatic
- 305.5 Gastrointestinal
- 305.6 Genitourinary
- 305.7 Endocrine
- 305.8 Organ of special sense
- 305.9 Other type

VII. SPECIAL SYMPTOMS
- 306.2 Tic
- 306.3 Other psychomotor disorder
- 306.4 Disorders of sleep
- 306.9 Other special symptom

VIII. TRANSIENT SITUATIONAL DISTURBANCES
- 307.3 Adjustment reaction of adult life
- 307.4 Adjustment reaction of late life

X. CONDITIONS WITHOUT PSYCHIATRIC DISORDER AND NONSPECIFIC CONDITIONS

Social maladjustment without manifest psychiatric disorder
- 316.0 Marital maladjustment
- 316.1 Social maladjustment
- 316.2 Occupational maladjustment
- 316.3 Dyssocial behavior
- 316.9 Other social maladjustment

Nonspecific conditions
- 317 Nonspecific conditions

No mental disorder
- 318 No mental disorder

XI. NONDIAGNOSTIC TERMS FOR ADMINISTRATIVE USE
- 319.0 Diagnosis deferred
- 319.1 Boarder
- 319.2 Experiment only
- 319.9 Other

Fifth-digit qualifying phrases

Section II	Section III
.x1 Acute	.x6 Not psychotic now
.x2 Chronic	

Sections IV through IX	All disorders
.x6 Mild	.x5 In remission
.x7 Moderate	

REFERENCES

Allen, E. B.: Functional psychoses in the aging simulating organic syndromes, Geriatrics **2**:269-279, 1947.

Allen, E. B., and Clow, H. E.: Paranoid reactions in the aging, Geriatrics **5**:66-73, 1950.

Birren, James E., Butler, Robert N., Greenhouse, Samuel W., Sokoloff, Louis, and Yarrow, Marian R.: Human aging: a biological and behavioral study, Washington, D. C., 1963 (reprint 1971), U. S. Government Printing Office.

Busse, E. W., Barnes, R. H., Silverman, A. J., Thaler, Margaret, and Frost, L. L.: Studies of the processes of aging. X. The strengths and weaknesses of psychic functioning in the aged, American Journal of Psychiatry **111**:896-901, 1955.

Camus, A.: The myth of Sisyphus, New York, 1959, Vintage Books, Inc.

Cannon, W. B.: Voodoo death, American Anthropologist **44**:169-181, 1942.

Choron, J.: Death and Western thought, New York, 1963, Collier Books.

Clausen, John A.: The sociology of mental illness. In Merton, R. K., Broom, L., and Cottrell, C. S., Jr., editors: Sociology today: problems and prospects, New York, 1959, Basic Books, Inc., Publishers.

Cohen, Mabel B., Baker, Grace, Cohen, R. A., Fromm-Reichman, Frieda, and Weigert, Edith V.: An intensive study of twelve cases of manic-depressive psychosis, Psychiatry **17**:103-137, 1954.

Committee on Nomenclature and Statistics of the American Psychiatric Association: Diagnostic and statistical manual of mental disorders, ed. 2 (DSM II), Washington, D. C., 1968, American Psychiatric Association.

Cumming, Elaine, and Henry, W. E.: Growing old: the process of disengagement, New York, 1961, Basic Books, Inc., Publishers.

Dovenmuehle, R. H., and Verwoerdt, A.: Physical illness and depressive symptomatology. I. Incidence of depressive symptoms in hospitalized cardiac patients, Journal of the American Geriatric Society **10**:932-947, 1962.

Dovenmuehle, R. H., and Verwoerdt, A.: Physical illness and depressive symptomatology. II. Factors of length and severity of illness and frequency of hospitalization, Journal of Gerontology **18**:260-266, 1963.

Durkheim, E.: Suicide (originally 1847), London, 1952, Routledge & Kegan Paul, Ltd.

Faris, R. E. L., and Dunham, H. W.: Mental disorders in urban areas, Chicago, 1939, The University of Chicago Press.

Feifel, H., editor: The meaning of death, New York, 1961, McGraw-Hill Book Co., Inc.

Fish, F.: Senile schizophrenia, Journal of Mental Science **106**:938-946, 1960.

Freud, S.: Mourning and melancholia. In Standard edition of the psychological works of Sigmund Freud, vol. 14, London, 1957, Hogarth Press.

Gallinek, A.: The nature of affective and paranoid disorders during the senium in the light of ECT, Journal of Nervous and Mental Diseases **108**:292-303, 1948.

Goldfarb, A. I.: Psychiatric disorders of the aged: symptomatology, diagnosis and treatment, Journal of the American Geriatrics Society **8**:698-707, 1960.

Goldfarb, A. I.: Prevalence of psychiatric disorders in metropolitan old age and nursing homes, Journal of the American Geriatrics Society **10**: 77-84, 1962.

Gorer, Geoffrey: Death, grief, and mourning, New York, 1965, Doubleday Anchor Press.

Gruenberg, E. M.: A mental health survey of older persons. In Hoch, P. H., and Zubin, J., editors: Epidemiology of mental disorders, New York, 1961, Grune & Stratton, Inc.

Havighurst, R. J., Neugarten, Bernice L., and Tobin, S. S.: Disengagement, personality and life satisfaction in the later years. In Hansen, P. F., editor: Age with a future: Proceedings of the Sixth International Congress of Gerontology, Copenhagen, 1963, Copenhagen Munksgaard, 1964.

Hollingshead, A. B., and Redlich, F. C.: Social class and mental illness: a community study, New York, 1958, John Wiley & Sons, Inc.

Inglis, J., Colwell, Catherine, and Post, F.: Evaluation of the predictive power of a test known to differentiate between elderly functional and organic patients, Journal of Mental Science **101**:281-289, 1955.

Jaco, E. Gartly: The social epidemiology of mental disorders, New York, 1960, Russell Sage Foundation.

Kaplan, O. J.: Mental disorders in later life, ed. 2, Stanford, Calif., 1956, Stanford University Press.

Kassel, Victor: Psychosis in the aged, Journal of the American Geriatrics Society **5**:319-337, 1957.

Kay, D. W. K., Beamish, P., and Roth, M.: Old age mental disorders in Newcastle upon Tyne. I. A study of prevalence, British Journal of Psychiatry **465**:146-158, 1964.

Kay, D. W. K., and Roth, M.: Environmental and hereditary factors in the schizophrenias of old age ("late paraphrenia") and their bearing on the general problem of causation in schizophrenia, Journal of Mental Science **107**:649-685, 1961.

Kral, V. A.: Psychiatric observations under severe chronic stress, American Journal of Psychiatry **108**:185-192, 1951.

Kramer, M., Taube, C., and Starr, S.: Patterns of use of psychiatric facilities by the aged: current status, trends and implications. In Simon, A., and Epstein, L. J., editors: Aging in modern society, Psychiatric Research Report No. 23, Washington, D. C., 1968, American Psychiatric Association.

Kutner, B., Fanshel, D., Togo, Alice M., and Langner, T. S.: Five hundred over sixty: a community survey on aging, New York, 1956, Russell Sage Foundation.

Lindemann, E.: Symptomatology and management of acute grief, American Journal of Psychiatry **101**:141-148, 1944.

Lowenthal, Marjorie Fiske: Lives in distress: the paths of the elderly to the psychiatric ward, New York, 1964, Basic Books, Inc., Publisher.

Lowenthal, Marjorie Fiske, Berkman, P., et al.: Aging and mental disorders in San Francisco, San Francisco, 1967, Jossey-Bass, Inc., Publishers.

Marris, P.: Widows and their families, London, 1958, Routledge & Kegan Paul, Ltd.

Menninger, K. A.: Man against himself, New York, 1938, Harcourt Brace, & World.

Mental health problems of aging and the aged, sixth report of the Expert Committee on Mental Health, WHO, Geneva, 1959, World Health Organization Technical Report Series, No. 171.

New York State Department of Mental Hygiene Mental Health Research Unit: A mental health survey of older people, Utica, 1960, New York State Hospital Press.

Parkes, C. M., Benjamin, B., and Fitzgerald, A.: Broken heart: a statistical study of increased mortality among widows, British Medical Journal **1**:740-743, 1969.

Patterson, R. D., Freeman, L. C., and Butler, R. N.: Psychiatric aspects of adaptation, survival and death. In Granick, S., and Patterson, R. D., editors: Human aging. II. HSM 71-9037, Washington, D. C., 1971, U. S. Government Printing Office.

Perlin, Seymour, and Butler, Robert N.: Psychiatric aspects of adaptation to the aging experience. In Human aging: a biological and behavioral study, Washington, D. C., 1963 (reprint 1971), U. S. Government Printing Office.

Post, F.: The significance of affective symptoms in old age: a follow-up study of one hundred patients, London, 1962, Oxford University Press, Inc.

Resnik, H. L., and Cantor, J. M.: Suicide and aging, Journal of the American Geriatrics Society **18**:152-158, 1970.

Roth, M.: The natural history of mental disorders in old age, Journal of Mental Science **101**: 281-301, 1955.

Sainsbury, P.: Suicide in later life, Gerontologica Clinicia **4**:161-170, 1962.

Schmale, A. H., Jr., and Engel, G. L.: The giving up-given up complex illustrated on film, Archives of General Psychiatry **17**:135-145, 1967.

Shanas, Ethel: The health of older people: a social survey. Cambridge, Mass., 1962, Harvard University Press.

Sheldon, J. H.: The social medicine of old age: report of an inquiry in Wolverhampton, London, 1948, Oxford University Press.

Shneidman, E. S., and Farberow, N. L., editors: Clues to suicide, New York, 1957, McGraw-Hill Book Co., Inc.

Shreber, D. P.: Memoirs of my nervous illness, London, 1955, Dawson.

Stenback, A.: On involutional and middle age depression, Helsinki, Finland, XIII. Nordiska Psykiaterkongressen, 1962.

Stengel, E.: Suicide and attempted suicide, Baltimore, 1964, Penguin Books, Inc.

Stern, K., and Menzer, Doris: The mechanism of reactivation in depression of the old age group, Psychiatric Quarterly **20**:56-73, 1946.

Stern, K., Williams, Gwendolyn M., and Prados, M.: Grief reactions in later life, American Journal of Psychiatry **108**:289-294, 1951.

Strömgren, E.: Epidemiology of old-age psychiatric disorders. In Williams, R. H., Tibbitts, C., and Donahue, Wilma, editors: Process of aging, vol. 2, New York, 1963, Atherton Press.

Vispo, Raul H.: Pre-morbid personality in the functional psychoses of the senium. A comparison of ex-patients with healthy controls, The Journal of Mental Science **108**:790-800, 1962.

Weisman, A. D., and Kastenbaum, R.: The psychological autopsy (monograph), New York, 1968, Community Mental Health Journal, Inc.

Weiss, J. M. A.: Suicide in the aged. In Resnik, H. C. P., editor: Suicidal behaviors, Boston, 1968, Little, Brown & Co.

Williams, R. H., and Wirths, Claudine G.: Lives through the years, New York, 1965, Atherton Press.

Williams, W. S., and Jaco, E. G.: An evaluation of functional psychosis in old age, The American Journal of Psychiatry **114**:910-916, 1958.

5
ORGANIC BRAIN DISORDERS

PROBLEMS IN NAMING DISORDERS (NOMENCLATURE)

Prior to the twentieth century, the organic brain disorders of late life were grouped together in a category known as organic senile dementia. But at the turn of the century, with an increasing number of older people, neuropathologists in examining the brain at autopsy began separating arteriosclerotic conditions from senile dementia and both of these from neurosyphilis. Kraepelin, in emphasizing description and symptomatology while ignoring the person's inner life, described five signs of an organic brain disorder. He failed to note the affective reactions to brain diseases as well as the reversible brain disorder.

Senile dementia, now separated from arteriosclerotic processes, became divided by symptoms in the older textbooks, as follows: (1) simple dementia, (2) delirium, (3) paranoid states, (4) depressed and agitated types, and (5) presbyophrenic types; but these subdivisions did not differentiate between the mental conditions themselves and the affective reactions to and in connection with such mental changes. In England, work has been done on hospital admission, following up patients when discharged until the time of their death. It was realized that everything could not be explained on an organic basis and Roth, one of England's foremost clinical investigators, devised a more sophisticated classification by dividing all the disorders of old age into the following: (1) affective psychoses, (2) senile psychoses, (3) arteriosclerotic psychoses, (4) delirious states, and (5) late paraphrenia.*

The Diagnostic and Statistical Manuals I and II of the American Psychiatric Association have further complicated the picture. DSM I presents the acute and chronic brain disorders, with qualifying psychotic, neurotic, and behavioral reactions; DSM II reverses the emphasis by describing psychotic and nonpsychotic disorders, with a single introductory remark distinguishing acute from chronic conditions. In addition no clinician specializing in the field of aging has ever served on the Committee on Nomenclature and Statistics of the American Psychiatric Association—which perhaps accounts for such age-prejudicial and invalid statements as the following definition of senile dementia: "Even mild cases will manifest some evidence of organic brain syndrome: *self-centeredness,* difficulty in assimilating new experiences, and *childish emotionality.*"† The student and practitioner will need to refer to the DSM II for hospital diagnoses, insurance forms, etc., but should not take the definitions and classification too seriously, since they do not clearly reflect reality for the older person. DSM I is actually better in this respect. (We have included

*Paraphrenia is a diagnosis used by some investigators to apply to paranoid-hallucinative disturbances in late life. Others deny the existence of the late-life schizophrenia implied in this description.

†From Diagnostic and statistical manual of mental disorders (DSM I), Washington, D. C., 1952, American Psychiatric Association, p. 24.

pertinent sections of the DSM II classification in Chapter 4.)

In clarifying one last major confusion, it can be observed that senile dementia and senile psychosis have been used interchangeably in some texts. In the past, however, senile dementia meant that the five basic signs of the chronic brain syndrome were more or less present; senile psychosis was used when obvious psychotic behavior was also manifested. This may be particularly important to know in reading old patient charts.

For the purposes of this book, the reader needs to keep in mind the general characteristic of organic brain syndromes found in older persons.

1. Organic brain syndromes may be either reversible (acute) or chronic.
2. The two most common chronic brain syndromes (CBS) in older people are (a) CBS associated with senile brain disease and (b) CBS associated with cerebral arteriosclerosis.
3. The organic brain syndromes may be complicated by psychotic, neurotic, and behavioral disorders.

DESCRIPTION OF ORGANIC BRAIN SYNDROME (OBS)

The organic brain disorders are mental conditions caused by or associated with impairment of brain tissue function. The distinctive features of such disorders are (1) disturbance and impairment of memory, (2) impairment of intellectual function or comprehension, (3) impairment of judgment, (4) impairment of orientation, and (5) shallow or labile affect. These five mental signs may not all be seen at the same time or to the same degree but they represent the core elements of organic brain disorder, particularly in full-blown and advanced states. The signs range in severity from barely perceptible changes to a profound loss of functioning and may be reversible (acute brain syndrome) or irreversible (chronic brain syndrome) with gradual or

Table 5-1. Prodromal characteristics of organic brain syndrome*

Early characteristics	Potential signs and symptoms†
Cognitive	
"Intellectual" decline	Perseveration
Reduced tempo of stream of thought	Increasingly impaired comprehension
Impoverishment of ideas	
Concreteness: impaired abstraction	Increasing memory loss (recent and remote)
Decline of recent memory	
Registration, recall, organization‡	Confabulation
Difficulty in maintaining attention set	Perseveration, irrelevance
Behavioral and affective	
Reduced attentiveness	Progressive withdrawal and self-isolation
Reduced responsiveness	Apathy
Decreased interpersonal interaction	Pseudo-depression vs. depression
Less direct, immediate affective expression	
Liability to "disintegration" during stress	"Inappropriate" affect
Later characteristics	
Emotional liability	Emotional incontinence
Impaired orientation	Confusion
Impaired judgment	

*Modified from Perlin, Seymour, and Butler, Robert N. In Human aging: a biological and behavioral study, Washington, D. C., Publication No. (HSM) 71-9051, 1971.

†A one-to-one relationship between presenting characteristic and potential symptom is not implied. Other symptoms may include irritability, apathy, suspiciousness, slovenliness, etc.

‡Impaired organization refers to the inability to remember (and utilize) items in a time-related sequence.

precipitous decline of mental abilities. Table 5-1 delineates the early warning (prodromal) characteristics of organic brain syndromes.

In some older persons with OBS, the brain impairments may represent the only disturbance observed, with basic personality and behavior remaining unchanged. These cases are uncomplicated in the sense that the person attempts to make suitable adjustments to disorders and has insight into what has happened to his intellectual abilities, especially in early stages.

Mrs. J, a hearty, good-natured woman of 83, compensated for her waning memory in a variety of ways. She made lists of things to remember, she tied letters to be mailed to the doorknob so she would see them when she went out, she attached her wallet and keys onto her belt or slip strap. She asked friends to call and remind her of appointments and she made deliberate efforts to read and talk about the daily newspapers "to keep my brain active."

Such a person can function fairly adequately with little assistance. Even when impairment has progressed to a more severe stage, the person can live at home if proper supports are given. In contrast, some persons realize that they can no longer remain at home and seek institutional care on their own.

Sam B was a 79-year-old farmer who appeared sad, anxious, and perplexed. He was garrulous, agitated, and occasionally irritable and contentious. He showed flight of ideas and was distractable, with difficulties in maintaining attention and set. Affect was usually appropriate and of sufficient depth, yet he had marked shifts of mood.

He had definite cognitive losses resulting in severe impairment. There were defects in remote memory, judgment was unreliable, and orientation was somewhat shaky. Performance on the Mental Status Examination was patchy. His appearance was sloven. Mr. B lacked insight into his cognitive losses and denied both these losses and his aging state.

Mr. B was diagnosed as having chronic brain syndrome, with senile brain disease, moderate and of seven years duration. His second diagnosis was personality trait disturbance, passive-aggressive personality, passive-dependent type, chronic and severe. His lifelong pattern was one of indecisiveness, dependency, and helplessness.

In spite of the severity of his losses and his dependent personality, Mr. B made a decision completely on his own to seek admission to an old age home. He decided he would prefer to do this rather than live with a nephew. Mr. B predicted a good home adjustment for himself and did in fact adjust well.

When OBS is accompanied by emotional symptoms, the situation of course becomes more complex. Behavioral reactions associated with OBS fall into several categories: first are the reactions caused by the deficit itself, as in the senile dementias; second are emotional reactions and adaptations to the deficits; and third are reactions termed release phenomena. The latter are shown in the appearance of latent personality traits and tendencies as a result of brain damage. Both neurotic and psychotic behavior may be present. It is now generally agreed that not only the organic disorder but also the individual's basic personality, his inherited or constitutional traits, and the environmental situation affect the kind and severity of symptoms that appear. People react to threats to their intellectual capacities in highly individualized ways, and this is most true in the beginning phases of decline. A conspicuous feature is often the presence of a successful social facade in which everything looks normal until one begins to examine responses more carefully, as in the case of the woman discussed below:

In a group of friends she enters into the conversation by taking an anecdotal role, discussing the older material that is well embedded in her memory. Only after one listens for a time does it become clear that she is circumstantial, slightly irrelevant, and telling the same stories over and over again to the same friends.

A leveling effect takes place as impairment increases, and at the final stages the effect is one of "look alike" or sameness in response as vital basic capacities drop away. There is also less immediate individuality of reaction when damage is sudden and massive (as with cerebrovascular accidents) rather than gradual.

Some clinicians feel that a pronounced emotional reaction is a hopeful sign, indicating that brain damage is minimal enough to allow the person energy and resources to elaborate on an emotional response. Goldfarb and others have observed that the presence of disorder of affect or thought content is indicative of a more favorable outlook for improvement, since the emotional reaction may be treatable. One must caution here that the emotional reaction itself can be intractable, particularly if it is associated with long-term personality problems. Actual treatment is the only reliable way to judge the reversibility of symptoms. We also wish to emphasize that organic disorders themselves are not necessarily the fixed conditions they first appear to be and may respond to treatment. Orientation, for example, may be improved by providing direct instruction and supplying orientation aids such as lights, signs, colors, sounds, etc. Chronicity is often used as an excuse for not doing anything when there may be many treatment techniques that could comfort, support, and even greatly increase the functioning of brain-damaged individuals.

Memory changes are one of the most obvious and noticeable symptoms of OBS, since memory so intimately affects interpersonal relationships with family and friends. Everyone has seen the older person whose memory for past events is clear although he is unable to remember who came to visit him today or what happened yesterday. It is a common notion that recent memory becomes destroyed in some manner by a deteriorative process in the brain, with memories from the past remaining intact longer. This conjures up a picture of a cranial filing system for memory storage, which protects its contents proportionate to the time elapsed since filing. Studies of the brain have not confirmed any such occurrence, nor are there reliable tests for remote memory, enabling us to judge how accurate past reminiscences are. A more relevant explanation for recent memory loss is the postulation that brain damage interferes with registration of incoming stimuli and affects the ability for retention and recall. In this event, an experience that ordinarily would become a memory either registers inaccurately or not at all.

I feel very often that Henry is simply not receiving new knowledge, that he does not retain the facts and experiences he does receive, that he is not registering visual experience. . . on a recent trip he tried to follow the instructions of tour guides ("on your left you see. . .") but would look straight ahead or turn to the left long after the scene had passed.

An added factor in memory loss is the possibility of emotional influence on recall capacities. Old people may need to deny, to disremember, or to distort that which is overwhelming or too painful to face; depression and preoccupation with problems may not be noticed yet can interfere with learning and memory.

Judge Grey has been experiencing slow, progressive organic changes but is only numbly aware of them. He cannot face up to the degree and the implications of what is happening to him. He seems to live in a state of constant fear, inadequate to even small demands on him, forgetting everything, missing trains, and becoming confused about schedules or well-rehearsed plans. I am never sure whether the confirmation of his fears that he will do everything badly is a true mental disability or a self-fulfilling prophecy.

Disorientation is a more easily and accurately tested symptom. Disorientation about time (the day, the hour, the year) is the first confusion to occur as a result of OBS. Loss of sense of place (where am I, what is this place, what country am I in) is likely to follow and, last, the person loses the ability to recognize other people and eventually cannot remember who he is. One sees this in individuals who do not recognize themselves in the mirror, do not know their own names or the names of loved ones, etc.

REVERSIBLE BRAIN SYNDROME (RBS)— ALSO KNOWN AS "ACUTE" BRAIN SYNDROME

The concept of "acuteness" as it applies to brain syndromes should be clarified, since it has been the traditional term used in this context. Acute carries with it the notion of rapid onset, dramatic symptoms, and short duration—none of which are reliably present in the brain syndromes of older people. The term "reversible" is a much more exact definition, since reversibility of the brain pathology remains the one consistent characteristic. Other names for the reversible brain syndromes are senile confusional states and senile delirium.

The reversible brain syndrome remains a frequently undiagnosed illness, more so in the United States than in some other countries, for example, England. The concept first began appearing in the literature in the 1930s and in a recent study of a large municipal hospital, 13% of the patients were found to have reversible brain syndromes while 33% exhibited mixed reversible and chronic disorders. One consequence of failure to identify the syndrome is that older people are often considered chronic patients and are sent to long-term institutional care facilities or nursing homes when active hospital care and return to the community would be the appropriate course of treatment.

Symptoms

A sign of reversible brain syndrome is a fluctuating level of awareness, which may vary from mild confusion all the way to stupor or active delirium. Hallucinations may be present, particularly of visual rather than auditory type. The person typically is disoriented, mistaking one person for another, and other intellectual functions can also be impaired. Remote as well as recent memory is lost. Behaviorally, restlessness, a dazed expression, or aggressiveness shows itself and the person can appear frightened either by the disorientation or as a result of the vivid visual hallucinations. Delusions of persecution may be present. Anxiety and lack of cooperativeness are other symptoms. The reversible brain syndrome should not be confused with transient behavioral disturbances, which can occur as a consequence of organic brain disease. Both may be reversible but the latter has a chronic, underlying cause not found in RBS.

Causes

Obtaining a detailed history from an observer (family, friend, acquaintance) is important, since the patient is unlikely to be able to supply it himself. Onset of the illness should be explored, with an account of preexistent disorders, and exposure to toxic substances should be carefully checked. Myriad possible causes for the reversible brain disorders exist, and we shall discuss the most prevalent.

Congestive heart failure

Congestive heart failure refers to decompensation resulting from the heart's declining capacity to pump blood. Thus oxygen, sugar, and necessary nutrients are undersupplied to the brain; 13% of acute myocardial infarctions come to medical attention primarily as confusional states.

Malnutrition and anemia

A large proportion of the elderly population is undernourished, although this is vehemently denied by some medical and lay people who share the illusion that the United States is the world's best-fed nation. Older people develop reversible brain syndromes associated with avitaminosis, pellagra,* and metabolic disorders. Malnourishment in the elderly has both social and economic associations. Poverty forces many to go hungry, while social isolation and depression from living alone can result in persons' simply not eating regularly or well. Older people may have problems in getting to stores for shopping, especially when physical infirmities are present. Appetites may decline as a result of depression, anxiety, or illness and the loss of teeth can interfere with eating solid foods. Therefore, even the middle- and upper-class elderly may be surprisingly malnourished.

Infection

Infection may not provoke the same level of effective bodily protection as in the young (fever, increase in blood white cell count, etc.). With infection come fatigue and some-

---

*Pellagra is a disease characterized by mental, neurological, cutaneous, mucous membrane and gastrointestinal symptoms. It is due to a severe deficiency of niacin (nicotinic acid) or its amide (niacin amide) along with their amino acid precursor, tryptophane. H. A. Meyersburg has reported cases of brain syndrome from pellagra in old people in his work in 1945. (Senile psychosis and pellagra: a report of two cases, The New England Journal of Medicine 233:173-176, 1945.)

times dehydration, which leave the individual vulnerable to mental confusion.

Cerebrovascular accidents

A temporary lack of blood supply to the brain (ischemic attack) can result in an undersupply of oxygen (hypoxia), followed by aphasia and paralysis. A common event among the elderly is a stroke; the person becomes unconscious and, upon regaining consciousness (if he survives), may pass through an acute state of confusion before a restoration of mental normality. If strokes are massive or repeated, chronic disorders eventually result.

Variations are described by Alvarez—the so-called "little strokes"—which probably occur much more frequently than realized. These produce transient confusion, nausea and vomiting, dizziness, and numbness of the extremities but not full-scale paralysis and aphasia.*

Drugs and other toxic substances

With increasing use of drugs of all kinds in the medical and psychiatric management of older people, drug reactions are a significant cause of reversible disorders. Suicide attempts through use of drugs or toxic materials are another factor. Barbiturates, tranquilizers, bromides, thiocyanates, gases, and hormones are not unmixed blessings: for example, both reversible and irreversible organic brain disorders can occur with use of the cortisone series; tranquilizers may cause damage if prescribed too long; steroids can affect mood, with manic or depressive manifestations. Old people who are undernourished or who have markedly reduced kidney function or arteriosclerosis may show greater negative response to even small amounts of drugs. The brain pathologies resulting from medications ordered by doctors are termed "iatrogenic" disorders, meaning they have resulted paradoxically from medical treatment itself and not from any usual physical dysfunction. Diuretics may lead to dehydration and mental confusion. L-Dopa (antiparkinsonian) and indomethacin (antiarthritic) may cause psychotic behavior.

Old people may also have exaggerated drug reactions that do not reach acute confusional proportions; examples are agitation from barbiturates, depression from tranquilizers. Such reactions can increase if the person is not clear about the side effects of various drugs and adds his own fears to the clinical picture. Thus a tranquilized person may become extremely depressed if he fears he is losing physical powers and is not aware that this is transitory. Doctors and medical personnel owe each person an exact description of what to expect from drugs, so unnecessary emotional complications can be avoided.

Head trauma

For people over age 65, 72% of all deaths due to falls and 30% of all pedestrian fatalities are a result of head trauma. Old people are more subject than younger ones to brain injuries in any type of accident, even minor ones. Nonfatal head injuries may leave the older person severely disabled (for example, by the subdural hematomas that occur after falls due to weakness, lack of coordination, or alcoholism). Tumor growths (neoplasms) and brain surgery are other traumas that can impair brain functioning.

A trauma can result in an acute syndrome followed by an irreversible disorder; for example, a head injury may lead to concussion and/or coma, traumatic delirium, and then to Korsakoff's syndrome with confabulation and fabrication.

Alcohol

Alcoholism is more common in old age than is generally recognized. Alcohol, as a central nervous system depressant, impairs intellectual functioning. Intoxication at any age results in a reversible brain syndrome.

Other causes

Diabetic acidosis, liver failure, dehydration, uremia, hypothyroidism, brain tumor, general surgery, blindfolding during eye

*One must always beware not to misread aphasia, when it is present, as intellectual deterioration. Aphasia may be transitory, partial, and responsive to treatment.

surgery, drastic environmental changes, and bereavements are some of the other common causes of reversible brain syndromes. Another cause is hypercalcemia due to metastatic carcinoma of lung or breast, primary hyperparathyroidism, multiple myeloma, or Paget's disease.*

It is important to note that there are no consistant or characteristic neuropathological findings in reversible brain syndrome. Old people show much the same reactions as younger people to exhaustion, vitamin deficiencies, and general disease—but they are likely to be more vulnerable.

Simon (1963) in a study of admissions at San Francisco General Hospital referred to the social-environmental aspects of reversible brain syndrome. Persons with reversible brain syndrome tended to be removed from family ties, were more often men than women, and in many instances were alcoholic. In a number of cases the reversible syndrome may be followed by, or occur simultaneously with, an irreversible disorder because of permanent damage done to the brain, as in cerebral embolism, arterial hypertension, cardiorenal disease, cardiac decompensation, or circulatory disturbances. In these situations, some improvement may be possible but residual disorders remain. In persons with mixed reversible brain syndrome and chronic brain syndrome, the environmental influence did not appear to be so prominent; physical deterioration, most often cardiovascular disease, was more evident.

Course of illness and treatment

Both a high immediate death rate and a high discharge rate from the hospital are typical of the reversible brain syndrome. Although mortality rates are substantial (an estimated 40% die, either from exhaustion or from accompanying physical illness), the person who survives the crises has a good chance of returning to the community. It appears that the reversible brain syndrome can result in complete recovery, although it must be noted that little follow-up work has been done on recovered patients to determine whether their health is maintained. Others are revealed to be only partially reversible, with an underlying chronic disorder. Finally, the reversible brain syndrome can lead to death, as a manifestation of a serious physical illness that caused the syndrome or complicated it. Psychiatric disorders can be a first signal pointing toward a developing physical illness, dehydration, and electrolyte disturbances.

Psychiatrically oriented medical facilities should be available to deal with the pathophysiological crisis that brings the person to the attention of others. Treatment must be intensive but can often be short-term, with malnutrition usually causing the longest hospital stay.

CHRONIC BRAIN SYNDROME (CBS)—IRREVERSIBLE

The chronic brain syndromes are the phenomena that many laymen and all too many medical personnel refer to by the inaccurate and emotion-laden term of senility. Many times, for lack of a thorough evaluation, the reversible brain syndromes also are subsumed under this category and the entire conglomeration termed untreatable. It was not until thirty to forty years ago that reversible and chronic disorders began to receive differential diagnosis and treatment. A realistic complication occurs in those cases where both disorders occur together, with one reversible and the other not. The prime characteristic of chronic brain syndrome is its irreversibility. Once brain damage has occurred, there is no full return to a normal physical condition. But even though damage is permanent and irreparable, many of the emotional and physical symptoms can be treated, resulting in support and actual improvement of functioning.

In older people there are two predominant types of chronic brain syndrome: senile psychosis (called senile dementia and senile

*Nonketotic hyperosmolarity syndrome, in which hyperglycemia and confusion occur without any ketosis, is not an uncommon cause of reversible brain syndrome.

brain disease) and psychosis associated with cerebral arteriosclerosis. These two disorders may look a good deal alike and thus, as mentioned earlier in the chapter, were not differentiated from each other until recent times.

An 80-year-old male state hospital patient was diagnosed as having chronic brain syndrome, but differentiation between senile psychosis and psychosis associated with cerebral arteriosclerosis was not possible. The patient was wizened, physically deteriorated, weak, and somewhat sloven in appearance. His sense of balance and direction was impaired, and his verbal productivity was increased although not to the point of garrulousness. He was distractable (as by noises in the hall or by room fixtures), occasionally irrelevant, delayed in reaction time, and at times perseverative.

It was not possible to obtain a history because of his confusion. But, confused as he was, he was able to maintain emotional contact with the nurse on the ward. He was disoriented with respect to time, place, and person and was unable to give his own name.

Some of his responses were seen as defensive (he denied his hospitalization and his age). He confabulated, weaving memory and fantasy into answers to questions which he either could not or would not answer in a more direct manner. He complained about his memory. There was some question as to his being at times aphasic rather than uncomprehending.

He was confused over once-familiar procedures, such as lighting cigarettes. On several occasions he would have placed the lighted end of a cigarette in his mouth had the interviewer not intervened.

In short, he had severe impairment in intellectual functioning, memory, judgment, and orientation; yet he retained occasional glimmers of insight and appropriate emotional response.

Pathological examination provides the most useful and reliable data on differences between the two, since clinical examination may be less precise and even contradictory. The two disorders occur simultaneously in about 20% of the cases.*

As Rothschild (1945) pointed out, early psychiatry attempted to link the cause of mental disorders with demonstrable cerebral changes. Because of the observable brain damage found in senile and arteriosclerotic brain syndromes, it was widely believed that such damage was the only cause of mental symptoms. However, later research found generally poor correlation between the degree of deterioration and neuropathological changes as it became evident that many inconsistencies existed between the extent of brain damage and the severity of mental symptoms. Grünthal and Rothschild, in the past, and recent studies have noted the discrepancies.* Persons who had little change neuropathologically sometimes showed serious mental and psychiatric change, while others with profound brain damage had only mild psychiatric disorders. Even normal elderly individuals can have brain changes which appear as marked as those in individuals with clinically obvious senile or arteriosclerotic disorders. Thus the anatomical brain changes are only part of the factors determining the psychiatric symptoms; one must consider the individual's own constitutional characteristics, personality, heredity, and environmental stress. Thus we repeat and reemphasize that the organic disorders, like so many other disorders in late life, must be viewed socially and psychologically as well as medically—in diagnosis, prognosis, and treatment—particularly in early stages before the damage is too global and leveling.

Senile psychosis

Senile psychosis refers to the chronic psychotic disorders in elderly people, who tend to show a progressive decline (particularly after 80 years of age) in mental functioning. This is associated with changes in the brain, primarily the dissolution of brain cells themselves. The disorder occurs

*Some investigators suggest an even higher association between the two disorders. (See Müller, C., and Ciompi, L., editors: Senile dimentia, Bern and Stuttgart, 1968, Hans Huber Publishers.)

*Corsellis, J. A. N.: Mental illness and the aging brain, London, 1962, Oxford University Press. Also Roth, M., Tomlinson, B. E., and Blested, G.: Correlations between scores for dementia and counts of "senile" plaques in cerebral gray matter of elderly patients, Nature **209**:109-110, 1966.

much more frequently in women than men, probably because of their longer life expectancy, with age of onset from 60 to 90 years, the average being 75 years. However, sex linkage itself may be a factor. Surveys indicate that although men have a shorter lifespan than women they are, when they do survive, generally healthier—both physically and mentally. Significant memory impairment is more frequently found in older women than in older men of the same age. The disorder may look similar to involutional melancholia, Korsakoff's syndrome, and many other mental disturbances caused by malnutrition, heart disease, toxemia, etc.

Brain pathology

The brain cells themselves atrophy and degenerate, independent of vascular change, most strikingly in the cerebral cortex. Other parts of the body's soft tissue may also atrophy but not as severely as the brain, which actually loses weight. Single nervous cells are destroyed in a widespread manner, without breaking down the structure of nervous tissue as a whole. Additionally, about 50% of patients also show changes caused by vascular disease with moderate atherosclerosis, but these changes usually are of minor importance.

Clinical symptoms

The older person may pass slowly from normal old age to senile psychosis with no abrupt changes (unless accompanied by arteriosclerotic disease). Friends and relatives gradually notice small differences in physical, mental, and emotional functioning.

> He has called our house, where we have lived for nearly five years, an "unhappy" one, comparing it unfavorably to the small, crowded house we had lived in previously where things had been all right. He thus comes close to realizing how long the present development has really gone on. I would say that I have been conscious of changes in him for perhaps six years. But only in the last two years could I have put my finger on definite differences, and the last year has unquestionably been the worse of the two.

Previous personality traits may become exaggerated.

> A patient's husband writes: "In areas where she has always deferred to me for either judgment or action, she is abdicating more and more, hardly participating even passively. This does not represent so severe a departure from the past pattern; I have always been the more practical and commonsensical of the two—but it now means that she depends on me wholly instead of heavily."

Early features of senile psychosis are errors in judgment, decline in personal care and habits, impairment of capacity for abstract thought, and lack of interest and apathy. Loosening of inhibitions can be an early sign. A host of emotional reactions are possible with depression, anxiety, and irritability being the most frequent, particularly in early stages. Depression is usually superficial rather than profound and is based on anxiety and loss. As the deterioration increases, mental symptoms proliferate and the traditional five signs of organic dysfunction become more evident (see earlier description of organic brain syndromes). Hallucinations can be present, especially at night. Poor orientation for time, place, and person as well as confused comprehension (for example, registering a single impression but not the whole picture), rambling incoherent speech, and fabrication may be seen. Sleeplessness and restlessness are common and the person may wander away from home. Paranoid tendencies may be exacerbated or appear for the first time, and one occasionally sees manic or hypomanic states.

Review of traditional types

We wish to review briefly the traditional but now outmoded classification of senile psychosis, since literature in the field of aging contains many references to it that might be otherwise confusing to the reader. Five types of senile psychosis were described in the following manner.

Simple deterioration. A progressive memory loss occurs, with loss of contact and initiative, combined with irritability and eventual mild stupor.

Depressed and agitated type. The usual senile changes are accompanied by restlessness, self-centeredness, depression, and hypochondriasis.

Delirium and confused type. A generally reversible process with acute onset, this represents a reaction to physical and/or social stress rather than a strictly senile process. However, chronic confusional states are sometimes seen.

Presbyophrenic type. Literally meaning "old brain," this term refers to psychosis that occurs more often in women than in men. It is marked by confabulation and by retention defect and is often thought of as a presenile disorder rather than a senile psychotic classification. The presbyophrenic patient seems alert on the surface, with normal appearing social manners and level of awareness. But in discussion or interview it soon becomes clear that there is much damage behind the normal facade, particularly in orientation and memory. The retention deficit is covered up by confabulation, in which the person fills in gaps in memory by fabricating and by accepting facts offered to him as his own ideas. The person sincerely accepts the fabrication as real and has no understanding of his memory impairment. Such a person may be jovial and good-natured, restless in an aimless fashion, talkative, and rambling. The picture is similar to that presented in Korsakoff's syndrome.

Paranoid type. Memory loss and other evidence of decreased mental functioning may be slight in early stages.* A delusional system is formed, often accompanied by hallucinations. An earlier, lifelong tendency toward suspiciousness and projection is a factor in the development of the paranoid type. The delusions are most often persecutory, grandiose, or erotic—with emphasis on money, personal harm, and wish-fulfillment. At first the personality may be quite intact, but intellectual impairment gradually develops.

*There are state hospital data comparing preservation of intellectual abilities among the subtypes of schizophrenia. The paranoid subtype appears to be relatively protected against deterioration, compared to other types. It has been surmised that this is due to the continued intellectual stimulation required to build paranoid defenses (Alpert, H. S., Bigelow, N. J. T., and Bryan, L. L.: Cerebral arteriosclerosis in the paranoid state, The Psychiatric Quarterly **21**:305-313, 1947).

• • •

These five types are really all variants of the same process and reflect personal, social, and other reactions and differences. For example, paranoid and depressed states are simply emotional reactions to underlying brain disorders. The classification is of limited practical application, since persons may present one or more types at once or may move from one to another in the course of illness. It is more useful to follow a classification that separates physical from emotional symptoms and reversible from chronic syndromes.

Causes

Little is known about the cause of senile brain disease. There is no general agreement on what the difference is between normal and pathological aging or what the aspects of pathological aging are. Similar changes to those seen in senile brain syndromes occur to a lesser degree in normal old age and to a greater degree in Alzheimer's disease. Some have argued that the senile brain syndrome is a quantitative increase in normal involutional change while others feel that it is qualitatively different. Dorken,* the NIMH human aging studies, and others have provided work which supports the latter view as does our own clinical experience. There also appears to be a strong environmental and personality factor, more so than in psychosis associated with arteriosclerosis. In fact some of what is seen as senile brain disease may be a massive defense against the reality of old age and death.†

Course of illness and treatment

Senile psychosis is eventually fatal, with a steady and progressive course. Persons may

*Dorken, H.: Normal senescent decline and senile dementia: their differentiation by psychological tests, Medical Services Journal **14**:18-23, 1958.
†Gillespie, W. H.: Some regressive phenomena in old age, British Journal of Medical Psychology **56**:303-309, 1962.

live ten years or more after onset of symptoms but average survival is five years. Emotional reactions may respond to treatment, and physical functioning can improve with proper support even though the physical loss itself is irreparable. Many persons would be able to remain in their own homes throughout most of the course of illness if adequate services and assistance were available.

Psychosis associated with cerebral arteriosclerosis

Arteriosclerotic psychosis is a chronic disorder that often shows an uneven and erratic downward progression, compared to the steady decline seen in senile psychosis. The disorder is associated with damage done to the cerebral blood vessels through arteriosclerosis (a term that includes both *arteriosclerosis*—a hardening of the vessel wall—and *atherosclerosis*—a narrowing and closing of the vessel itself).* The blood flow to the brain is interfered with and, as a result, insufficient oxygen and nutrients reach the brain. Table 5-2 compares the cerebral oxygen circulation† in various age groups and diagnostic categories.

The disorder is found in middle and later life because it is a progressive disease which may remain asymptomatic until that point. Age of onset is between 50 and 70 years, with an average age of 66 years. Men outnumber women by a ratio of 3 to 1.

*The presence of retinal arteriosclerosis does not establish the presence of cerebral arteriosclerosis, nor does its absence assure the absence of arteriosclerosis in the brain. (See Alpers, B. J., Forster, F. M., and Herbut, P. A.: Retinal cerebral and systemic arteriosclerosis, a histopathologic study, Archives of Neurology and Psychiatry 60:440-456, 1948.) Similarly, evidence of peripheral arteriosclerosis is not diagnostic of cerebral changes. Arteriosclerosis is not a generalized condition: not all organs and tissues of the body are uniformly affected.

†Using the technique of Kety and Schmidt (Kety, S. S.: Human cerebral blood flow and oxygen consumption as related to aging, Journal of Chronic Diseases 3:478-486, 1956).

Table 5-2. Mean values of cerebral oxygen metabolic rate in various groupings of aged subjects*

Groupings	Number	$CMRO_2$
Normal young	15	3.5
Normal healthy aged	28	3.3
Chronic brain syndrome without psychosis	2	2.7
Chronic brain syndrome with arteriosclerosis with psychosis	10	2.7

*Based on data from Butler, R. N., Dastur, D. K., and Perlin, S.: Relationships of senile manifestations and chronic brain syndromes to cerebral circulation and metabolism, Journal of Psychiatric Research 3:229-238, 1965.

Brain pathology

The brain typically shows areas of softening with complete deterioration of cerebral tissue over a circumscribed, limited area. The damaged area may be anemic or hemorrhagic resulting from the inadequate blood supply caused by blocked vessels.

Clinical symptoms

Early symptoms are dizziness, headaches, decreased physical and mental vigor, and vague physical complaints. Onset can be gradual or sudden, with over 50% occurring acutely in the form of a sudden attack of confusion. Cases with slower onset can look much like senile brain disease. There is usually a gradual intellectual loss, and *impairment of memory tends to be spotty* rather than complete. A person may be unable to remember one minute and regain total capacity the next. There may be a certain degree of insight and judgment, again in a spotty sense. The course is up and down rather than progressively downhill. (Note the "lucid interval" in forensic psychiatry; see Chapter 9.) The person may hallucinate and become delirious, indicating the insufficiency of cerebral circulation.

Paranoid reactions are often misdiagnosed as chronic brain syndromes. One of the authors (RNB) went into a state hospital to gain volunteers for research and requested the hospital to indicate definitive cases of cerebral arteriosclerosis with psychosis. In

30% of the cases referred, patients showed clear instances of paranoid reaction with minimal or no evidence of brain damage. An example was the following:

Diagnosis for this 74-year-old female hospital patient had been probable chronic brain syndrome with psychosis associated with cerebral arteriosclerosis. However her faculties were quite clear except for mild memory impairment and impaired judgment as a consequence of her delusional system (not a cognitive defect). She did not show the classic signs of a chronic brain syndrome. There was no disorientation, no substantial decline in intellectual functions, nor a lability of affect.

The woman had a hearing impairment and language difficulty (she was born in Europe), which made interviewing difficult and undoubtedly contributed to her poor performance on vocabulary tests. During the mental status examination she had good retention, logical memory, and minimal difficulty in abstracting. She adapted well to the interview, was not depressed, and was likeable and affable.

Her predominant symptoms were those of paranoia. Her delusional system concerned her admission to the hospital, and she implicated her daughter-in-law and other family members as conspirators in an elaborate plot to "put her away." (Her general sense of being abandoned by her family was built into a complicated delusional process which nevertheless had some roots in reality.)

The misdiagnosis of such cases is too often the result of careless examination and unclear diagnostic thinking.

Causes

The cause of arteriosclerosis is still unclear although many explanations have been offered. Lipid dysfunction, heredity, diet (especially cholesterol), smoking, environmental pollution, lack of exercise, and other elements have been held contributory. Some claim that a head injury may accelerate cerebral arteriosclerosis, but we have not seen examples of this.

Course of illness and treatment

There is great diversity from person to person and even with the same person at different times. A cerebrovascular accident causing confusion or clouding of the mental state can lead quickly to a fatal outcome or may produce an organic condition lasting as long as ten to fifteen years. The average survival of those admitted to a mental hospital has been estimated in the past to be three to four years.

The hospitalized cardiac patient or the patient with a general vascular disease may also develop psychosis due to cerebrovascular disease. A goodly number die but those who survive may experience subsidence of the problem, with varying amounts of intellectual impairment. Good remissions may be possible in a number of cases, when intellectual capacity is retained. If new attacks follow, each does additional damage. Often the person's physical condition is worse than seen in senile psychosis, because of the neurological or cardiac problem; many are bedridden, at least during acute stages. Death, when it occurs, is usually from cerebrovascular accidents, arteriosclerotic heart disease, or pneumonia.

In treatment there is a greater need for special medical care because of the critical physical involvement in arteriosclerotic psychosis. If and when remission occurs, the person can often benefit from psychotherapy, physical therapy, recreation, and all the usual therapeutic supports and services. Physical capacities are often a greater problem than intellectual capacities, although intellectual damage can be profound after massive or repeated cardiac attacks or strokes.

PRESENILE DEMENTIA

The presenile dementias are a group of cortical brain diseases that look clinically like the senile dementias seen in old people but occur earlier, in the 40- and 50-year age groups. Intellectual deterioration and personality disintegration are two predominant features, just as they are in senile psychosis. A successful social facade may be maintained in the early stages. These presenile conditions are unforgettable and tragic when seen clinically, for they so globally affect the lives of the middle-aged people who are the victims. Alzheimer's and Pick's diseases are the two common forms. While many regard Alzheimer's disease to be simply an early form of senile brain disease, all agree that Pick's disease is an independent entity.

With the present knowledge of these diseases, it is of little practical benefit to the patient to diagnostically differentiate among the various presenile dementias. Once it is clear that a chronic process rather than a reversible one is taking place, the clinical pictures of the presenile disorders are practically similar. But brain pathologies after death reveal rather distinct differences and thus may be useful for research and further knowledge into the aging process and the origins of organic disorders.

Alzheimer's disease

Alzheimer's disease is the presenile dementia seen most frequently although comprehensive data on incidence are not available. The clinical appearance is one of rapid mental deterioration, beginning with marked mental deficits and tendencies toward agitation. It proceeds toward more severe symptoms such as incoherence, aphasia, agnosia, apraxia, a parkinsonism-like gait, and convulsive seizures. Later the person becomes rigid and may be unable to stand and walk; eventually utter helplessness prevails, with incontinence and marasmus. Onset takes place in the forties and fifties, and an individual seldom lives longer than four or five years after illness begins. Remissions can occasionally occur. Treatment is limited to attention to symptoms and patient comfort.

In its early stages Alzheimer's disease can be mistaken for a behavioral disorder and also may be complicated by emotional reactions to the organic changes. One may see depression, denial, and anxiety as the person has not yet lost capacity for insight and attempts to deal with phenomena that begin to subtly manifest themselves. There is yet little known about the etiology of the disease; however, it is suspected that three elements play a part: the process of aging itself; constitutional and genetic factors (there is an occasional familial incidence of the disease); and pathogenic factors in the environment—perhaps toxins or infection.

Pathologically the brain as a whole shows atrophy, generally of a more severe nature than is found in senile brain disease. This may be due to the greater vigor of pathological processes in a younger person or simply a reflection of the fact that younger persons tend to live longer and the pathology has more time to progress.

Pick's disease

Pick's disease is clinically very similar to Alzheimer's and differentiation, as we have already stated, may be impossible until autopsy reveals the distinctive brain pathology. There is usually an earlier onset (in the fourth decade) although it may occur also after age 65. General behavior is most often a lack of initiative rather than the overactivity of the Alzheimer patient. Symptomatology includes early selective impairment of mental functioning with the memory reasonably intact except for new material. Focal signs begin to appear at a later stage (aphasia, aphrasia, apraxia, etc.), and eventually the person sinks into a vegetative existence before death. The cause is unknown, but genetic factors appear relevant. The prognosis is always fatal, with survival from two to fifteen years. The course of illness is steadily progressive, and treatment of symptoms is all that can presently be done.

Pathologically the brain shows a clear-cut and circumscribed rather then global atrophy, concentrating on the anterior portions of the frontal and temporal lobes of the brain.

OTHER MANIFESTATIONS OF ORGANIC DISORDERS

Pseudobulbar palsy

This condition is marked by poor control of emotions (laughing and crying), which is organically based. The labile emotionality must be differentiated from psychological behavior of a hysterical nature. There is almost always a history of strokes affecting each side of the body. The emotional instability is both inappropriate and uncontrollable and can occur in a less marked manner after even minor strokes.

Tremors

Tremors are involuntary movements occurring in one or more parts of the body and produced by alternate contractions of opposing muscle groups. They are symptoms rather than clinical entities in themselves.

In diagnosing a tremor, one should note the rate, rhythm, and distribution, and the effect of movement or rest. A rapid tremor is one that oscillates 8 to 10 times per second; a slow tremor is one oscillating 3 to 5 times per second. Tremors may be fine or coarse. Intention tremors appear during or are accentuated by a volitional movement of the affected part. Rest tremors are present when the involved part is at rest but diminish or disappear with active movements.

Tremors associated with organic disease

Organic diseases of the central nervous system

PARKINSONISM. The tremor is a coarse, alternating tremor of about 4 to 8 movements per second, usually present during rest and tending to diminish or disappear on movement and during sleep. It is most commonly present in the fingers, forearm, eyelids, and tongue. Rigidity, masklike facies, and slowness of movement are also noted.

DEMENTIA PARALYTICA (GENERAL PARESIS). A fine, rapid tremor involving the face (especially periorally), tongue, and hands is an early symptom of this syphilitic disease. It is probably due to damage to the frontal lobe and its connections with the brainstem and cerebellum. It may be increased by voluntary movements.

CEREBRAL ARTERIOSCLEROSIS. The tremor in this condition may either be of the intention type or resemble that of parkinsonism, depending on the part of the central nervous system involved. The tremors associated with "senility" probably fall into this group.

INTOXICATION. Tremor is a prominent symptom. Opiate addicts show a fine tremor of the facial muscles and fingers. The most common toxic state in which tremor is seen is alcoholism. In this condition, there is a rapid, coarse tremor involving the fingers, tongue, limbs, and head.

Tremors associated with functional disease

The tremors appearing in functional disorders may simulate those of organic, central nervous system disease. A psychiatric evaluation helps in making a diagnosis. Tremor is a fairly common symptom in both chronic and acute anxiety states. Tremor may be seen in anxious depressions and in hysteria.

General paresis

General paresis is a form of central nervous system syphilis and is characterized by ideas of grandeur, often of gigantic proportion. With recurrent episodes of venereal disease in the general population, we can expect to see much more of this disorder in the future. Many contemporary elderly received forms of therapy that were not as effective as penicillin (which began to be available only in 1941). Some were treated with arsenicals, whereas others with paresis were treated by the fever therapy of Wagner von Jauregg. Thus syphilis must always be given diagnostic consideration in older people.

Anosognosia

Anosognosia is an interesting symptom, which may be viewed as a defensive denial of severe organic change. The person "does not know *and* he does not know that he does not know the nature of his condition."

A 64-year-old black engineer had a residual paralysis of his right side (hemiparesis). He refused to admit that he could not move either extremity. When confronted by his doctor on this point, he would lift his right arm or leg with his left arm and say "See, I can move them."

CONCLUSION

Even the so-called organic disorders in late life are multicausal—with social and personal as well as organic roots.

We have emphasized in this chapter both the possibilities of treatment in the reversible brain syndromes and the personal and social components associated with the chronic conditions. In Chapter 9 we shall detail methods of making these important diagnostic distinctions, and in Part II we shall be dealing extensively with treatment.

REFERENCES

Alpers, B. J., Forster, F. M., and Herbut, P. A.: Retinal, cerebral and systemic arteriosclerosis, a histopathologic study, Archives of Neurology and Psychiatry **60**:440-456, 1948.

Butler, Robert N., Dastur, Darab K., and Perlin, Seymour: Relationships of senile manifestations and chronic brain syndromes to cerebral circulation and metabolism, Journal of Psychiatric Research 3:229-238, 1965.

Cosin, Lionel Z., Post, Felix, Westropp, Celia, and Williams, Moyra: Persistent senile confusion: study of 50 consecutive cases, The International Journal of Social Psychiatry 3:195-202, 1957.

Diagnostic and statistical manual of mental disorders (DSM I), Washington, D. C., 1952, American Psychiatric Association.

Diagnostic and statistical manual of mental disorders (DSM II), Washington, D. C., 1968, American Psychiatric Association.

Goldfarb, Alvin I.: Prevalence of psychiatric disorders in metropolitan old age and nursing homes, Journal of the American Geriatrics Society **10**:77-84, 1962.

Kallman, F. J.: Genetic differences in aging: comparative and longitudinal observations on a senescent twin population. In Hoch, P. H., and Zubin, J., editors: Psychopathology of aging, New York, 1961, Grune & Stratton, Inc.

Kay, D. W., and Roth, Martin: Environmental and hereditary factors in the schizophrenias of old age ("late paraphrenia") and their bearing on the general problem of causation of schizophrenia, Journal of Mental Science **107**:649-686, 1961.

Libow, L. S.: Pseudo-senility: acute and reversible organic brain syndromes, Journal of the American Geriatrics Society, 1973. (To be published.)

Müller, C., and Ciompi, L., editors: Senile dementia, Bern and Stuttgart, 1968, Hans Huber Publishers.

Noyes, Arthur P., and Kolb, Lawrence C.: Modern clinical psychiatry, ed. 5, Philadelphia, 1958, W. B. Saunders Co.

Post, Felix: The clinical psychiatry of late life, London, 1965, Pergamon Press, Inc.

Roth, Martin: The natural history of mental disorders in old age, Journal of Mental Science **101**:281-301, 1955.

Rothschild, David: Senile psychoses and psychoses with cerebral arteriosclerosis. In Kaplan, O. J., editor: Mental disorders in late life, Stanford, Calif., 1956, Stanford University Press.

Simon, Alexander, and Cahan, Robert: The acute brain syndrome in geriatric patients. In Mendel, W. M., and Epstein, L. J., editors: Acute psychotic reaction. Psychiatric Research Reports of the American Psychiatric Association, Washington, D. C., 1963, American Psychiatric Association.

Sjögren, H.: Neuropsychiatric studies in presenile and senile diseases, based on material of 1,000 cases, Acta Psychiatrica Scandinavica **106** (supp.):9-36, 1956.

Ullman, Montague: Behavioral changes in patients following strokes, Springfield, Ill., 1962, Charles C Thomas, Publisher.

Weinstein, Edwin A., and Kahn, Robert C.: Denial of illness: symbolic and physiological aspects, Springfield, Ill., 1955, Charles C Thomas, Publisher.

6

SPECIAL CONCERNS

Racism, sexism, retirement, crime, alcoholism, deafness, blindness, and sexuality

Do old people like to make love? Can they? How does racism affect the lives of the elderly? Should older women join the women's liberation movement? Do alcoholics live long enough to become old? Are there "geriatric criminals"? We will be considering in this chapter some of the important human issues that are part of old age. Misunderstandings abound in the folklore created around aging.

RACISM AS IT AFFECTS MENTAL HEALTH CARE

The elderly are a multiracial and multicultural group. Many are immigrants from other countries. At least 1.6 million are persons of minority group background—blacks, Indians, Cubans, Mexican-Americans, Puerto Ricans, Asian-Americans. A nation as diverse as the United States needs transcultural studies of the elderly within its own borders; different cultural and racial groups have different conceptions of the life cycle; each has been treated somewhat differently by the majority white culture. Research on the black elderly has become more active in recent years and attention has been focused on them through the National Caucus on the Black Aged, formed in 1970.* But the same is not yet as true for other minority groups. The United States Senate Special Committee on Aging under the leadership of Senator Frank Church has established special advisory groups for blacks, Indians, and Cubans and has also published a report from delegates of the 1971 White House Conference on Aging, which deals with older blacks, Indians, Asian-Americans, and Spanish-speaking people.*

There are two major and distinctly separate issues regarding minority-group elderly. First are the unique cultural elements found in each minority group, which have bearing on the lives of its elderly members; second are the effects imposed upon the elderly as a result of living in a majority white culture. We would like to touch on both of these issues but it is clear that most available research centers around vital statistics, social and economic conditions, and the effects of racism rather than the cultural life of individual groups. In Chapter 1 we have presented some of the facts and figures of minority old age in America. This chapter will deal with the direct effects of racial prejudice on the mental health care of older people. We look forward to the time when more will be known about the varied and distinctive life styles inherent in each culture. One would hope such variety could be preserved, protected, and used as a primary consideration in physical and mental health treatment. A richer diagnostic and treatment picture would result.

*Hobart C. Jackson, Chairman, National Caucus on the Black Aged, 4400 West Girard Avenue, Philadelphia, Pa. 19104.

*Report to the Delegates from the Conference Sections and Special Concerns Sessions, 1971 White House Conference on Aging, Washington, D. C., 1971, U. S. Government Printing Office.

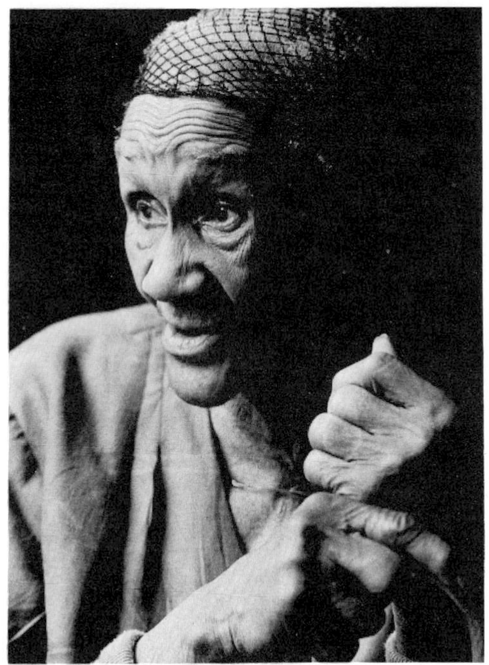

Multiple jeopardy: age, blackness, poverty, widowhood, womanhood.

Courtesy Zebra Associates, Inc., Advertising, New York. Photographer, Hugh Bell.

Black elderly

Black psychiatrists at the annual meeting of the American Psychiatric Association, May, 1970, called racism the number one mental health problem in America. This was echoed by the black caucuses of the American Orthopsychiatric Association and the National Association of Social Workers. The National Urban League in 1964 published a significant study called "Double Jeopardy," which described the dual discrimination of ageism and racism experienced by the black aged.* Black people who face racial prejudice all their lives are met with the added burdens of age prejudice when they grow old. Dr. Jacqueline Jackson, who has contributed much to the understanding of the black aged, has added a third "ism"—sexism—to the jeopardies confronting older black women, for they are in even worse circumstances than black men despite myths to the contrary.

Two of the most obvious effects of discrimination have been the overrepresentation of black elderly on Old Age Assistance and their shorter life expectancies. Whites often have Social Security and private pensions, while many jobs open to blacks were never or only recently covered by Social Security. And since black older people die at a younger age, they may never become eligible for retirement benefits even if they have them.

Outpatient mental health care

Racial prejudice and discrimination affect both the quality and the amount of mental health care available to the black elderly. Dr. William A. Reid, psychiatrist and leader of the Parkside-Arthur Capper Community Mental Health Team in Washington, D. C., has talked about a problem that is crucial in most community mental health centers:

> The majority of CMHC staff have at best only a superficial understanding of the culture, life experiences, and needs of their clients. It is a widely acknowledged fact that most psychiatric professionals, products of white middle-class America, are unable to bridge the cultural chasm between

*Double jeopardy, the older Negro in America today, New York, 1964, National Urban League.

themselves and proverty stricken Black people in the context of mental health work. Diagnosis and treatment are based on traditional psychiatric concepts of mental health and mental disorder. These in turn hinge on white middle-class norms and values. It is clear that traditional psychiatry cannot be applied to the situation of Black people. Effective mental health workers must be able not only to identify with the culture of their clients, but also to distinguish between the effects of societal pathology and individual psychopathology.*

In describing the experiences of his staff in the black community Reid states: "Clinically we are finding depression and reactions of anxiety, shame, and guilt. Some few show classical neuroses and psychoses." He emphasizes that too many mental health workers arbitrarily assign individual responsibility for misfortune rather than considering social factors. Successful treatment must challenge society's assumptions and not deny the reality of blackness. Psychoanalyst Franz Fanon† in 1967 wrote that any study of the psychology of a black person must include (1) a psychoanalytic interpretation of the life experience of the black man; and (2) a psychoanalytic interpretation of the Negro myth. Grier and Cobbs‡ make similar points. A body of theory and treatment techniques designed especially for the black population has begun to emerge.

The amount of outpatient care offered to the black aged is small. Hospital emergency rooms give minimal attention to psychiatric problems, particularly if the patient is old and poor. Voluntary nonprofit hospitals tend to refuse admission at the gate, a practice that now segregates by income rather than strictly race, with almost the same effect. Old people of all races make up only 4% to 5% of community mental health clientele, so one can see that only a small fraction of the total are black. Day hospitals and day care center accommodations are equally rare. These services receive little priority in municipal and county hospital budgets, and private sponsorship is difficult to obtain.

*Personal correspondence with Dr. Reid.

†Fanon, F.: Black skin, white masks, New York, 1967, Grove Press, Inc.

‡Grier, William H., and Cobbs, Price M.: Black rage, New York, 1968, Basic Books, Inc.

Home care

It is a commonly held view that the black community does not readily seek admission of its elderly for institutional care. Some explain this as indicative of a greater tolerance for abnormal behavior and a view of mental illness as a weakness or stigma. Others, such as Carter,* feel that it may represent a basic distruct of institutions because of previous life experiences. It is also apparent that there simply are not many institutional facilities other than state hospitals available for the elderly black person.†

Home care services are scarce, and families have been forced to provide care by themselves. Some studies suggest that the older person is more respected and considered less of a burden than in white families. True or not, this is no defensible reason for failing to provide supportive services in black homes.

Institutional care

It appears that staying out of institutions is not as big a problem for older blacks as is getting into them when they are needed.

Nursing homes and homes for the aged. These homes remain largely segregated even though segregation is usually not openly stated as a policy. Less than 3% of residents are black. Whites do not apply for admission to black homes, and white homes claim they have not received any "qualified" black applicants. Carter refers to the difficulty of finding homes for black males, who appear to be even more discriminated against than black females. Black-owned facilities having difficulty in meeting health,

*Carter, James H.: Psychiatry, racism and aging, paper presented at the Research Conference on Minority Group Aged in the South, Durham, N. C., Oct. 12, 1971.

†Jackson, Hobart C.: Alternatives to institutional care for older Americans: practice and planning: "Planning for the specially disadvantaged," presentation for the Conference on Alternatives to Institutional Care, Duke University, June 3, 1972.

fire, and building standards may be closed rather than given assistance and encouragement.* Many nonprofit, church-sponsored homes avoid integration by restricting admissions to their own parishioners, already a self-selected group in term of race and social class.

Mental hospitals. When a black older person requires institutional care, state hospitals are the only facilities routinely available. The integration of mental institutions has occurred relatively recently in most cases. St. Elizabeths Hospital in Washington, D. C., one of the well-known hospitals in the nation, was segregated until 1955; the hospitals in North Carolina were segregated until 1966. Segregated black hospitals were underfinanced and consequently in worse condition than the already inadequate white hospitals. With integration and the sharing of facilities, blacks fared somewhat better than before in terms of physical accommodations but it is doubtful that their medical or psychiatric treatment improved, since custodial care rather than active treatment is still customary. White aides and attendants are frequently unknowledgeable and insensitive to the cultural aspects of black life. They may not wish to provide personal services like giving baths, carrying out bedpans, giving enemas, etc. Open neglect can occur. White doctors and other professionals may share in the same insensitivity, lack of knowledge, and, at times, directly racist attitudes. Black aides and attendants who accept the "servant" role tend to be overly solicitous of older white patients, infantilizing them, while others may be passive-aggressive, ignoring patient needs. Thus aggression, passive and active, flows between white and black staff members to white and black patients.

Lifetime attitudes and conditioning often persist in old age, even after mental impairment occurs. An aged white woman with strong racial prejudices managed in spite of brain damage and incoherence to consistently call black staff members, including her psychiatrist, "niggers." Sometimes elderly black patients are seen waiting on white patients by performing personal services, while the whites give orders. There may be rebellion in older blacks; in one case an elderly black man spent his last years giving verbal vent to his murderous feelings toward whites, which had been stored up for a lifetime. Older blacks may share the belief that black professionals are inferior. It is not unusual in an integrated institution for them to confuse a white social worker as their doctor and relegate the black doctor to an attendant status, for as Pinderhughes* has observed, we all have shared a "pro-white, anti-black group-related paranoia."

Community-resident black elderly

Because of joint poverty the aged of both races tend to inhabit the inner city. It is a dangerous area for both groups, particularly since they are vulnerable to robberies, muggings, and fraud. The shared sense of danger can bring them together against the young. Both groups in Washington D. C.'s Project Assist program expressed a fear of the young men who menaced them, and both willingly accepted help from black and white staff. On the other hand elderly whites may attempt to compensate for their own loss of social status by expressing outspoken hatred of the black community, including older blacks.

Research is beginning to explore some of the specific psychological and cultural implications of black old age. There are differences between rural and urban dwellers, Northerners and Southerners, upper- and middle-income citizens versus those with lower income, as well as the various age groups and professions. For example, very old blacks, according to Dr. Ira Reid, prefer

*Position statement on Sarah Allen Nursing Home in West Philadelphia by the Board of Directors, Stephen Smith Geriatric Center, 1972.

*Pinderhughes, C. A.: The universal resolution of ambivalence by paranoia with an example in black and white, American Journal of Psychotherapy **24**:597-610, 1970.

the name "colored," while younger people are most comfortable with "Negro" and the very youngest demand "black." The "black revolution" has not escaped the aged. They may admire the young and support them, or they may be confused, isolated, and labeled by the young as "Uncle Toms." The concept of retirement may be meaningless for poor blacks who cannot afford to stop work. Thus "retirement crisis" does not apply to people who are in a "survival crisis." The black church has proved to be a stabilizing force, providing the elderly with social participation, prestige, and power in the internal life created by parishioners.

Mexican-American elderly*

Racial discrimination has had many of the same social and economic effects on all racial minorities. The Mexican-American population is heavily weighted with the young, because of high fertility, low life expectancy, and the return of some elderly to Mexico. There are great cultural differences from region to region in the United States,* and such diversity leads to questions about any given situation in aging as well as relationships with family and community. The notion of close family support is challenged because many elderly have become isolated physically and emotionally by the mobility and poverty of their children. The elderly have experienced strong anti-Mexican discrimination, particularly in the 1920s and 1930s when mass deportations occurred. Inability to speak English is a common handicap. As with blacks, many Mexican-Americans never live to retirement age.

*See for data on Mexican-Americans: Reich, J. M., Stegman, M. A., and Stegman, N. W.: Relocating the dispossessed elderly: a study of Mexican-Americans, Philadelphia 1966, University of Pennsylvania, Institute for Environmental Studies; and see Steglich, W. G., Cartwright, W. J., and Crouch, B.: Survey of needs and resources among aged Mexican-Americans, Lubbock, Texas Technological College, 1968.

*Examples of this are shown by the names people prefer. Spanish-Americans, Latins, Mexicans, and Chicanos are names that apply in specific regions, and to use them incorrectly may be offensive to older people.

American Indian elderly

An estimated 600,000 Indians live in the fifty states, speak some three hundred lan-

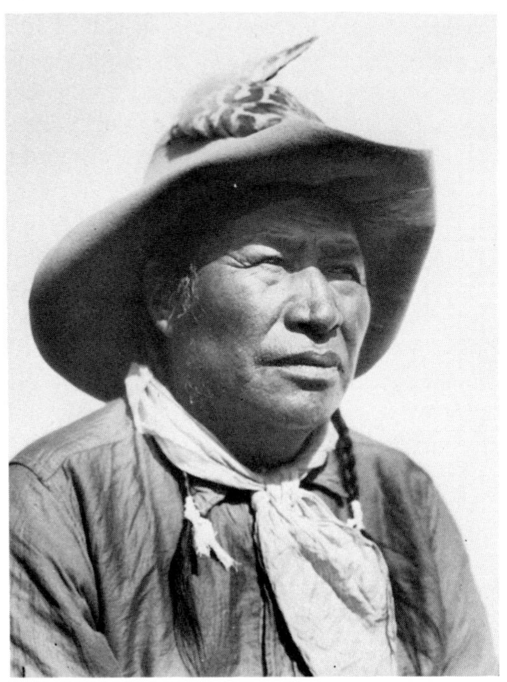

The first American: old age and poverty.

Courtesy H. Armstrong Roberts, Inc., Philadelphia.

guages, and have different customs and traditions from each other. The sole source of income for many of the elderly is welfare, with a minimum level of Social Security at age 72. The federal government through the Bureau of Indian Affairs did not set up retirement programs so that the elderly could participate in company retirement plans, insurance plans, private investments, and in many cases Social Security. State public assistance programs have pressured the elderly Indians to sell their allotted reservation land, even though the federal government has claimed it supports the Indians' desire to retain their tribal property. Because of jurisdictional questions, some states have refused to license nursing homes on reservations; therefore, federal funds, which must be given only to state-licensed homes, are not authorized. Indian spokesmen have stated that federal funds should be released to them directly, administered as part of the Indian Health Service. We have discussed the elderly Indians' plight in Chapter 1. They have suffered much, receiving very little in return, and the emotional effects can only be described as incalculable.

Asian-American elderly

Cultural barriers, language problems, and discrimination have added to the old age burdens of yet another group, the Asian-Americans. Spokesmen point to a pervasive myth that has excluded these elderly from services:

> This emasculating myth that discriminates against Asian-American elderly is that Asian-American aged do not have any problems, that Asian-Americans are able to take care of their own and that Asian-American aged do not need nor desire aid in any form. Such assertions which are generally accepted as valid by society are false. . . . it is impossible for Asian-Americans to look only to their families for help.*

There are five basic groups (Chinese, Filipino, Korean, Japanese, and Samoan)—all with their own languages and cultures; yet they are often lumped together as Orientals.* Most of the elderly are immigrant and many are literate in their native language although they may not speak English. There is need for a diverse number of services that cannot be met solely by families.

Basic differences exist among the elderly of each cultural group, which reflect not only their inherent uniqueness but also the patterns of racial discrimination they have faced in this country.

Many elderly Chinese were brought to the United States in the late nineteenth century as "coolies," and whites became frenzied by the imagined threat of inundation from Chinese hordes. Therefore, Chinese men were prohibited from bringing their wives and children with them, and they were forbidden to intermarry in America. "This produced the sex ratio which has plagued Chinese communities ever since. In most areas with large Chinese-American populations there are groups of single males who have been derailed, as it were, from the normal cycle of life."* It is considered a great misfortune for a Chinese man to fail to produce sons who will care for him in old age and in afterlife. But racism has caused the breakdown of these traditions. Many elderly men live isolated lives, addicted to opium and uncompensated for their years of hard labor. Perhaps for similar reasons, the Filipino population has an unusually large proportion of men in psychiatric hospitals.

Early Japanese immigration policies were not so devastating and dehumanizing. Women and children were allowed to accompany men, and this has had a profound effect upon the lives of present-day elderly. Family structure is much more stable and supportive. The Japanese elderly were able to survive the World War II internment in relocation centers with the loss of jobs and their roles in American society because their children could carry on for them. Many of

*From White House Conference on Aging, 1971, Asian American elderly, Report on Special Concerns, p. 61.

*From Kalish, R. A., and Yuen, S.: Americans of East Asian ancestry; aging and the aged, The Gerontologist 11:41, 1971.

the children have become highly educated and successful while retaining patterns of loyalty to parents.

What can be done to improve mental health care for minority-group elderly?

1. Income maintenance is a prime requirement. Social Security age-eligibility rules should reflect the life expectancies of minority groups. For example, a rural, migrant Mexican-American should be eligible for benefits at age 45. Private and government pension plans should be portable from job to job. A system of income maintenance that is not related to earnings and is available to all on an equal basis would do much to provide a base of support. Old Age Assistance, tied to a "means test" and costly in administration, should be replaced by a minimum guaranteed annual income.

2. Minority professionals and the elderly themselves should be in key-decision–making and advisory positions in any actions affecting the elderly.

3. Mental health staffs should reflect the racial composition they serve. Training in the mental health field should be widely available for minority-group members.

4. At present, treatment cannot be handled by minority personnel alone, since there are so few of them. White personnel should have special training and supervisory monitoring by minority-group professionals if they work with nonwhite clientele.

5. Research from the minority perspective should be funded and encouraged. Problems pertinent to minority elderly (e.g., hypertension among blacks) need emphasis.

6. More alternative methods of care must be made available—home care services, nursing homes and homes for the aged, psychiatric hospitalization outside of state hospitals, day care, day hospitals. Techniques of individual and group psychotherapy relevant to minority needs should be developed. Meals-on-wheels could supply ethnic foods, and food stamps should be usable in ethnic groceries. Recreation and leisure therapy should be aimed at cultural interests. Information systems, service workers, legal assistance, and psychiatric therapy should all be provided on a bilingual basis for the elderly who do not speak English.

SEXISM AND THE PROBLEMS OF OLDER WOMEN

Eleven million women in the United States are 65 years of age and older. Sexism and ageism are the twin prejudices directed against them. They have experienced sex discrimination all their lives, but age discrimination begins only after they have lost their youth and accelerates as they age. The end result is a greater rate of poverty and social unacceptability than for men, combined ironically with a longer life-span. The cultural denigration of the older woman is taught at an early age through fairy tales that depict old hags, evil crones, scary old witches, and nasty biddies of all sorts. Mother-in-law stories abound. Doctors and medical students call older female patients "crocks." Unmarried aunts are scorned as "old maids." Even grandma becomes a family nuisance as she outlives grandpa and experiences and expresses the emotional and physical facts of aging. Thus the message comes across that a woman is valuable for bearing and rearing children, and perhaps to nurse her husband in his dotage, but after that it is clearly useless and even burdensome to have her around. The mistreatment of old women is a national habit that has yet to be challenged even by older women themselves. They are defined as "old" and "women" (in the traditional sense) but rarely as viable, valuable human beings.

Low visibility of the elderly woman

One of the traditions of the American social system is to keep its "undesirables" out of sight. For years we pretended to know little about the poor or the blacks until they were "discovered" with great alarm. But how many old women do you see on television or in the newspapers or hear on radio? The elderly condition in general is rarely seen as newsworthy unless something extraordinary occurs. Elderly women must be truly exceptional to be noticed—Helena Rubenstein at 92 running a business empire, Grandma Moses painting primitive art, Martha Graham still dancing at 76, or Helen Hayes performing on the stage at 70. To be less than remarkable is to be invisible.

Profile of the elderly woman

What is the life of an *average* older woman like? In many cases it means being widowed and living alone, on a low or poverty-level income, perhaps in substandard housing, with minimal medical care and little chance of employment to supplement resources.

Income

A small proportion of older women are well off financially and some few have inherited enormous wealth. At the other end of the spectrum are those women who have been poor all their lives and who can expect even greater poverty in old age. But in between these two groups are a multitude of women who have lived comfortably throughout their lives and first experience poverty after they are old: the newly poor. Poverty is not reserved for women alone, since old men too are often in dire financial condition. Yet whenever poverty is found, it is generally more profound and of greater consequence for women. In 1967 the average Social Security benefits for a retired man were $95 a month while women averaged $72. Retirement benefits for women workers in general averaged 76% of the amount for men. Nonwhite women averaged only $56 monthly.

Even women with sufficient income have problems because many of them do not know how to handle money for their own benefit. It is here, particularly, that societal patterns of passivity and accedence to masculine financial management show themselves. Women are encouraged to turn their money over to men to manage—to bank representatives, guardians, lawyers, male children, etc.—and those women who do take care of their own finances are often untrained and ill prepared to make sound decisions. A study of business and professional women found that they were good savers but suffered badly from inflation because of the way they invested.* These were women who were well above average in income, job level, education, and years of experience; but they knew little about investments or how to increase capital. Money management was for them a passive activity in which they preferred the false security of savings, cash, and annuities over a sounder investment program that required an understanding of economics and finance.

Employment

About 1 million or 10% of older women are employed, often out of necessity. Many never worked outside their homes until their children left home and they are employed in dead-end and unskilled jobs. Others were employed all their lives but usually earned much less than men of comparable talent and initiative. All of this results in lower Social Security and private retirement benefits and, combined with a longer life-span for women, produces lower income that must be stretched over a greater number of years.

Employers are reluctant to hire older women because of stereotyped attitudes that they are not adaptable to today's jobs and technology; old women are seen as cantankerous, sexually unattractive, overly emotional, and unreliable due to health problems. Yet studies indicate that they make exceptionally good employees, with lower turnover, higher productivity, and less absenteeism than men or younger women. At one point in 1969 the Department of Health, Education, and Welfare itself closed the door on women over 35 years of age as potential appointees for high-level jobs in the department.

Social Security discriminates against older women in a number of ways. We have mentioned that women earn less and therefore receive less in benefits. Many jobs held by

*Erb, Charlotte: Do women invest wisely? A study of savings for retirement. Summary of research, Washington, D. C., 1970, Business and Professional Women's Foundation.

women have only recently been covered under Social Security—agriculture, hotel and restaurant work, hospital jobs, and domestic work (the latter is still frequently uncovered). Much work done by women, primarily work as housewives and mothers, has earned them nothing. Until 1973 a widow received only 82.5% of her husband's benefits even though she has worked all her life as a full-time employee in her home. If a man and woman are married, they may get less Social Security than if they were not married. Thus some old couples live together without marrying in order to obtain the benefits they both have earned. The Social Security "means test," which limits the amount of income that can be earned, is especially hard on women, since they live longer and use up their resources; many are reduced to doing bootleg work to hide their income from the government because they need to survive. Finally, Social Security is a regressive tax with a base rate of $10,800 (1972, 1973), $12,000 (after 1974); therefore women pay proportionately more than men because of their lower incomes.

Marriage

Of the 11 million older women, more than 6 million are widows and an additional 1.2 million are divorced or single. (Approximately 7% of all women never marry.) Thus 65% of older women are on their own, an interesting fact when one remembers that they, more than any younger group, were raised from childhood to consider themselves dependent on men.

Why so many widows? Women outlive men their own age and also tend to marry men older than themselves. The difference in life expectancy seems to be a rather recent and poorly understood occurrence. In 1920 men could expect to live 53.6 years and women a year longer, but by 1970 a seven-year spread was evident with a life expectancy of 67.5 for men and 74.9 for women.

Old men have a tremendous advantage over old women when it comes to marriage. Because they tend to marry younger women who will outlive them, they are much less likely to be widowed. More than that, they can count on a fairly healthy spouse to nurse them as they age. Should their wife die prematurely, they have endless options for remarriage. At age 65 when men number 8 million, the 11 million women already outnumber them by 3 million and the odds improve as men grow older. In remarrying, men can bypass their own age group altogether and marry women from 65 all the way down to girls in their twenties or teens. One can readily see what is happening to older women in all of this; their chances for remarriage are small, and only 16,000 each year find a second husband. It is socially frowned upon for an older woman to date or marry a man much younger than herself, a blatant form of discrimination when men are freely allowed this option.

Living arrangements

Currently, 34% of elderly women live alone, 18% live with husbands, 39% with relatives, 4% with nonrelatives, and only 5% in institutions. Many women have never lived alone until old age. It is estimated that up to 60% live in substandard housing.

Health

Old women cannot count on the medical profession. Few doctors are interested in them. Their physical and emotional discomforts are often characterized as "postmenopausal syndromes" until they have lived too long for this to be an even faintly reasonable diagnosis. After that, they are assigned the category of "senility." Doctors complain about being harassed by their elderly female patients, and it is true that many are lonely and seeking attention. Yet more than 85% have some kind of chronic health problem, and both depression and hypochondriasis commonly accompany the physical ailments.

Emotional results of prejudices against older women

The phenomenon of "self-hatred" is found in most groups of people who are the victims of discrimination. If enough people tell you something bad about yourself for a long enough time, you end up believing it. Thus older women typically discredit themselves in both obvious and subtle ways. A successful film star of 72 admits that men are favored as actors over women in old age. Yet she insists she has no use for Women's Liberation: . . . "No, no, no. I want a man to know more . . . Physically I want him stronger, mentally I want him stronger." A representative of the Department of Labor's Women's Bureau said many older women have a "Uriah Heep" attitude about employment, feeling they must appear obsequious and obedient because they feel they have little of value to offer an employer.

There are women who profit from and exploit the insecurities of their contemporaries. Helena Rubenstein, one of the world's wealthiest self-made women, is a fascinating example of a female who maintained her own power and influence until age 92 but made millions off the cravings of women to stave off inevitable aging.

A pervasive theme in the efforts of older women to find a meaningful life is the preference for male company and the downgrading of female companionship. Many cannot see themselves as fulfilled unless they have a husband or at least some male to whom they can relate, and this becomes more frustrating as the male population thins out. Some women compensate with an overbearing idolization of a son or grandson. Others make sad, futile efforts to appear young and thus recapture the lost rights of their youth and early adulthood. The top-heavy ratio of women to men encourages an already culturally established pattern of competition with fellow females for the few remaining men. The mother-in-law syndrome is another way women may express their disdain toward their own sex (their daughters-in-law) as well as the envy an older woman can feel toward a younger woman. The harsh experiences of women during the aging process make it understandable that they may see the young as rivals, not only for the attention of males but also for the very economic resources necessary for their survival in old age.

Some elderly women turn to religion, in a passionate excessive manner that seems less a spiritual search than a way of filling the void of their former family. If a man is not available, then perhaps a masculine God-figure may give some sense of comfort and meaningfulness. Religion can be truly beneficial, but it can also serve as a cover-up for terribly lonely women who have no relevant human beings in their lives.

The "club and charity" set is a further example of the attempt to find meaning. Club and charity organizations reveal an effort to extend mothering to the whole world of orphans, the sick, poor, blind, and halt; yet noble as this sentiment appears, it is quickly evident in many cases that the real purpose is to fill empty time and lend a sense of importance—not to get down to the task of relieving the suffering of others. There are, of course, remarkable exceptions but most older women were conditioned to the lesser role and thus congregate together in dilettante fashion to fill up their lives.

What's good about being an older woman?

We have detailed some of the difficulties of older women. But there is more. Many older women have learned much about the double whammy of sex and age discriminations and have a great deal to teach the young. Their experiences give us guidelines for combating prejudice and supporting older women in their efforts to find a satisfying life. Some of the present and future possibilities of old age for women will be discussed.

Older women today have the potential for being the most liberated group of American women in terms of personal expression. In addition to their increasingly good records of health and longevity, they do not have to fight the conflicts between mothering and careers which, even with day care, plague younger women. They can function as the only adult females who are truly free of the demands of child responsibility and, in many cases, marital responsibility. Widowhood and lack of males need not carry the stigma of failure. The idea of dependency on a male is deeply ingrained in white and in many minority cultures, but older women may be responsive to challenges of this tired stereotype. Many women who were forced into marriage by cultural and family pressures might have been happier single, as career or professional women. Educational programs should be designed especially for them to explore late-life careers. Other older women are homosexuals who have been hiding as "heteros" for a lifetime and might be willing to "come out" if the climate were favorable. Numbers of others could have satisfied heterosexual companionship and maternal needs without marriage or children and still can. They could challenge the sex-age prejudice and obtain the sexual options now reserved for men. We might, for example, be surprised at the number of secret liaisons between young males and older females, which could surface if they became socially acceptable.

Older women by example could give younger women confidence to resist the youth trap, with the knowledge that a rich life can await them as they age. Women of all ages may begin to refuse to be discarded and demand recognition as human beings. Young women and even the middle-aged are floundering for viable female models to follow. A considerable number of old women have forged unique positions for themselves in terms of identity, personal achievement, and even financial and political power; but they need to be located and made visible.

Another unique asset of age is that most older women have adjusted in some way to the idea of personal death. It is characteristic of the elderly to fear death much less than the young do. They may attain a certain degree of extra objectivity from this vantage point. There is a possibility for a greater sense of moral commitment and flexibility beyond their own egos. Old people are often thought of as conservative, but in truth they are inclined to be dovish on war and liberal on political and social issues. In terms of flexibility this is the generation which indeed has, as Nikita Khrushchev so aptly put it, gone "from the outhouse to outer space" in one lifetime.

Politically the older woman is in an advantageous position and it is likely to improve. With a voting strength of 11 million, 90% of whom are registered voters and most of whom vote regularly, they represent a major and fast-growing constituency that already could elect their own congresswomen in those states where they reside in high proportions. They have the available time and energy to lobby, campaign, and promote candidates, since 90% are retired from active employment. There is reason to suppose that women as candidates for the presidency and as appointees to the Supreme Court may come from this age group, since older people often fill these positions.

In spite of widespread poverty for many women, there are tremendous sums of money in the hands of widows and female heirs. It is time that women took up their own financial management instead of entrusting it to male husband-surrogates. Women of wealth could exert much greater influence in economic, social, and artistic spheres if they used the resources they already have. They could provide backing for the women's movements and specifically for their own age group problems.

Many elderly women have lived out their last years in the way thus characterized by Edna St. Vincent Millay: "Life must go on —I forget just why." But there is a sturdy and hopefully growing group of old women who are undaunted and look to life with enthusiasm. An 83-year-old former suffragette who recently became excited by the Women's Liberation movement states, "I don't want to leave the world without being a part of this."

RETIREMENT

Everyone "reacts" to retirement but not everyone goes through a "retirement crisis." Retirement does not mean the same thing for everybody. Some view it as the end of their worthwhile life and think that anything beyond is downhill. This is particularly true of men who tend to identify strongly with their jobs. Some are "workaholics" who are addicted to continuous laborings. Other people see retirement as a relief from hard work, a chance to rest, a period of passive emjoyment and relaxation. Still others feel that it marks the completing of their commitment to society and the beginning of their active commitment to themselves and all the things they have been waiting and wanting to do. It is not unusual to see second and even third careers occurring in late life, creative ventures begun, whole new personalities emerging as people discover and rediscover themselves. Max Lerner once said that retirement should enable people to move into work they love to pursue, after leaving work that has pursued them. The emotional quality of retirement is dependent on the individual personality, income, health, social circumstances, and sense of worth.

Work has long been recognized as a useful defense that occupies minds and bodies and keeps feelings in control. This brings to mind the individuals who get sick, anxious, or upset on Sundays, holidays, or vacations and feel fine once they are back at work. In retirement, these symptoms can become everyday occurrences unless work-substitutes and a satisfactory new life style are found; otherwise perfectly healthy men and women may develop headaches, depression, gastrointestinal symptoms, and oversleeping. These disorders can begin even in anticipation of retirement. Irritability, loss of interest, lack of energy, increased alcoholic intake, reduced efficiency are all familiar and common reactions. Many people have work dreams in which they dream of being back on the job. In many cases these feelings are transitional as the retired person adjusts to a new life and new associations. Consideration must be given to the tremendous changes that take place over a relatively brief period of time, including the absence of structured work and one's role as a producer of work, the removal from working colleagues, the absence of travel to and from work, the change in daily scheduling, and the reduction in income—usually to about one half its former level.

Retirement comes in three phases: the actual day itself is perhaps a day of celebration or commemoration. Then comes the longer period of working through feelings and adjusting to a new life. Finally the person arrives at a state in which he thinks of himself as "retired." At this point the adjustment has been made and he has identified with a new life condition.

The phenomena of both over and under preparation for retirement can be observed. The overly prepared are those people who anxiously begin to plan ahead in early middle age, with elaborate attentions to the details of their future life. Such overachievers are usually indicating that they are unhappy or insecure in their present life and are trying desperately for something better in the future. On the other extreme are those who do not even conceive of, let alone prepare for, retirement and who are sadly surprised when it catches them unaware. The most successful retirees are those who take reasonable precautions for their old age but enjoy living in the present rather than expecting some future "golden age."

Many women have dual roles, as homemakers and career working women, which may be an unfair burden in earlier years but can serve them well as they retire from employment. Keeping a home always provides a familiar pattern of life to fall back on. The majority of men have no such diverse identity (which may also be true of unmarried women). In Chapter 3 we have described the need for male as well as female liberation to allow men a sense of themselves apart from their work. The present overidentification with work may be a factor in the high rate of suicide in older white men.

We wish to reemphasize that not everyone dreads retirement. Many people never identify personally with their jobs but use them only to survive financially. Countless numbers are only too delighted to get rid of jobs that have been boring, dead-end, demeaning, or demanding. And there are numerous older people who truly look forward to and enjoy the freedom and possibilities of a new way of life.

CRIME

Older people commit very little crime. There are few "geriatric criminals." But they are the victims of crime, especially robbery.

> Traditionally the older person in the community had a role in that he had lived longer, he therefore had more experience, he was wiser. . . . he knew where the tigers were in the jungle.
>
> NATHAN W. SHOCK

Experience can do little to protect the elderly person today, particularly the urban dweller in the inner city and other low-income areas. Crime in cities is widespread, as is the fear of crime. Except for the *District of Columbia Report to the 1971 White House Conference on Aging,* subtitled "Metropolitan Police Contact with the Elderly,"* there is no document of recent date that shows the degree to which crimes are committed against elderly persons. In *Project Assist* Brostoff pointed to "a large group of old people (over 60). . . a depressed underclass . . . who are particularly vulnerable to crime, easy victims of street robbery, unable to move out of high-crime neighborhoods . . . and likely to have no other community resource to turn to other than the police if trouble occurs. . . ." Police reports often do not indicate the ages of victims. However, the incidence of crime that is recorded against the elderly suggests that crimes occur primarily where large numbers of older people are concentrated. Public housing complexes are a prime target, since almost 20% of people in such housing are 65 or more years of age. Bus and subway stops, basement laundry rooms in apartment buildings, dark halls, back doors, elevators, and shortcuts (paths, passageways hidden from view) can all be dangerous places for older people. Mailboxes in unguarded apartment vestibules are the province of thieves who know when Social Security and welfare checks arrive. Food stamps are a frequently stolen item. The disabilities of old age—deafness, slowness, blindness, spotty memory—make elderly people more vulnerable.

In Washington, D. C., about 90% of crimes against the elderly were robberies and 8% were assaults. Most robberies take place on the streets rather than at home. The methods used are purse-snatching, frightening, and strong-arming. The amount of money stolen is often under $5, and little is ever recovered. Stolen checks and food stamps are recoverable, but the delay can mean having no food or rent money when it is needed. Many of the poor elderly have no phone on which to notify police of crime. Crimes committed by relatives, landlords, etc. against older people rarely are prosecuted because they get lost in the law enforcement system.

The elderly seek police help with social problems as well as those due to crime; for example, 15% of telephone calls to the police during Project Assist were about crimes while 40% came from people asking for help and information (how to get an ambulance, heat in an apartment etc.). Thus the police are excellent sources for referral and

---

*In June, 1970, the Office of Services to the Aged, Human Resources Adminstration, D. C. Government, awarded a contract to the Washington School of Psychiatry to study the relationship between older people and the metropolitan police department. The purposes of the research contract were as follows:

1. To determine the extent to which older persons are victims of crime in the District of Columbia
2. To discover what social or health problems result from such victimization and how they are dealt with
3. To ascertain under what circumstances older persons come to the attention of the police when no crime has been committed, but aid of police is sought because other community resources are unknown or not available
4. To explore methods and techniques for quick and appropriate referral for service by police in disposing of problems of older persons encountered as victims of crime or as persons needing or seeking help

Project Director Mrs. Phyllis Brostoff, M.S.W., conducted the study, called *Project Assist,* and compiled the above-mentioned document for the White House Conference. (For additional information see Brostoff, Phyllis, Brown, Roberta, and Butler, R. N.: The Public Interest: Report no. 6: Beating up on the elderly: police, social work, crime, Aging and Human Development 3:319-322, 1972.)

for location of the isolated elderly. They are contacts for people with chronic brain syndromes who wander from home, elderly alcoholics, and acute brain syndrome victims who are in difficulty on the street or at home.*

But the main responsibility of the police is considered to be law enforcement and their focus is on prevention of crime and apprehension of criminals. Many object to providing social services and want a "magic number" they can call for referral of social problems. Social agencies could work more closely with the police than they now do. Multiservice senior centers would be an ideal resource for the variety of problems older people bring to the police.

Protection of older people from crime should be improved.† Escort services could be arranged by volunteer groups; dead bolt locks should be provided for the older person's residence; federal government and welfare agencies could arrange to send checks directly to banks free of charge for those persons who would prefer this, thus reducing the theft of checks. Special low-cost checking account service might encourage people not to carry cash but to establish credit and to pay by check whenever possible. It has been said that if it were generally known that old people no longer dealt in cash the incentive for criminal attack would be markedly reduced. Vertical policing throughout all the floors in high-rise buildings should be done by police on the beat or by volunteers. Police could perform security audits of buildings to spot crime hazards. Tenants themselves could guard mailrooms at the beginning of each month to protect against check thefts. The older woman might carry an old empty purse for use as a decoy to be given up under attack.

A plan of protection that has kept the crime rate at 1% in an entire low-income public housing project is used by the Cuyahoga (Ohio) Metropolitan Housing Authority. Harry Atkins, chief of safety and security for the Authority's vast complex of twenty high-rise buildings (in which 3,000 elderly and disabled people live), describes its Guide Program. Five hundred volunteers, mostly women, monitor buildings on a two-hour per day basis. They report the presence of strangers, check security devices such as buzzers, locks, and alarms, and send for ambulances or police if needed. A training seminar is held each month for participants. In addition to the volunteers there are two coordinators, trained in law enforcement and licensed to carry guns, who patrol the buildings at regular intervals. Security guards are on duty in some of the buildings until 1:30 A.M., and state patrol cars drive through the area from dusk until early morning. All residents have a telephone number to reach either the security guard or police.

A safe environment (versus one of fear and genuine danger) is crucial to the mental health of older people. No one can live under threat of harm, without physical and emotional repercussions. The elderly need protection also when they get into trouble (forgetfulness, getting lost, home accidents, isolation, and self-neglect) because of their own disabilities. And finally, they need protection against the fraud (e.g., medical quackery) or deceit that preys on their vulnerabilities.

ALCOHOLISM*

Alcoholics do indeed live to old age in greater numbers than ever. In addition, some older people become alcoholics only after becoming old. *Alcoholism* is a condition due

*Matthews, R., and Rowland, L.: How to recognize and handle abnormal people—a manual for the police officer, New York, 1960, The National Association for Mental Health, Inc., Chapters 6 and 10.

†See Elderly are crime targets, SOS, Senior Opportunities and Services Technical Assistance Bulletin 2(4):1-3, Feb.-March, 1972, Also a useful booklet entitled "Your Retirement Safety Guide" has been prepared by the American Association of Retired Persons, 1225 Connecticut Avenue, N.W., Washington, D. C.

*The National Council on Alcoholism estimates that there are some 5 million alcoholics in the United States. The Langley Porter studies under Simon and Lowenthal provide information on alcoholism in old people.

to excessive ingestion of or idiosyncratic reaction to alcohol. *Acute* alcoholism is a state of acute intoxication with temporary and reversible mental and bodily effects. *Dipsomania* refers to periodic or "spree" drinking. *Chronic* alcoholism is the fact and consequence of habitual use.

Alcohol is a central nervous system depressant. It is not, as many believe, a stimulant except as it indirectly inhibits cortical control (higher intellectual functions are associated with the cerebral cortex) and thereby releases emotional reactions. With inhibition and impairment of intellectual functions comes failure in judgment, which adds to impairments that may already exist as a result of cerebral arteriosclerosis and senile brain disease. Alcohol can affect muscular coordination and bodily equilibrium, causing falls and accidents in old age. Families tend to be more negative and less supportive to the older person who drinks.

Chronic alcoholism usually involves poor nutrition primarily due to vitamin and protein deficiencies and liver dysfunction. In addition to a general deterioration of the personality, one may see delirium tremens followed by Korsakoff's psychosis. Confabulations or fabrications of memory and inability to retain new information are the latter's most striking symptoms.

Alcoholism in old age is of two types insofar as duration is concerned, lifelong and late-life. The former used to result in death far before old age, but because of antibiotics, better nutritional care, and hospital management many alcoholics now live to grow old. In addition, some older people first turn to alcohol in old age becaues of grief, depression, loneliness, boredom, or pain. Grief stricken widows who drink are an example of this. Another pattern in alcoholism is a lifelong habit of drinking, which becomes even more severe as life stresses pile up.

Mr. D, the black gardener and handyman in a white, wealthy neighborhood, was only 65 years old but he looked much older. His eyes were tired and sometimes vacant. He worked at hard, backbreaking tasks and each family in the neighborhood expected him to do the bulk of the work on their property. There was no sick leave, no paid vacations, no retirement pension beyond the Social Security based on payments that were subtracted from his already meager pay checks. He had become arthritic, with painful, swollen joints. But none of his employers relaxed their expectations of him as he aged and grew more feeble. In fact, one employer called all the others when the worker became eligible for Social Security and said "We must be sure Billy doesn't take advantage of Social Security and earn more than he is supposed to." Mr. D had drunk steadily for years, on weekends, but now began coming to work drunk. His employers wondered "What has come over Billy?"

One sees a high proportion of alcoholism among older patients, mostly men, in Veterans Hospitals and Domiciliaries. It has been suggested that war experiences and exposure to the cultural drinking patterns of the Armed Services played a causative role.

Treatment of older chronic alcoholics usually consists in detoxification or "drying out," followed by vitamins, meals, and medical care. Many who are poor or isolated from their families come to medical attention through the police. Therapy for alcoholics at any age is often unsuccessful. In our view one must go to the roots of the problem when alcoholism is secondary to depression, for example, or a reflection of social conditions such as poverty or variations in drinking patterns of ethnic cultures. In addition, Alcoholics Anonymous, individual and group therapy, family therapy, and recreation and social therapy may be helpful.

DEAFNESS

Hearing is so crucial to mental health in old age that we wish to give it special emphasis. Hearing loss is more common than visual loss and in 1964 the National Health Survey found significant hearing loss in about 30% of the 65-plus population, compared to 10% in the general population. In the older age group 450,000 people were profoundly deaf and totally isolated from any sound. Depression and paranoid ideation are the most common severe emotional consequences of hearing loss.

> When a person becomes deaf through disease . . . not knowing what his fellow men are saying he becomes doubtful of auditory memories and images; he misinterprets auditory sense impressions which have been distorted by disease, and incorporates tinnitus caused by such disease into his world of inner phantasy. He projects his inner feelings of inferiority caused by his deafness onto his environment and develops ideas of reference. Systematization soon follows, with active delusions of persecution. If the personality is sufficiently unstable a psychotic illness results.*

In Chapter 3 we discussed the relationship between hearing loss and depression. Hearing defects create irritation in others because they interfere so markedly with communication. The loud, badly articulated speech of the deaf person and the need to shout and speak slowly make simple conversations frustrating. The hard-of hearing are often mistakenly thought to be retarded or mentally ill. The dramatic story of Ludwig van Beethoven notwithstanding, the deaf receive much less empathy than the blind and are more subject to depression, demoralization, and psychotic symptomatology.

In the late years one is likely to observe nerve as well as conduction deafness.† Another source of hearing impairment involves the cochlea, a spiral tube of the inner ear, which resembles a small shell. The cochlea contains about 20,000 hair cells at birth, which gradually die off and cannot be replaced. Loss of these ganglion cells is called *presbycusis* and is believed to be associated with the aging of the body and/or brain. The central nervous system also is very important in hearing loss because it is the analyzing mechanism for sounds. Older people may be able to hear sounds but not understand them. Immigrants who have learned a second language appear to have special difficulty in this respect with their second language as they age. It is important not to overlook impacted wax (cerumen) in the ear as a cause of reduced hearing, although wax secretion probably diminishes with age. Since infections, diabetes, cancer, and many other conditions can also cause ear problems, referral to the ear-nose-and-throat specialist is always indicated.

Hearing impairment produced by aging is noted first in the higher sound frequencies and begins to be observed after age 50. This does not in itself interfere with normal speech, but the person may miss the song of birds, a distant telephone ring, or the ticking of a watch. Noise pollution is increasingly a factor in hearing loss. The decibel level of one's environment can become great enough to permanently damage the tiny hairs in the inner ear. (The decibel, named after Alexander Graham Bell, is the smallest difference in loudness the human ear can detect.)

Normal breathing	10 decibels
Leaves rustling in the breeze	20 decibels
Whisper	30 decibels
Quiet restaurant	50 decibels
Normal speech	60 decibels
Busy traffic	70 decibels
Niagara Falls	90 decibels
Subway	100 decibels
Pneumatic riveter	130 decibels
Jet takeoff (discomfort)	140 decibels

Many experts are predicting hearing loss for young people who listen to loud rock music with high decibel levels. The increasing noise of city life portends hearing problems for the population in general. Studies of the Mabaans of Sudan, a tribe so isolated that they do not even use drums, show very clearly how lack of noise protects hearing, for they live with a background noise of 40 decibels and experience very little hearing damage. Hospitals themselves have a high decibel level in spite of their "Quiet, please" signs.

BLINDNESS

The four most common causes of blindness in people over 65 years are macular degeneration, cataracts (lens opacities),

*From Houston, F., and Royse, A. B.: Relationship between deafness and psychotic illness, The Journal of Mental Science **100**:990-993, 1954.

†Conduction deafness is due to middle or external ear pathology, whereas nerve deafness results from interruption of the auditory nerve pathway. (See Ruben, R.: Aging and hearing. In Clinical geriatrics, Philadelphia, 1971, J. B. Lippincott Co., Chapter 14.)

glaucoma, and diabetic retinopathy.* These account for 20%, 17%, 13%, and 12%, respectively, of all blindness in people over 65.† According to Harlin,‡ there are an estimated 380,000 blind elderly in the United States and four to five times that many with some impairment of vision. This involves 1.9 million or approximately 10% of the elderly population. Nearly half of the legally blind§ population is 65 years of age or older.

Nonmedical members of mental health teams should learn the common physical symptoms of eye problems, to avoid putting a psychiatric label on a physical process and to increase empathy and understanding. For instance, if a person reports colored halos around lights, this could be one of the classic prodromal symptoms of glaucoma and not an illusion due to psychological processes. Such knowledge can result in quicker and more accurate diagnosis and treatment.

Nearly all older people wear glasses because of presbyopia (a form of farsightedness occurring after middle age, caused by diminished elasticity of the crystalline lens). But other than this, about 80% of older people have reasonably good sight until age 90 and beyond. In many cases at least one eye functions well even though the other may lose vision. Psychologically the elderly fear going blind and tend to overestimate the possiblities of this. But actual vision impairment can be devastating, in terms of both psychological isolation and physical immobilization. With many people vision loss is gradual and they are able slowly to compensate and adjust. A sudden loss of vision or loss occurring when the person is feeble and unable to muster resources is usually the most difficult.

SEXUALITY IN OLD AGE

Societal attitudes toward sexuality in old age

Many people, young and old, are astonished at the idea of human beings making love in their seventies, eighties, and even beyond. It is assumed that (1) old people do not have sexual desires; (2) they could not make love even if they *did* want to; (3) they are too fragile physically and it might hurt them; (4) they are physically unattractive and therefore sexually undesirable; (5) anyway, the whole notion is shameful and decidedly perverse. There may also be anxieties on the part of young people related to Oedipal connections with parents (we all know that, God forbid, *our* parents were not interested in sex). Yet, in work with older people it is clear that sex is a major concern in late life. Fear about loss of sexual prowess is a common preoccupation for the older man and can reach devastating proportions. Elderly women will often describe sexual desires, but many regard such feelings as undignified, if not depraved. Some older persons can freely accept their interest in sex, but their children and grandchildren may disapprove and make them feel guilty.

The elderly become the butt of jokes. Old men are frequently ridiculed as impotent or as "dirty old men." (A California bumper sticker protesting this idea read "I'm not a dirty old man. I'm a sexy senior citizen.") Old women fare even worse in the public eye. They are the neuters of our culture, who have mysteriously metamorphosed from desirable sexy young things to mature and sexually "interesting" women; finally, at about age 50, they steadily decline into sexual

---

**Macular degeneration* affects a vital part of the retina and leads to loss of central vision, leaving peripheral vision intact. *Glaucoma* involves increased tension within and hardening of the eyeball due to increased fluid. There are two basic types: acute congestive (narrow-angle) and chronic (wide-angle). *Diabetic retinopathy* is a deterioration of the retina caused by chronic diabetes.

†Moorhead, H. B., et al.: Causes of blindness in 4,965 persons whom it stated were added to their MRA registers in 1966. In Proceedings of 1960 Conference of Model Reporting Area for Blindness, U. S. Public Health Service, Washington, D. C., 1969.

‡Harlin, R. G.: Estimated prevalence of blindness in the United States, 1952, Social Security Bulletin 16:8-11, 1953.

§In legal blindness, central visual acuity does not exceed 20/200 in either eye with corrective lenses, or the visual field is less than an angle of 20 degrees.

oblivion. This is the way society sees it. But this is not the way a lot of older women see it.

Homes for the aged, nursing homes, and mental institutions all add to the impression that the elderly are sexless. There are no provisions for privacy; in fact, there seems to be an agreement that the aged must be prevented from having *any* sexual contacts. They are often rigidly segregated, men from women, with no visting in each other's rooms. Conjugal visits with spouses are seldom provided for. Nursing staffs become anxious and upset when the elderly, understandably, resort to masturbation. The problem is often no less difficult for older people who live with their children or in other people's homes.

Curiously enough, even the Social Security system has been a barrier to remarriage, and consequently sex, because widows who remarried were forced to give up their husbands' Social Security benefits. A reporter for the Miami News in 1965 described the practice known as "Social Security sin" wherein thousands of old people were living together in common-law arrangements to preserve their pensions. The problem was finally alleviated when Congress passed legislation allowing a widow to retain her previous pension or choose her new husband's benefits, whichever sum was greater.

The fear of death is another factor affecting sexuality. There are many symbolic associations between sexual activity and death —as in the French word for intercourse, "petit mort" or little death. Fears of the occurrence of heart attacks or strokes during the course of sex may lead couples to acquire twin beds, separate bedrooms, and a habit of abstinence that may or may not be justified medically. Currents of anxiety, depression, and hostility can accompany these fears as sexuality is inhibited.

Female longevity creates another baffling situation. Since 7% of women never marry, many others are widowed relatively early, and still others have husbands who are older than they and perhaps sickly, there are many women without partners. What alternatives do they have? Women do not have the cultural prerogatives of men to socialize with younger members of the opposite sex. There are not enough older men available. Extramarital affairs are difficult for many to reconcile religiously or morally. Masturbation, although increasing in old age, is still considered shameful or harmful. Thus women legitimately complain that society has not provided suitable sexual expression or even information that is relevant to sexual needs in late life. Someone has half-seriously, half-facetiously suggested that polygamy legalized after age 60 might be a sensible solution to the undersupply of men. Older women reacted sharply. One said "I am lonesome, but not that lonesome!" Better solutions might be the equalizing of the lifespan through research, the equalizing of sex roles to give women the same opportunities as men, the encouragement of dating and marriage with younger men, and the development of more lenient attitudes toward the homosexuality that already exists.

Research findings

The data which have been accumulating on the sexuality of the elderly have generally supported the view that sexual capacity has been underestimated except where illness or lack of sexual partner is a factor. Kinsey can be considered the pioneer in modern-day studies of sexuality in older people. The aged constituted only a small part of his sample, but his findings were useful in beginning to demolish the notion of termination of sexuality in late life. It was found that most men at age 60 were sexually capable and that there was little evidence of sexual decline in women until late in life.

Masters and Johnson's contributions have been exceedingly useful, since they include direct clinical observations of sexual performance as well as interviews. The Duke longitudinal studies examined 250 people between ages 60 and 94 every three years. Interestingly, these studies found that about 15% of older persons actually *increased* their patterns of sexual activity and interest as they aged.

Physical characteristics of sex in old age

Older men

Changes which occur with aging are often misinterpreted as evidence that older men are becoming impotent. "From a psychosexual point of view, the male over age 50 has to contend with one of the great fallacies of our culture. Every man in this age group is arbitrarily identified by both public and professional alike as sexually impaired."*

For a variety of causes associated with chronological aging there are age-related sexual changes. The older man ordinarily takes longer to obtain an erection but, as Masters and Johnson point out, "One of the advantages of the aging process with specific reference to sexual functioning is that, generally speaking, control of ejaculatory demand in the 50-75 year age group is far better than in the 20-40 year age group."* Translated, this means the older man can remain erect and make love longer before coming to orgasm. There is also the advantage of lovemaking experience gained throughout a lifetime.

Older men experience a reduction in the volume of seminal fluid, which explains the decrease in the pressure to ejaculate. Orgasm begins to be experienced in a shorter one-stage period, compared to two stages in earlier life, but it remains pleasurable. There is, after age 50, a physiologically extended refractory period, meaning that the capacity for erection following ejaculation cannot be regained as quickly as in younger men. It may be twelve to twenty-four hours before sex is again possible. Couples who are aware of this may want to delay ejaculation in order to make love as long as they wish. No panic is called for when the male's penis becomes flaccid more promptly upon ejaculation. This is natural and not a sign of impairment.

A vital point to remember is that the older man does not lose his facility for erection as he ages unless physical or emotional illness interferes. Most men over 60 are satisfied with one or two ejaculations per week but can enjoy sex and satisfy a partner more frequently than that because erections are possible whenever stimulated. A consistent pattern of sexual expression helps to maintain sexuality.

Older men are usually able to continue some form of active sex life until their seventies, eighties, and perhaps beyond. If they lose interest or become impotent, there can be a number of factors involved: boredom, fatigue, overeating, excessive drinking, medical and psychiatric disabilities (impotence can be one of the first signs of depression), and fear of failure. The latter is common and often based on misinformation about what is normative in old age. Among physical causes of impotence are arteriosclerotic, cardiorespiratory, endocrine, genitourinary, hematological, neurological, and infectious disorders. Frequently perineal prostatectomy and occasionally suprapubic and urethral prostatectomy can be factors. Drugs are also responsible. Chlordiazepoxide (Librium), imipramine (Tofranil), phenothiazines (especially thioridazine, known as Mellaril), alpha-methyl-dopa (used in parkinsonism), and alcohol have all been reported an inducing impotence. For women also, any tranquilizing drug can act as a depressant for sexual feelings.

Older women

Biologically the older woman experiences little sexual impairment as she ages. If she is in reasonably good health, she can expect to continue sex activities until late in life, assuming she has maintained a frame of mind that encourages this and has a sexual partner with whom to enjoy it. Menopause, also called "change of life" or "climacterium," occurs with the cessation of menstruation, usually between the ages of 45 and 50. Certain myths have surrounded menopause, including a fear of insanity, the ending of sexual desire and attractiveness, and the myths of inevitable depression, adverse physical symptoms, and defeminiza-

*From Masters, W. H., and Johnson, Virgina E.: Human sexual inadequacy, London, 1970, J. & A. Churchill, Ltd., pp. 316 and 318.

tion. These have been disputed by Helene Deutsch, Therese Benedek, Bernice Neugarten, and others who have written about the female climacterium. It is generally concluded that most women experience minimal physical problems; but because of cultural expectations and varying amounts of misunderstanding, there can be adverse psychological reactions. These are, however, not inevitable.

The physiological situation of older women during and after menopause requires review. They commonly suffer from the effects of gradual steroid insufficiency that causes a thinning of the vaginal walls. Cracking, bleeding, and pain (dyspareunia) can result during sexual intercourse. There may be vaginal burning and itching (so-called "senile" vaginitis*). The urethra and bladder become more subject to irritation as they are less cushioned by the atrophied vaginal walls, and there can be burning or frequency of urination for several days after sex. The loss of sex steroids also reduces the length and diameter of the vagina and may shrink the major labia. However, sex-steroid replacement therapy can substantially reduce many of these menopausal symptoms. The natural estrogen complex (conjugated estrogens, U.S.P.) has been in use for more than twenty-five years.† It is inexpensive and can be immeasurably helpful against osteoporosis (chronic backache, compression fractures, and "dowager's hump"), estrogen-deficient vaginitis, pruritus, and other aggravating symptoms.

Bartholin's gland secretions that lubricate the vagina may decrease with age. But this does not seem to occur in women who were sexually stimulated on a regular basis once or twice a week from youth on. As with men, a consistent pattern of sexual activity is beneficial to women in maintaining their sexual capacities.

Sex and chronic physical conditions

The realization that people with chronic illnesses have sexual interests may be unexpected and even unwelcomed. It complicates the medical picture for doctors. The well spouse may not know how to respond. Yet patients may live for years with the help of medical treatment and want as normal a life as possible, including sex. Most current studies of sex concentrate on healthy populations rather than including people with disabling conditions. Sexual activity may be both therapeutic and preventive medicine. There is some evidence, for example, that sex activity helps arthritis, probably because of adrenal gland production of cortisone. The sexual act is itself a form of physical activity, helping people stay in good physical condition. It helps to reduce tensions, which are both physical and psychological.

Cerebrovascular accidents and coronary attacks cause concern, in that it is not yet clearly documented if and when sex can be safely resumed. The oxygen cost in sexual intercourse is equivalent to that in climbing a flight of stairs or walking briskly. The heart rate ranges from 90 to 150 beats per minute, with an average of 120 beats—about the level for light to moderate physical effort. There is not yet a conclusive mass of data regarding sudden death during sex, but it probably occurs much less often than patients fear and somewhat more than the reported incidence (due to reluctance to report accurately). A conservative estimate is that 1% of sudden coronary death occur during intercourse. Potency may be affected psychologically because heart disease is not only frightening but also tends to undermine confidence in physical capacities. For some people the anxiety and tensions caused by restricting sex may be greater than the actual physical risk from participating in it.

Diabetes mellitus is common in old age

---

*We believe this term is demeaning and prefer "estrogen-deficient vaginitis."

†The dosage for menopausal and postmenopausal estrogen deficiency, including atrophic vaginitis and pruritus vulvae, is 1.25 to 3.75 mg, daily, three weeks on and one week off. Estrogens in a vaginal cream can also be used. Some public hospitals and clinics discriminate against the poor by not prescribing estrogens after 60 or 65 years of age. The general use of testosterone replacement therapy in men is presently not justified on the basis of reliable knowledge.

and causes impotence two to five times as often as in the general population although sex interest and desire may persist. Impotence from poorly controlled diabetes usually disappears when control is established. But the adequately controlled diabetic man who develops impotence usually has a more permanent problem. The effects of diabetes on the sexuality of women is unknown.

Pelvic surgery must be carefully planned to avoid unnecessary sexual impairement. Of men who have had prostatectomies, 70% remain potent. Three types of prostatectomy are listed.

1. *Transurethral resection,* or TUR. A wire stainless steel tube is inserted in the penis, a knife is maneuvered through the tube, and the gland is reamed. The tissue may grow back; therefore, TUR is indicated for men in their seventies or if other severe disease is present.
2. *Perineal.* An incision is made between the scrotum and anus, removing most of the prostate.
3. *Suprapubic.* The incision is made through the abdomen.

After a prostatectomy the semen is deposited in the bladder rather than ejaculated. Potency is rarely affected with the TUR and suprapubic approaches, and some men even have increased potency. Impotence may occur for psychological reasons. Nonpsychological, physical impotence is most often associated with the perineal approach.

There is no evidence that hysterectomy, with or without ovariectomy, produces any change in sexual desire or performance in women. If change does occur, it is usually psychological. The fear of sexual impairment, fear of loss of sexual desire, and fear of becoming unattractive to men are most commonly seen. People tend to become upset about any subtractive surgery, especially if it is a major subtraction like hysterectomy.

Peyronie's disease can interfere with sexual activity in men unless it responds to treatment or regresses spontaneously. The symptoms are an upward bowing of the penis, with a shift angled to the right or left. Hard tumors in the corpora cavernosa cause the symptoms, but the etiology of these tumors is unknown. Intercourse may be difficult and painful or completely impossible. A variety of treatments may be used and the disease itself may regress in about four years.* This disease has been thought to be rare, but judging from our own clinical experience, we suspect it is more common than is believed.

Mental health treatment considerations

Sex, self-esteem, and self-image are closely related. A task of the mental health specialist is to help older people deal with their personal feelings, fears, and possible misunderstandings about sex in old age. If sexual activity and potency decline while interest remains high, the therapist must decide whether improvement is possible or some divergent activities can be substituted. Marital counseling, individual and group psychotherapy, and family counseling may be indicated and can be quite successful.†

Masters and Johnson treat older people in their clinic. They report a higher incidence of referrals of men with sexual dysfunction than women, probably because of the need for erective capacity in male sexuality. They report a higher failure rate with their older patients, which they attribute to the length of time the problem has existed and not the ages of the patients. Nonetheless, there was more than 50% success rate even when the problem may have existed twenty-five years or longer. They state "The fact that innumerable men and women have not been sexually effective before reaching their late fif-

---

*McDonald, D. F.: Peyronie's disease, Medical Aspects of Human Sexuality 6:64-70, May, 1972.

†A bachelor participating in the NIMH Human Aging Studies undertook intensive psychotherapy four times a week at age 65 and married for the first time. The English sexologist Havelock Ellis overcame lifelong impotence in his old age with the help of a loving and responsive woman. (Calder-Marshall, Arthur: The sage of sex, a life of Havelock Ellis, New York, 1959, G. P. Putnam's Sons.)

ties or early sixties is no reason to condemn them to continuing sexual dysfunction as they live out the rest of their life span. The disinclination of the medical and behavioral professions to treat the aging population for sexual dysfunction has been a major disservice perpetrated by those professions upon the general problem."*

Sex education for old people is important. Normal age changes need to be understood so that neither men nor women mistake such changes for loss of sexuality. Techniques of sexual intercourse especially pertinent to old age should be clarified. (For example, sex in the morning may be preferable for those older persons who fatigue easily.) The importance of masturbation when sexual partners are unavailable should be emphasized for those who do not find its practice personally upsetting. Masturbation helps preserve potency in men and the functioning of Bartholin's gland in women, releases tensions, stimulates sexual appetite, and contributes to general well-being. It must be remembered that many older people were brought up to believe that masturbation is harmful physically and mentally. Such cultural and historic viewpoints cannot be lightly dismissed, but people may be responsive to new information.

Another cultural element is seen in the reluctance of some older women to go to a doctor for help with gynecological problems. Women with even advanced carcinoma of the vulva may delay asking for medical care. Some elderly women tolerate general prolapse of the uterus for long periods of time, and it is not unusual to find infection and edema from such untreated conditions. Women may need encouragement in accepting examinations on a regular basis.

Regular physical examinations, proper medical treatment, adequate diet and exercise all help to preserve sexual capacities. As Masters and Johnson have so encouragingly reported, the two major requirements for enjoyable sexual activity until late in life are reasonably good health and an interested and interesting partner.

*From Masters, W. H., and Johnson, Virginia E.: Human sexual inadequacy, London, 1970, J. & A. Churchill, Ltd., p. 344.

REFERENCES

Burgess, E. W., editor: Aging in Western societies, Chicago, 1960, University of Chicago Press.

Clark, Margaret, and Anderson, Barbara G.: Culture and aging. An anthropological study of older Americans, Springfield, Ill., 1967, Charles C Thomas, Publisher.

Davis, M. E.: Estrogens and the aging process. The detection, prevention and retardation of osteoporosis, The Journal of the American Medical Association **196**:219-224, 1966.

Double jeopardy, the older Negro in America today, New York, 1964, National Urban League.

Elderly are crime targets, SOS, Senior Opportunities and Services Technical Assistance Bulletin **2**(4):1-3, Feb.-March, 1972.

Fanon, F.: Black skin, white masks, New York, 1967, Grove Press, Inc.

Feigenbaum, E. M., Lowenthal, M. F., and Trier, M. L.: Aged are confused and hungry for sex information, Geriatric Focus **5**:174-177, 1967.

Ferenczi, S.: Sunday neurosis (1919). In Rickman, J., editor: Theory and technique of psychoanalysis, New York, 1952, Basic Books, Inc.

Finkel, A. L., Moyers, T. G., Tobenkin, M. I., and Karg, S. J.: Sexual potency in aging males, Journal of American Medical Association **170**: 1391-1393, 1959.

Ford, Amasa, and Orfirer, Alexander: Sexual behavior and the chronically ill patient, Medical Aspects of Human Sexuality **1**:51-62, Oct., 1967.

Freeman, J. T.: John S. ——— widower, Journal of the American Geriatrics Society **18**:736-746, 1970.

Gaitz, C. M.: Characteristics of elderly patients with alcoholism, Archives of General Psychiatry **24**:372-378, 1971.

Gochros, Harvey L.: The sexually oppressed, Social Work **17**:16-24, March, 1972.

Grier, William H., and Cobbs, Price M.: Black rage, New York, 1968, Basic Books, Inc.

Houston, F., and Royse, A. B.: Relationship between deafness and psychotic illness, The Journal of Mental Science **100**:990-993, 1954.

Jackson, Hobart C.: Alternatives to institutional care for older Americans, practice and planning: planning for the specially disadvantaged. Presentation for the Conference on Alternatives to Institutional Care, Duke University, June 3, 1972.

Jackson, Jacqueline J.: The blacklands of gerontology, Aging and Human Development **2**:156-172, 1971.

Kalish, R. A., and Yuen, S.: Americans of East Asian ancestry: aging and the aged, The Gerontologist **11**:36-47, 1971.

Kastenbaum, Robert J., editor: Special issue–Black aging, Aging and Human Development **2**: 155-231, 1971.

Kent, D. P.: The elderly in minority groups: variant patterns of aging, The Gerontologist **11**:26-29, 1971.

Kinsey, A. C., Pomeroy, W. B., and Martin, C. R.: Sexual behavior in human male, Philadelphia, 1948, W. B. Saunders Co.

Kinsey, A. C., Pomeroy, W. B., Martin, C. R., and Gebhard, P. H.: Sexual behavior in human female, Philadelphia, 1953, W. B. Saunders Co.

Kupperman, H. S.: The menopausal woman and sex hormones, Medical Aspects of Human Sexuality **1**:64-68, 1967.

Lewis, Myrna, I., and Butler, R. N.: Why is Women's Lib ignoring old women? Aging and Human Development **3**:223-231, 1972.

Masters, W. H., and Johnson, Virginia E.: Human sexual response, Boston, 1966, Little, Brown & Co.

Masters, W. H., and Johnson, Virginia E.: Human sexual inadequacy, London, 1970, J. & A. Churchill, Ltd.

McDonald, D. F.: Peyronie's disease, Medical Aspects of Human Sexuality **6**:64-70, May, 1972.

Moore, Joan W.: Mexican-Americans, The Gerontologist **11**:30-35, 1971.

Neugarten, Bernice L., and Kraines, Ruth J.: "Menopausal symptoms" in women of various ages, Psychosomatic Medicine **27**:266-273, 1965.

Newman, G., and Nichols, C. B.: Sexual activities and attitudes in older persons, Journal of American Medical Association **173**:33-35, 1960.

Pfeiffer, E.: Geriatric sex behavior, Medical Aspects of Human Sexuality **3**:19-29, July, 1969.

Pinderhughes, C. A.: The universal resolution of ambivalence by paranoia with an example in black and white, American Journal of Psychotherapy **24**:597-610, 1970.

Ruben, R.: Aging and hearing. In Clinical geriatrics, Philadelphia, 1971, J. B. Lippincott Co.

Rubin, Alan: Sexual behavior in diabetes mellitus, Medical Aspects of Human Sexuality **20**:23-26, Dec., 1967.

Rubin, Isadore: Sexual life after sixty, New York, 1965, Basic Books, Inc.

Streib, G. F., and Schneider, C. J.: Retirement in American society, New York, 1971, Cornell University Press.

U. S. Senate Committee on Aging: Proceedings of the ninetieth and ninety-first Congress, Availability and usefulness of federal programs and services to elderly Mexican Americans. Parts 1-4, Washington, D. C., 1969, U. S. Government Printing Office.

U. S. Senate Committee on Labor and Public Welfare: The education of American Indians, Washington, D. C., 1969, U. S. Government Printing Office.

U. S. Senate Special Committee on Aging: A working paper. Advisory Council on the Elderly American Indian, Washington, D. C., 1971, U. S. Government Printing Office.

U. S. Senate Special Committee on Aging: The Multiple hazards of age and race: the situation of aged blacks in the United States. (Working paper by Inabel B. Lindsay, D.S.W.), Washington, D. C., 1971, U. S. Government Printing Office.

White House Conference on Aging, 1971: A report to the delegates from the Conference Sections and Special Concerns Sessions, Nov. 28-Dec. 2, 1971, Washington, D. C., 1971, U. S. Government Printing Office.

Wylie, F. M.: Attitudes toward aging among black Americans: Some historical perspectives, Aging and Human Development **2**:66-70, 1971.

7

OLDER PEOPLE AND THEIR FAMILIES

The American elderly have been pictured as isolated and rejected by their families. Adages such as "one mother can raise ten children but ten children cannot care for one old mother" are solemnly cited as typical of the attitudes of American children toward their aging parents. The urban, industrialized society, which thus far indeed has placed little value on the virtues of old age, has been singled out as the annihilator of the extended family and its network of mutual assistance. But is there evidence to support this generally accepted view of American family life? Can a culture so institutionalize its prejudice against the old that ties of affection and loyalty between parent and child are discarded? The tenacity of kinship bonds throughout history—in spite of wars, conquest, slavery, immigration, political ideology, and cultural change —would lead one to doubt easy assumptions concerning demise of the parent-child relationships. From the standpoint of mental health it is questionable whether young human beings can ever function or grow in a reasonably healthy manner without emotional and interactive bonds with adults who care about them. This drive for emotional sustenance is not likely to dry up as people reach adulthood. Survival in a productivity-minded society may in fact make kinship support *more* necessary and meaningful as human beings are buffeted by constant challenges and reexaminations of their worth in the outside world.

FAMILY LIFE CYCLE*

Four fifths of all older people have living children. A family may span three to five living generations, complete with a past reaching farther back than one can trace and a future stretching beyond the lives of any present family members. Each person experiences his own individual life cycle from birth to death while at the same time participating as an integral part of a family with a collective life cycle of its own. It is rare to find an older person who truly has no "family," even if it means only distant relatives. The closeness of kin in terms of blood relationships and the numbers of kin give no clear indication of the amount of meaningful contacts. But they do indicate the kin potential, implying usually an emotional tie, whether positive or negative. A person cannot easily "divorce" his blood relatives, since his or her own identity is intricately bound up with those to whom he is related. (For example, adopted children seem to inevitably yearn at some point in their lives for knowledge of their kin and may actively search for them even though their lives may be otherwise satisfactory.) A feeling of kin relatedness is probably an essential element in orienting oneself in time and space as a significant human being.

The number of people who are considered "family" by an older person may change markedly throughout a lifetime. Some older people have grown up with brothers and sisters but never married and therefore have no "immediate" family of children and

*Models of the developmental processes of families are as important as models of individual personality development. Sociology, anthropology, psychiatry, and social work all have valuable experience in this area, which they do not often share with each other.

grandchildren. Others may have expanded from a small childhood family unit to produce a large number of sons, daughters, grandchildren, and great-grandchildren with their assorted in-laws. Some older people relate closely to distant kin and others even adopt as kin people to whom they are not related at all. One should never be deceived by statements from older people claiming they have broken off contact with a family member (e.g., not speaking to a brother or sister for thirty years). Such relationships usually have as much emotional content as more directly active ones—or even more—as demonstrated by the concerted effort to avoid contact.

DO AMERICAN FAMILIES "ABANDON" THEIR ELDERLY?

Research evidence

Urbanization and industrialization have led to theories about changes and/or breakdown in family structure.* The nuclear family consisting of mother, father, and children has been postulated as the most functional family unit in a society that requires mobility, compactness, and emotional self-sufficiency to be built in and carried along. Older people and other extended-family members are seen as not fitting into this streamlined picture, so the nuclear family supposedly closed its ranks and its heart, determined to go it alone. Older parents and grandparents have been pictured as left to shift for themselves. This may *sound* plausible, but it has not happened and is not likely to. The emerging pattern of family life is one of separate households for all but the very old or sick, while at the same time maintaining a complex pattern of family relationships that are viable and supportive. Sussman calls this the "modified and extended" family system in which the nuclear family is not isolated but is part of "an extended kin-family system, highly integrated within a network of social relationships and mutual assistance that operates along bilateral kin lines and vertically over several generations."* Aid to the elderly takes the form of economic help, living arrangements with families when this is imperative, and affection and companionship. Brothers, sisters, children, aunts, uncles—even nephews, nieces, and cousins—may be involved in the flow of mutual aid. When families do not offer help to their older members, a whole range of personal, social, and economic forces are usually at work rather than an attitude of neglect and abandonment.

*Parsons, T., and Bales, R.: Family, socialization and interaction process, New York, 1955, Free Press of Glencoe, Inc.

Many studies have verified the continuing existence of strong family ties in the United States and elsewhere. A World Health Organization report states:

> Wherever careful studies have been carried out in the industrialized countries, the lasting devotion of children for their parents has been amply demonstrated. The great majority of old people are in regular contact with their children, relatives, or friends. . . .Where distance permits, the generations continue to shoulder their traditional obligations, of the elders toward their children, and the children to the aged.†

Townsend, in England, found that the families of institutionalized aged showed ". . .much more evidence of genuine affection and loyalty than the reverse. . ."‡

Approximately two out of every ten older people in the United States live alone. Most of these are single, widowed, or divorced and a large proportion are women. Many have children but prefer to live separate from them. Naturally a greater proportion of the very old (over 80) live with family

*From Sussman, Marvin B.: Relationships of adult children with their parents in the United States. In Shanas, Ethel, and Streib, Gordon F., editors: Social structure and the family, generational relationships, Englewood Cliffs, N. J., 1965, Prentice-Hall, Inc.

†From World Health Organization: Mental health problems of the aging and the aged, Technical Report Series, No. 171, Geneva, 1959.

‡From Townsend, P.: The effects of family structure on the likelihood of admission to an institution in old age: the application of a general theory. In Shanas, Ethel, and Streib, Gordon, editors: Social structure and the family, Englewood Cliffs, N. J., 1965, Prentice-Hall, Inc., pp. 163-188.

members because of declining capacities. Unmarried people may live with siblings and friends. Studies indicate that the majority of older people choose independent living quarters with a spouse or alone as long as this is possible and then expect to move in with family members.

In spite of the desire for separate households on the part of both parents and children, Shanas has observed:

> The physical separation of older people and their children in the United States is more apparent than real. Despite extensive internal migration in that country, older people and at least one of their children still maintain a close physical relationship. Four of every ten older unmarried people with children live in the same household with at least one child and an additional three of every ten are ten minutes or less distant from their nearest child. In all, 82 percent of all unmarried old persons in the U.S. who have children are less than 30 minutes distant from at least one of these children. In time of illness, older parents turn to their adult children for help. Parents expect that their children will be available to help them, children on their part expect to give whatever assistance is needed.*

She feels that the "myth of alienation" has been created and perpetrated by two groups: *professional workers* in the field of aging, who tend to see those elderly who do not have normal family supports, and *childless old people,* who constitute one fifth of all old people and are likely to believe that the aged are neglected by their children. In our experience, gross negligence of parents by children has been exaggerated, but there is no doubt of its existence. Subtle and open disparagement and cruelties are not uncommon even though they may not be the norm.

Three-generational household

In 8% of United States families, three generations live together under one roof. Such arrangements generally occur when the older person has become too infirm or impoverished to live alone. Because of the advanced age at which most people move in with their relatives, the average length of the stay is not a long one, because of the death of the older person or serious illness requiring hospital or nursing care. In most instances the pattern is one of an older mother moving in with her daughter and family. The manner in which these two women relate is often the key to success or failure of the living arrangement. Most families manage the problems quite well, perhaps realizing that precedents are being set for the next generation of children and parents. Genuine affection combined with a sense of ethical responsibility motivates many children to voluntarily assist their elderly parents.

"Filial" economic responsibility

Filial responsibility* includes more than just law and custom (Schorr, 1960), since it refers also to the personal attitudes of responsibility toward parents: the ethical and emotional responses of children to their mothers and fathers. But we shall be discussing here the legal and social requirements and expectations. Children were held accountable for the care of their parents under medieval Church Law and it was not until the Elizabethan Poor Law that the concept of community assistance was introduced. However, families were expected to do everything they could before receiving outside help. During the early part of the twentieth century filial responsibility versus governmental aid began to be tested to a greater degree. There were greater numbers of older people, sometimes two generations of them in one family, and the preindustrial, agricultural society was disappearing. In its place came industrialization, separating wages from the ownership of the means of production. Older people no longer had the

*From Shanas, Ethel: The unmarried old person in the United States: living arrangements and care in illness, myth and fact, paper prepared for the International Social Science Research Seminar in Gerontology, Markaryd, Sweden, Aug., 1963.

*Schorr, A. L.: Filial responsibility in the modern American family, U. S. Department of Health, Education, and Welfare, Social Security Administration, Washington, D. C., 1960, U. S. Government Printing Office.

power of ownership of land, tools, animals, etc. or the sustenance of the agricultural community; therefore, they became more vulnerable economically as they aged. Their children were forced to take on more responsibility for them or look to the government for assistance. Social Security, beginning in 1935 in the United States, provided basic economic maintenance for increasing numbers of older people. Instead of individual families paying for their own older members, Social Security is based on a concept of intergenerational support whereby the entire middle-aged generation in the labor force supports the older generation.*

Although governmental agencies are necessarily and increasingly providing financial support and services for the elderly, some policies still reflect the earlier traditions of total filial or family responsibility. The "responsible relative" clause in many welfare programs is the most obvious example. Families usually turn to welfare for help with older persons only when they are already in desperate straits. But many localities insist that close relatives must exhaust their own resources before their elderly can receive assistance. Such requirements force a lower standard of living not only on the elderly but also on their families. Savings may be completely used up, endangering the family's future. Families may have to deny other family members' needs in order to finance the older person's care. The spouses of older persons may lose the accumulated resources of a lifetime and have to also accept welfare themselves to survive. (We have seen this happen with applications for welfare assistance with nursing home placements.) Middle-aged persons may have as many as four parents and up to eight grandparents who are living; thus they simply cannot afford to be financially "responsible" relatives to all. The government and welfare agencies must remove the financial burdens from families so that they can attend to the many other emotional and personal needs of older people. In Denmark, for example, the elderly are completely independent financially from their children because of the comprehensive welfare structure; yet they maintain a high degree of interaction and mutuality with their families in every other respect.

*Kreps, Juanita M.: The economics of intergenerational relationships. In Shanas, Ethel, and Streib, Gordon F., editors: Social structure and the family: generational relationships, Englewood Cliffs, N. J., 1965, Prentice-Hall, Inc.

Are old people "dumped" into institutions?

This is another of the myths that confuse the realities of life in old age. There are, of course, some families who do unload their responsibilities to elderly family members despite ensuing guilt. In addition, isolated, family-less old people may be placed in an institution when they become ill or feeble, simply because there is no other place for them to go. But most people who have families move in with their relatives when they can no longer live independently. Old people shudder at the thought of institutions, as do their children. Institutions are reserved as the last recourse after everything else has been tried, and families will often go through unbelievable hardship before giving in to placement. The following is a letter we received from a son seeking help for his mother:

> My 84-year-old mother lives with me in my four-room apartment. Her senility has become worse and she is totally confused, unable to sit still, care for herself, or even remain continent. Three years ago I had to quit my job in order to stay home with her, as she used to wander the streets and get lost. I lived on my savings; I am unmarried. I am 52 years old, still unemployed and have passed up two good jobs. Three weeks ago I placed her in an expensive, beautiful nursing home but she became more confused, totally dependent, and over-medicated. She lost 7 pounds and her bowels became impacted. In desperation I took her back home. I am at my wit's end. What should I do? I love the poor woman. But I cannot enjoy life at all. What is the best thing for her? and me?

Families such as this one may be forced to accept permanent institutional care simply because there are no other alternatives

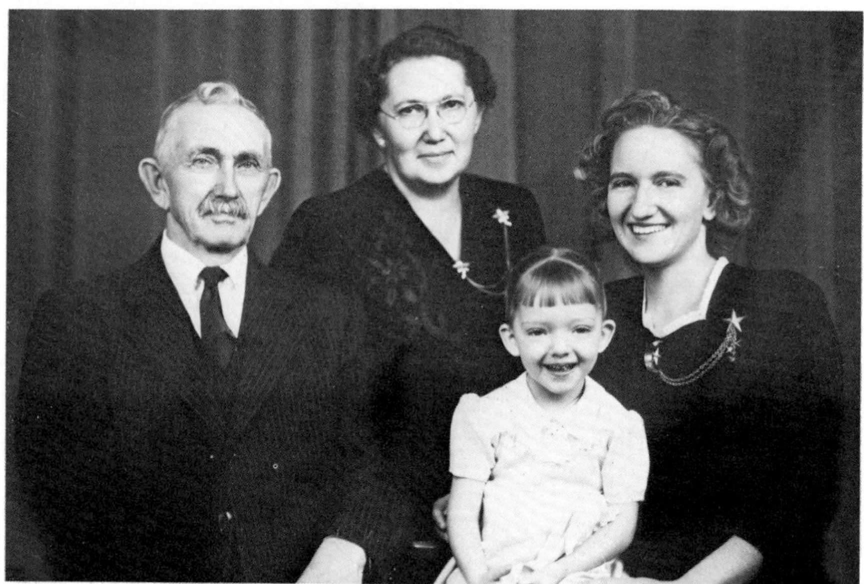

A four-generation family.
Courtesy Cora Kohlmeyer.

available. (See Chapter 10 on home care.) And in this particular case, an enormous amount of money was expended, for very poor care, during a brief trial placement. Families should have a whole range of services to assist them in keeping the older person at home, including economic aid. When institutional care is absolutely necessary, it should be reliable, therapeutic, and reasonably priced.

MULTIPLE GENERATIONS

Longer life-spans have increased the likelihood of families with three, four, or even five generations. A sizeable number of persons over 65 years of age have one or two living parents. Likewise, aging parents may have with them their aging children. We have seen parents in their eighties who were caring for aging and ailing children in their sixties. Townsend calls attention to the existence in Western nations of increasing numbers of elderly persons with great-grandchildren.* The implications of these new phenomena in human societies have yet to be understood.

*Townsend, P.: The emergence of the four-generation family in industrial society. In Neugarten, B. L., editor: Middle age and aging: a reader in social psychology, Chicago, 1968, University of Chicago Press.

GRANDPARENTS

In the United States 70% of older people have living grandchildren,* and 32% of persons over 65 are great-grandparents, according to a 1962 national survey.† Grandparenthood, like many of the other aspects of late life, has received only meager research attention, primarily in the form of small pilot studies, which may or may not be generalizable to grandparents as a whole. But they do add intriguing pieces of clarifying information about a function so familiar to us.

Early psychoanalytic interpretations of grandparenthood were rather grim and villainous, reflecting patriarchal values. Ferenczi pictured the grandfather as either an imposing, authoritarian old man who frightened and challenged his grandchild or a

*Kahana, Eva, and Kahana, B.: Theoretical and research perspectives on grandparenthood, Aging and Human Development 2:261-269, Nov., 1971.
†A pre–White House Conference on Aging: Summary of developments and data. A report of the Special Committee on Aging, U. S. Senate, Nov., 1971, p. 25.

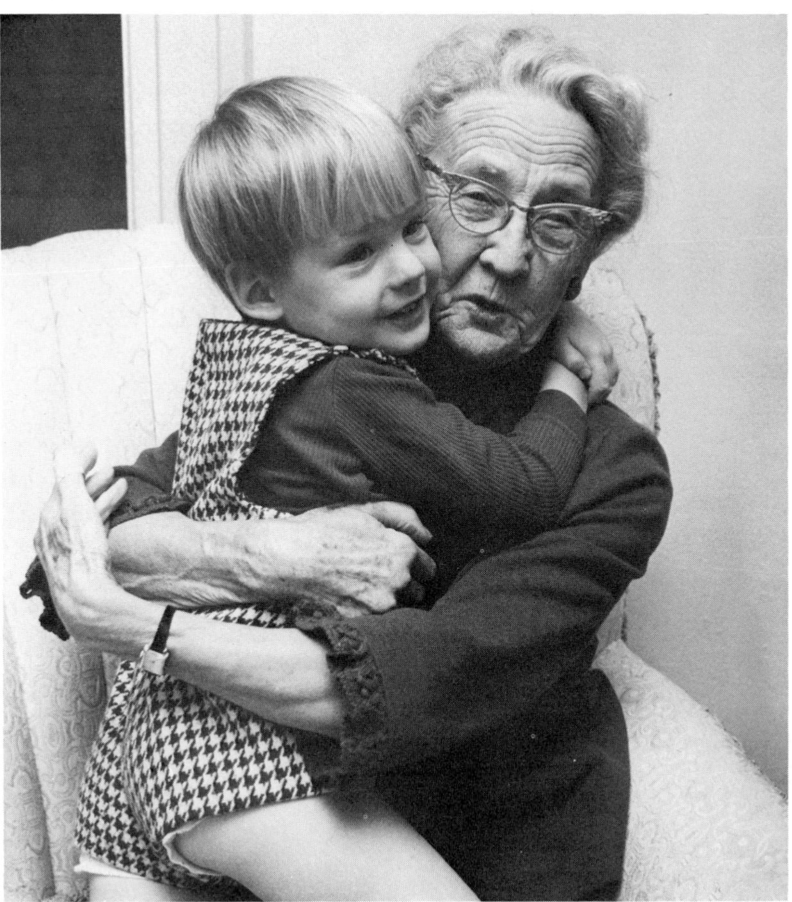

Grandparentage.
Courtesy H. Armstrong Roberts, Inc., Philadelphia.

helpless, feeble person who invited the grandchild's disparagement because he was weak and near death.* Ferenczi conceded that boy children may learn about death for the first time through contacts with grandfathers, but he viewed this essentially in an Oedipal context as an opportunity to learn a new way of getting rid of father.

Grandmothers likewise received stern treatment from scholars and practitioners (e. g., Abraham, 1955). An overly earnest social worker defending children from the evils of grandmothers wrote an article in 1942 titled "Grandma Made Johnny Delinquent," in which the author self-righteously argued that grandparents "interfering with the raising of a child" should be removed from the home. LaBarre, Jessner, and Ussery (1960) wrote in the same vein in their paper, "The Significance of Grandmothers in the Psychopathology of Children."* Actually, evidence shows that few grandparents (less than 10%) function as surrogate parents, and there is little reason to doubt that many of these have been lifesavers rather than evildoers in the lives of grandchildren.

In a more positive mood, Benedek has

*Ferenczi, S.: The grandfather complex. In Rickman, J., editor: Theory and technique of psychoanalysis, New York, 1926, Basic Books, Inc.

*Presented at 1958 annual meeting, University of North Carolina School of Medicine, Chapel Hill.

identified the grandparent role as one available universally to most older people:

> Grandparenthood is a new lease on life because grandparents—grandmothers more intensely than grandfathers—relive the memories of the early phase of their own parenthood in observing the growth and development of their grandchildren. Grandparenthood is, however, parenthood one step removed. Relieved from the immediate stresses of motherhood and the responsibilities of fatherhood, grandparents appear to enjoy their grandchildren more than they enjoyed their own children. Their instinctual wish to survive being gratified, they project the hope of the fulfillment of their narcissistic self-image to their grandchildren. Since they do not have the responsibility for raising the child toward that unconscious goal, their love is not as burdened by doubts and anxieties as it was when their own children were young.*

Neugarten and Weinstein (1964) have differentiated types of grandparents in their study of seventy middle-class, older couples: the formal grandparent, the fun seeker, the surrogate parent, the reservoir of family wisdom, and the distant figure who arrives only on holidays and family occasions. They found the fun seeker and the distant figure most common of the types. It was noted that not all older people wanted the grandparent role, although most expressed satisfaction with it. Some felt exploited by their children (as babysitters, etc.); others expressed negative attitudes toward their own children through their grandchildren. Some joined forces with the young in secret struggles against the middle generation. Biological continuity, emotional self-fulfillment, vicarious accomplishment, teaching, and helping in various ways were some of the meaningful roles in grandparentage.

Kahana and Kahana (1970) have studied grandparenthood from the grandchild's perspective (white, middle-class sample). The feelings of grandchildren depend on the amount of contact, grandparents' behavior toward them, parents' relationships with grandparents, and the child's perceptions of old people in general and grandparents in particular. Children's responses to grandparents change as the youngsters develop; very young children react to gifts, favors, and open affection whereas slightly older ones prefer sharing activities and having mutual fun.

Grandparenthood now occurs in middle age as well as old age and great-grandparents are not uncommon. When grandparents have power and responsibility (as in the role of surrogate parents), they are likely to be more formal and perhaps authoritarian. But when removed from responsibility, they tend to be indulgent, enjoying the grandchildren but not feeling burdened. Some volunteer to be surrogate grandparents to other people's children as in the Foster Grandparent Program (a component of Action). Youthful grandparents may avoid any element of the traditional grandparent role, preferring to be called by their first names and functioning as friends. The image of the white-haired, elderly grandpa and grandma may eventually have to be reserved for great-grandparents.

ELDERLY MARITAL COUPLE

Care during illness, household management, and emotional gratification are three expectations found in older marriages. The older couple married for many years will find they have a different marriage in old age than they had in middle or early life. Each of them has been changing and experiencing life individually as well as together. They may have grown more different or more alike. Conflicts between them can intensify or dissipate as they age, with more tolerance or, on the other hand, more rigidity in their expectations of each other. One study has shown some degree of deterioration in up to one third of elderly marital relationships.* It is difficult to assess an adult in his total environment because it

*From Benedek, T.: Parenthood during the life cycle. In Anthony, E. J., editor: Parenthood, Boston, 1970. Little, Brown & Co., p. 201.

*Yarrow, Marian R., Blank, P., Quinn, Olive W., Youmans, E. G., and Stein, Johanna: Social psychological characteristics of old age. In Human aging, Washington, D. C., U. S. Government Printing Office Pub. No. (HSM) 71-9051, 1971.

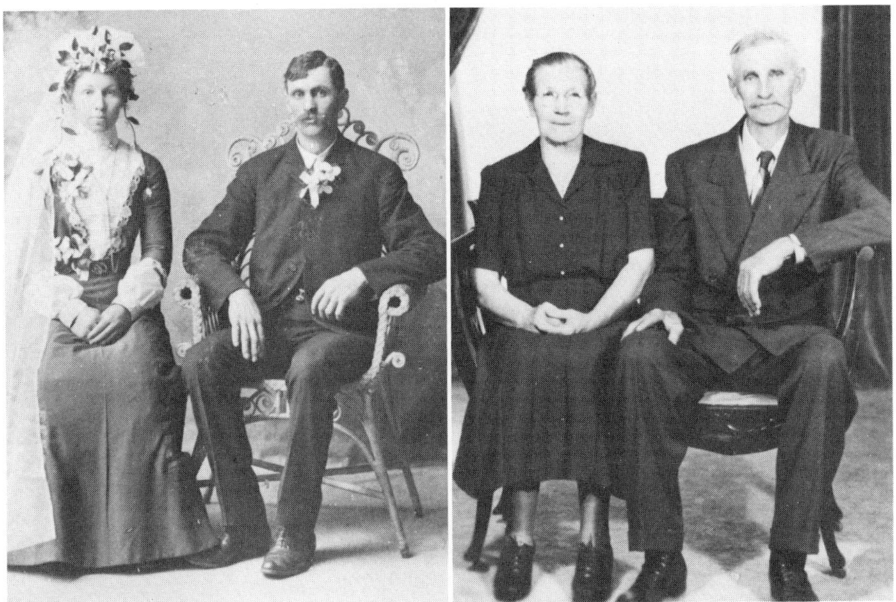

An elderly couple's wedding and fiftieth wedding anniversary pictures.

Courtesy Emil and Irene Eickhoff.

is much more complicated than for a child. Many more people, life experiences, accidental happenings, stresses, losses, and accomplishments are involved, and prediction of eventual individual outcome is precarious. It requires an innocent and hopeful faith to promise in marital vows to love and honor someone "until death do us part," for in twenty, thirty, or forty years the partner one married may have become quite a different human being, and that same partner may be equally surprised at changes in his spouse. Often the life cycle itself offers revealing aspects of human adaptability or lack thereof. Men, for example, who married "sweet young things" may not accept the fact that women age just as they themselves do. Women who doted on their roles as wives and mothers may rebel at the thought of being nursemaid to an ailing and aging husband. Of course there are people who expect and accept change with dignity and constructive response, having reached maturity with relatively few personality handicaps that would impede adaptability. Environmental influences, physical and mental health, and the historical period of time in which one is living are other variables affecting marriages over a long span of time.

Most older marriages are broken by death rather than divorce. Divorce can be more easily risked in youth or middle age when resources and options are greater. Children and grandchildren serve as a strong bond between marital partners. Couples who reach old age have usually adapted to each other in a way that each finds supportive or at least more acceptable than the unknown. And when so many other losses are occurring naturally, marriage may be one of the more familiar and comfortable patterns remaining. Older people can become intensely dependent on each other for intimacy, personal services, and mutual support; a major psychological blow then occurs when one partner dies. As we have said before, factors of the immediate environment are *very* closely related to the older person's behavior and attitudes, with significant persons being the most important of these factors. Thus, in general, divorce occurs before old age, if it is to occur at all, and older people perceive threats to themselves emanating from outside the marital relationship as more significant than those from within. Marriage becomes a more valued human relationship by the very fact of powerful outside forces and eventual death.

Older marriages, although less likely to dissolve, do have problems that carry over from the past or develop as a result of current stress.

Mr. and Mrs. H had been married forty years. They had arrived at serious disagreements and mistrust early in the marriage but had stayed together because of the children. They reached a state of truce in which there was as little contact between them as possible. Mr. H obtained employment that required him to travel about 80% of the time. For thirty years he devoted his energy and interest to his work and to impermanent, extramarital relationships. After retirement at 65 he returned to their loveless home. He became depressed and thought often of death. Finally he developed numerous hypochondriacal symptoms, which occupied his time and energy in much the same manner as had his former job. He and Mrs. H continue to live together, each obviously unwilling to leave the other.

A common difficulty in older marriages is the disequilibrium caused by the physical or emotional illness of either spouse. Major chronic changes occurring with senile brain disease, for example, can drastically alter the marital relationship. One partner may become the caretaker or nursemaid for the other, often with little help from elsewhere. Illnesses can drain the physical, emotional, and financial capacities of the caretaker spouse. Anger and depression may occur, and it is not unusual to find the formerly well spouse develop physical or psychiatric symptoms of his or her own.

Patterns of dominance may shift in old age, with the female assuming a more active and responsible role than formerly. Many of today's elderly were brought up in a male-dominant, female-subordinate culture. But with shorter life expectancies for men and their practice of marrying women younger than themselves, they are usually older than their mates and consequently less capable physically. Gold (1960) in studying age and sex patterns of familial dominance in 24 preliterate societies found a shift to female dominance in later life in 14 of these. She states "Although old women did not gain the upper hand in all societies studied, aging in no instance led to the husband's gaining in authority."* She suggests that husbands may be willing to accept female domination as the price of security as they age. We submit that some females, having been deprived of equal cultural status all their lives, may even enjoy the opportunity to exert their influence as males become more dependent and infirm with age. Unfortunately their taste of greater status is frequently mitigated by the need to provide nursing services to their husbands. When that is accomplished and their husbands die, they are left to nurse themselves through old age or accept help from someone else. The ascendance to dominance may be short-lived and unrewarding. Mutuality and equality (e.g., in sex roles and age of marriage) throughout life might be a better pattern and carry over to a more consistently mutual relationship in old age.

There seems to be some interdependence between the life-spans of husband and wife; studies have shown an association between the length of life of husband and wife (e.g., the early study of Ciocco, 1941). It has been suggested that this is due to selection (healthy people may select other healthy people as partners, while frailer men and women may not marry) or to the marital environment itself, which supposedly encourages a moderate, temperate life. Suicide rates are lower for married men and higher for divorced. In old age the mutual aid and support in a marriage can become a crucial factor in the health of each partner, just as depression and loss of support can contribute to the deterioration of the health of a surviving spouse during widowhood. For many people the maintenance of closeness with another is the center of existence up to the very end of life.

---

*From Gold, S.: Cross-cultural comparisons of role change with aging, Student Journal of Human Development, Spring, 1960, p. 11a.

Remarriage, after death or divorce of a spouse, does occur with some frequency. There are May-December marriages in which an older man marries a much younger woman; but marriages between people of approximately the same age are more usual. Children from an earlier marriage may or may not bless the new union. Their negative attitudes may be voiced strongly, particularly if they feel a parent is being taken advantage of, is acting foolishly, or is endangering their inheritance; on the other hand, children may actively encourage parents to find new lives for themselves through remarriage.

IN-LAWS

Sooner or later almost everyone becomes an in-law. Each person who marries gets an average of six members of the spouse's family as in-laws. Ask almost anyone and he will tell you that "in-law" means "trouble," especially if it happens to be a mother-in-law and she happens to be involved with her son or daughter's life. Although no one knows for sure, our guess is that the mother-in-law "problem" stems from the cultural encouragement of competition among women from the time they are small girls. Added to this are the stresses facing the older woman because of her longer life-span and low social status. Over-involvement with children is another possible factor. But the entire problem is very likely exaggerated, since numbers of people manage to get along reasonably well with in-laws, including mothers-in-law. In-laws can be supportive as well as trouble-making. Personality factors are probably more critical than the social roles as in-laws in establishing relationships.

ELDERLY "ISOLATES"

Isolation as we are defining it here refers to individuals who have minimal or no contact with other human beings. Some people become isolated in old age because of life circumstances and would choose to live differently if they could. Others isolate themselves by choice, often following a lifelong pattern of existence as "loners." Townsend distinguishes between isolates and "desolates": "Those who are secluded from family and society, as objectively assessed on the basis of defined criteria, are the isolates. Those who have been recently deprived by death, illness or migration of someone they love—such as a husband or wife or child—are the desolates. A major conclusion of the present analysis is that though the two are connected, the underlying reason for loneliness in old age is desolation rather than isolation."* The emotional meaning of isolation depends on whether it is a habitual life style or whether it has come about or been exacerbated by emotional loss.

Shanas (1963) makes much the same point when she comments that isolation is not synonymous with loneliness nor is it a direct causative factor in mental illness.† Some older people have lived alone so long they have lost the notion of what loneliness means. Shanas found that the loneliest and most isolated people appear to be those widowed persons who have no children and live alone. On the other hand, isolation and loneliness of people are not necessarily relieved by closeness of children or frequent contact with them. In this case isolation is a state of mind rather than actual social alienation.

Attempting to explain the fact that a greater number of single or widowed people over 65 are admitted to mental hospitals, compared to married people, Shanas feels the blame cannot be placed on social isolation. Instead, she postulates that serious illnesses

---

*From Townsend, P.: The emergence of the four-generation family in industrial society. In Neugarten, B. L., editor: Middle age and aging: a reader in social psychology, Chicago, 1968, University of Chicago Press.

†Shanas, Ethel: The older person at home—a potential isolate or participant. Reprinted from National Institute of Mental Health. In Research utilization in aging, an exploration, Proceedings of a conference sponsored by Community Research and Services Branch, April 30-May 3, 1963, Washington, D. C., 1964, U. S. Government Printing Office.

can devastate the person who is alone because there is no one to care for him; thus continuation in the community becomes impossible when this would not be the case for someone with family or friends. Lowenthal (1968) in tracing the connection between social isolation and mental illness in old age states:

> Lifelong extreme isolation (or alienation) is not necessarily conducive to the development of the kinds of mental disorder that bring persons to the psychiatric ward in their old age; lifelong marginal social adjustment may be conducive to the development of such disorder; late-developing isolation is apparently linked with mental disorder but it is of no greater significance among those with psychogenic disorders than among those with organic disorders, and may be more of a consequence than a cause of mental illness in the elderly; finally, physical illness may be the critical antecedent to both the isolation and the mental illness.*

The choice to be a loner must be respected. As we have seen, people who isolate themselves are not all frail, dependent, lonely persons. We must be able to differentiate this group from those older people who truly want and need assistance in making changes in their lives. Above all, both loners and those isolated unwillingly by circumstance should have the needed help they require in order to maintain the kind of life most satisfactory to them.

INHERITANCE AND THE FAMILY

The issue of who gets the inheritance, if there is any, is a sensitive one for many families and the manner in which this is handled is a good indicator of family problem solving. Some older people make their wills early and in secret. Others fully inform each child. For many people, making a will is such a painful process that it is put off and they die intestate (without a will). Children who are used to sharing with each other and who have resolved their major conflicts with parents may be able to settle an estate amicably with no will. But for others this is precisely the time for angry, hurt, and disappointed feelings to come to the fore, and a royal battle ensues.

The making of a will can be therapeutic for several reasons. The older person, by his own action, takes the potential for conflict out of the hands of his children. His estate will be handled according to his own wishes. And the disposing of the burden of possessions through a will can free the older person and simplify his life; many give things away even before they die. The will tells a great deal about the relations of the legator to his or her legatees (children, charitable interests, etc.). The nature of wills varies according to the stage of life of the testator. For example, if one has young children, trusts may be set up. Selection of executors and trustees is important: the executor is appointed to execute the will; the trustees are persons or agents, such as a bank, holding legal title to property in order to administer it for a beneficiary.

In some states a person may make an oral or nuncupative will; in others a holographic will—one written in the testator's own handwriting and unwitnessed—is acceptable. Old people may need to know that there are two main classes of property: real and personal. The former refers to such immovable objects as land, houses, and trees. The latter includes all other kinds of property (called legacy). If no will has been made, the property descends to lawful heirs, as legally prescribed, or to the state. Property passes into the hands of the executor who sells it and divides the proceeds among the next of kin: If a will has been made and the person dies, the will must be probated, or proved to be authentic. The executor brings the will before the court (probate or surrogate's court), and any possible heir is given the opportunity to object to the probate of the will.*

*From Lowenthal, Marjorie F.: Social isolation and mental illness in old age. In Neugarten, Bernice, editor: Middle age and aging, Chicago, 1968, University of Chicago Press, p. 234.

*For information on wills, see Siegel, Edward: So you're wondering about a will. How to avoid lawyers, New York, 1969, Fawcett Publications, Inc.

It is likely that the future will bring changes in laws of inheritance, since many question the right of ownership in fee simple—that is, absolute ownership—in a complex society providing many goods and services funded through public revenues.

*Prenuptial agreements** are a time-honored method in most states of allaying the fears of children when their parents remarry in old age. Such agreements also protect older people themselves by keeping their resources intact and unavailable to anyone but designated persons. Wealthy people are inclined to use prenuptial agreements even in earlier marriages to protect family estates. With people now living longer, with more late-life marriages, and with more inherited wealth, prenuptial agreements are increasingly common. Legal consultation is necessary. The agreement customarily describes what will *not* be available to the opposite spouse. Trusts can be alternatives to prenuptial agreements.

FAMILY INVOLVEMENT IN MENTAL HEALTH CARE OF THE ELDERLY

Family therapy

Empirical evidence has made it clear that most older people are *not* alienated from their families; therefore, one must go further and assume that any problems, crises, and changes affecting an older person also affect his family. The newly forming field of family therapy, begun fifteen to twenty years ago, has recognized that the problems of the elderly have impact on the entire kinship network. Even the youngest family members will be reacting emotionally to the events in the life of grandmother and grandfather. It is through these experiences that they learn firsthand about late life, and many of their attitudes toward the elderly and their own eventual aging will be modeled after the situations and attitudes in the family circle. Family therapy involving everyone from young to old can be a way of helping to understand what is happening to the older person, clarify feelings, review and deal with old conflicts (which may be surprisingly undiluted by the passage of time), and mobilize every one in the care and concern for the older member. (See Chapter 12 for discussion of family counseling.)

"Filial maturity"

Blenkner* has used the term *filial maturity* to describe a middle-aged developmental stage beyond the usual Freudian framework. (The latter encompasses development from birth through early adulthood, with little theoretical consideration given to middle and late life.) The adult in his forties and fifties experiences a *filial crisis* when it becomes evident that his parents are aging and that he will be called upon to provide the support and comfort which they need. This may contrast with his childhood visions of his parents as powerful and nurturing individuals who assist and support their offspring rather than vice versa. In view of the vicissitudes of early parent-child relationships, there is often unfinished developmental work to be done in freeing middle-aged adults from hostile, ambivalent, or immature parental ties that impede a healthy relationship. Maturity for the middle-aged child "involves being *depended on* and therefore being dependable insofar as his parent is concerned," with full recognition of the parent as an individual with his own rights, needs, limitations, and life history. "It is often necessary to assist the child to complete his unfinished emancipation from the parent *in order that he may then be more free to help his parent.*" Neurotic guilt toward parents must be differentiated from the real guilt of failure to assume filial responsibility.

*We are indebted to Newton Frohlich, Washington lawyer and author of "Making the best of it," Harper & Row, Publishers, New York, 1971, for his help on discussion of prenuptial agreements.

*For an excellent summary on family relationships in old age, see Blenkner, Margaret: Social work and family relationships in later life with some thoughts on filial maturity. In Shanas, Ethel, and Streib, Gordon F., editors: Social structure and the family: generational relations, Englewood Cliffs, N. J., 1965, Prentice-Hall, Inc.

Blenkner reminds us that much psychiatric and social work literature treats the interactions between older people and their children in a negative, patronizing fashion. The term *role-reversal* has become a favored concept because it fits so comfortably with the negative stereotypes depicting the aged as dependent or regressed; the child supposedly becomes the parent to his own parents as they slip from self-sufficient adulthood to a state of childish dependency. Surely a more derogatory interpretation of the realities of old age could not be imagined, especially when dependency in this society is consistently equated with laxness and moral decline. Certain other societies have managed a very different view:

> An Igbo elder (Eastern Nigeria) is no more productive than his American counterpart, but can demand care in his old age as his publicly acknowledged right, without any sense of guilt, ego damage, or loss of face. Whoever fails in giving such care is culpable and subject to scorn and ridicule, and runs the risk of being cut off from the ancestors.*

Thus the elderly Igbo has the powerful authority of the ancestor world to back his claim to respect and care, while the elderly American must rely on the good will of his children and/or society.

Some of the more practical matters of helping older family members can be easily learned.† Indeed, several rehabilitation centers now teach families how to perform required therapies. Visiting nurses and home health specialists perform a teaching function within the family. (See Chapter 10.) Many more older people could be treated at home if their problems were detected early and prompt psychiatric, social, medical, and economic resources were made available. Families could then be free to provide the blend of affection and personal services so essential to mental health in old age.

---

*From Wylie, Floyd M.: Attitudes toward aging and the aged among black Americans: some historical perspectives, Aging and Human Development **2**:68, Feb., 1971.

†See Stern, Edith M., with Ross, Mabel: You and your aging parents, New York, 1952, Harper & Row, Publishers; also see U. S. Department of Health, Education, and Welfare: The older person in the home, Public Health Service Publication No. 542, Washington, D. C., 1957, U. S. Government Printing Office.

REFERENCES

Abraham, K.: Some remarks on the role of grandparents in the psychology of neuroses. In Abraham, H., editor: Selected papers: clinical papers and essays in psychoanalysis, vol. 2, New York, 1955, Basic Books, Inc.

Adam, Ruth: The role of grandmother today. In Owen, R., editor: Middle age, London, 1967, British Broadcasting Corp.

Anthony, E. J., editor: Parenthood, Boston, 1970, Little, Brown & Co.

Benedek, Therese: Parenthood during the life cycle. In Anthony, E. J., editor: Parenthood, Boston, 1970, Little, Brown & Co.

Blenkner, Margaret: Social work and family relationships in later life with some thoughts on filial maturity. In Shanas, Ethel, and Streib, Gordon F., editors: Social structure and the family: generational relations, Englewood Cliffs, N. J., 1965, Prentice-Hall, Inc.

Brody, Elaine M.: Aging is a family affair, Public Welfare **25**:129-141, April, 1967.

Brody, Elaine M., and Spark, G. M.: Institutionalization of the aged: a family crisis, Family Process **5**:76-90, 1966.

Ciocco, A.: On the interdependence of the length of life of husband and wife, Human Biology **13**:505-525, 1941.

Duvall, Evelyn M.: In-laws in your life, Pastoral Psychology **52**:39-47, Dec., 1954.

Farrar, Marcella S.: Mother-daughter conflicts extended into later life, Social Casework **36**: 202-208, 1955.

Ferenczi, S.: The grandfather complex. In Rickman, J., editor: Theory and technique of psychoanalysis, New York, 1926, Basic Books, Inc.

Kahana, B., and Kahana Eva: Grandparenthood from the perspective of the developing grandchild, Developmental Psychology **3**:98-105, April, 1970.

Kahana, Eva, and Kahana, B.: Theoretical and research perspectives on grandparenthood, Aging and Human Development **2**:261-268, 1971.

Kreps, Juanita M.: The economics of intergenerational relationships. In Shanas, Ethel, and Streib, Gordon F., editors: Social structure and the family: generational relations, Englewood Cliffs, N. J., 1965, Prentice-Hall, Inc.

LaBarre, M., Jessner, L., and Ussery, L.: The significance of grandmothers in the psychopathology of children, American Journal of Orthopsychiatry **30**:175-185, 1960.

Lowenthal, Marjorie F.: Social isolation and mental illness in old age. In Neugarten, B., editor: Middle age and aging, Chicago, 1968, University of Chicago Press.

Lowenthal, Marjorie F., and Haven, Clayton: Interaction and adaptation: intimacy as a critical variable. In Neugarten, B., editor: Middle age and aging, Chicago, 1968, University of Chicago Press.

McKain, Walter C.: Retirement marriage, Storrs, 1969, University of Connecticut.

Neugarten, Bernice: Continuities and discontinuities of psychological issues into adult life, Human Development **12**:121-130, 1969.

Neugarten, Bernice L., and Weinstein, Karol K.: The changing American grandparent, Journal of Marriage and the Family **26**:199-205, May, 1964.

Parsons, T., and Bales, R.: Family, socialization and interaction process, New York, 1955, Free Press of Glencoe, Inc.

Schorr, A. L.: Filial responsibility in the modern American family, U. S. Department of Health, Education, and Welfare, Social Security Administration, Washington, D. C., 1960, U. S. Government Printing Office.

Shanas, Ethel: The health of older people: a social survey, Cambridge, Mass., 1962, Harvard University Press.

Shanas, Ethel: The unmarried old person in the United States: living arrangements and care in illness, myth and fact. A paper prepared for the International Social Science Research Seminar in Gerontology, Markaryd, Sweden, Aug., 1963.

Shanas, Ethel: The older person at home—a potential isolate or participant. Reprinted from the National Institute of Mental Health. In Research utilization in aging, an exploration, Proceedings of a conference sponsored by Community Research and Services Branch, April 30-May 3, 1963, Washington, D. C., 1964, U. S. Government Printing Office.

Shanas, Ethel, and Streib, Gordon F.: Social structure and the family: generational relations, Englewood Cliffs, N. J., 1965, Prentice-Hall, Inc.

Sheps, J.: New developments in family diagnosis in emotional disorders of old age, Geriatrics **14**:443-449, 1959.

Stern, Edith M., and Ross, Mabel: You and your aging parents, New York, 1952, Harper & Row, Publishers.

Sussman, Marvin B.: Relationships of adult children with their parents in the United States. In Shanas, Ethel, and Streib, Gordon F., editors: Social structure and the family: generational relationships, Englewood Cliffs, N. J., 1965, Prentice-Hall, Inc.

Sussman, M. B., and Burchinal, L.: Kin family network: unheralded structure in current conceptualization of family functions. In Neugarten, B. L., editor: Middle age and aging: a reader in social psychology, Chicago, 1968, University of Chicago Press.

Townsend, Peter: The family life of old people, London, 1957, Routledge & Kegan Paul, Ltd.

U. S. Senate Special Committee on Aging: Summary of developments and data, a pre-White House Conference on Aging report, Nov., 1971.

World Health Organization: Mental health problems of the aging and the aged, Technical Report Series, No. 171, Geneva, 1959.

PART II

Evaluation, treatment, and prevention

8
GENERAL TREATMENT PRINCIPLES

We are writing the treatment section of this book on two levels: one describing what we consider to be appropriate and ideal mental health care of older people and the other dealing with contemporary realities, far from ideal. Our aim is to keep in sight the direction for improvements while also advising mental health personnel, older people themselves, and anyone involved in their welfare on how to make the best of what is now available.

NEW ATTITUDES TOWARD MENTAL HEALTH TREATMENT OF THE ELDERLY

There have been no such exciting and dramatic new directions in the psychiatric treatment of the elderly as there have been and will continue to be in the physical aspects of aging (e.g., treatment for atherosclerosis, cancer, and other diseases). But there has been a steady growth in theory and practice, which emphasizes the importance of active as well as restorative and rehabilitative possibilities. Most importantly, the potentiality of reversibility has been demonstrated, especially in the functional disorders and the reversible (acute) brain syndromes.* Prevention, comprehensive evaluations, and genuine therapeutic efforts have begun to be accepted as worthwhile activities on behalf of the old.

Changes in psychiatric perspectives

Psychiatry, at the turn of the century, had a detached view of abnormal behavior—observing and cataloging exterior behavior. Later, dominated by Freudian thinking, it moved to the interior and the inner life of humans—probing subjective experience and internalized modes of adaptation. Since World War II, psychiatry has moved out somewhat (but only *somewhat*) into the community—examining the influences of institutions and environmental conditions on human behavior, inner experience, and adaptations. Recently some attention has turned to the inherent changes of the individual as he progresses through the life cycle. Thus in about eighty years, psychiatry has looked at man's outward behavior, his inner life, his environment, and finally at his passage through his finite existence—the life cycle. This includes a new interest in the psychology of old age.* However, psychiatry as a practicing specialty has not kept pace with the theoretical aspects of the discipline. It is the private psychotherapy and analytic practice that remains psychiatry's chief preoccupation, with little active participation in the broader field of community psychiatry. The financial opportunities in private practice have militated against the application

*Private mental hospitals demonstrate the correlation between financial capacity and reversibility. In studies done in private institutions, Dr. Robert Gibson and Dr. J. M. Myers stressed the reversibility of the psychiatric conditions of old age. From 54% to 75% of patients over 65 were able to be discharged to their own homes in two months. Thus if one can afford private care, the chances are greater for reversibility. Unfortunately only 7,000 elderly patients received treatment in private hospitals in 1969, compared to 50,000 patients treated in state and county hospitals. See Gibson, Robert W.: Medicare and the psychiatric patient, Psychiatric Opinion 7:17-22, 1970.

*Berezin, Busse, Goldfarb, Greenleigh, Grotjahn, Linden, Rothschild, Simon, Thompson, and Weinberg are but a few of the American psychiatrists whose work has stimulated research into the psychopathology and psychodynamics of aging as well as developing treatment approaches.

of new understanding in the area of human behavior. Other disciplines have become more involved than ever in mental health work. Nurses, social workers, psychologists, paraprofessionals, and members of still-forming specialties are doing much of the work traditionally thought of as "psychiatry" in the past.

Life cycle theory—what is it?

A science, or perhaps more humbly, a perspective and body of knowledge of the life cycle, is barely born. Social, biological, medical, and other changes have led to longer life and increased visibility of the stages of the life cycle. Sanitized and medicated survival and death control without birth control have increased the number of children and old people. The middle years of life stand as a fulcrum and largely support the two ends of the life cycle—namely, childhood and old age. This is true individually when parents are responsible both for their children and for their own parents; it is true also in society, where middle-aged people hold the power, make the decisions, and produce the goods. We do not yet know to what extent normative, modal features of the life cycle account for the varying patterns of change and adaptation we see. A handful of investigators are engaged in endeavoring to disentangle the features of the successive phases of the life cycle from the contributions of social change, medical disease, historical variation, etc. Butler (1968) has used the term "average expectable life cycle" as a counterpart of Heinz Hartmann's concept "average expectable environment" to bring focus to the notion that there are average, normative experiences against which to measure individual patterns. If, for example, we see correlations of conservative behavior with age, are these due to the conditions of youth carried forward in time or are they intrinsic to aging? If we observe preoccupation with bowel function in aged persons, is it a result of the popular lore of the turn of the century or a consequence of the inherent character of old age? Are the declines in memory associated with aging to be interpreted as a consequence of brain disease, educational obsolescence, social anomie, depression, and/or the mysterious, inevitable, irreversible process(es) called aging?

There is not yet a sufficiently sensitive methodology to weigh the relative significance of the many elements that are involved in the production of changes in man and adaptation to those changes. We believe the life cycle itself—the changes inherent in the rhythm of a life from birth to death—makes profound contribution to the variability. The study of human development has tended to stop with adolescence. It needs to start up again, this time continuing with fact gathering and theoretical formulations all the way through middle and late life, instead of losing interest after the "achievement" of adulthood. Contemporary personality and developmental theories need enlargement and expansion to provide a full account of man. Naturally such an effort would give further direction to the treatment of older people.

In clinical work and reflections Butler has come to speak of the development of an *individual inner sense of the life cycle,* which is neither the same as the average expectable life cycle nor the same as a personal sense of identity, although it is related to both. It is a subjective feel for the life cycle as a whole, its rhythm, its variability, and the relation of this to the individual's sense of himself. This inner sense seems to be a necessary personal achievement in order for the individual to orient himself wherever he happens to be on the life cycle. It becomes particularly important as the person ages and begins to comprehend his own eventual end.

In adolescents, the middle-aged, and the elderly, such a personal sense of the cycle of human life is a necessary adaptive mechanism. To understand the kinds of changes to be expected and face oneself with the reality and inevitability of these changes, including death itself, is important to individual security. It gives people the opportunity to prepare themselves, to plan and order their lives in more meaningful ways, and (perhaps most important), to be assured that they are not alone in their experiences. All generations and all of their fellow living human beings share the same basic realities. The understanding of all of this is part of what humans long for when they speak of searching for the meaning of life through religion or a personal philosophy of life. An inner sense of the life cycle—often unspoken—produces a profound awareness of change and evolution—birth, maturation, obsolescence, and death—and therefore a profound but nonmorbid realization of the precious and limited quantity of life. For old people it is not the same as "feeling old"; it is instead a deep understanding of what it means to be human.

One sees all kinds of people struggling for greater sensibility about life but, for various reasons, not being able to face what is there. There are adolescents who can comprehend the notion of suicide (perhaps because the person kills himself and thus has control over his death) but cannot imagine death in old age or even that they themselves will grow old. Middle-aged persons often develop anxiety symptoms about aging and try to turn the clock back to youth by dressing and acting young. Even in their old age one sees Peter Pans—those who have never grown up to face their age and the fact of death.

From our own work we have seen what an inner sense of the life cycle can mean in old age. It can portend adaptation to inevitable changes in the best manner possible; or its absence can guarantee maladaptation, wherein the older person reacts with terror, dependency, and prolonged grief to personal change. The following case examples are illustrative:

Case 1. A still handsome, warm, and magnetic 78-year-old former politician who had received many public awards called for a psychiatric consultation, his voice full of despair. He had always been healthy and unusually vigorous until the previous summer, at which time he developed glaucoma. Shortly thereafter he began to notice weakness of his left arm. By means of a myelogram, electromyelographic studies, etc., it was determined that the patient had anterior horn cell disease.

He had been an unusually healthy man all of his life, extremely vigorous, very proud of his sexual prowess and attractiveness. He had been married three times and had had many private affairs.

However, until his recent problems, he had never taken seriously the fact that he could become old. Moreover, his much younger brother was suffering from severe chronic brain syndrome and was residing in a nursing home; this fact began to preoccupy him.

Our patient remained somewhat busy in public life but had recently given up his last private love affair. During a warm and somewhat grief-stricken lunch together the two quoted Ecclesiastes to each other: "Everything in its season. . ."

Yet he never prepared for old age. He never thought about old age when he was younger; in fact he gave it little thought until his glaucoma. On the rare occasions when he did, he would say to himself "Why shouldn't I live to be 100?" Whenever he rarely thought about death, he wished for, and he thought that he would have, a quick sudden death. He had turned aside suggestions that he write his memoirs.

Now he felt helpless. His sense of omnipotence was under sudden seige and near collapse. He became extremely hypochondriacal. He not only went to physicians from a whole range of specialties but sought out possible quacks.

In summary, he had not experienced aging or the diseases associated with aging gradually. All was precipitous, with no stepwise intimations of mortality!

Although he had five children, he was not in any sense strongly involved with them, which suggests that he had not grown or fulfilled the life cycle task of parenthood.

He became very much dependent upon the therapist. Although the psychotherapist was obviously doing nothing "material," he felt the therapist was the only physician who was "doing anything" for him—in spite of the fact that the others had offered drugs and had conducted a variety of tests. Emphasis in psychotherapy was on consideration of the unfolding of the life cycle and on renunciation and restitution; that is, on grieving and accepting things as they are and finding other avenues for personal pleasure and development—particularly those pertinent to later life: teaching, counseling, leaving "traces," etc. It was necessary to reduce the number of sessions to help him resolve his sudden (but not unexpected) dependency. He improved, but any lengthy separations created setbacks.

Case 2. In 1965 an 87-year-old former schoolteacher sustained a stroke from which she recovered except for a residual right hemiplegia.

There was no aphasia. She had always been an extremely independent person and she was quite agitated and depressed over what happened to her. Unlike the first patient, however, she did not respond with helplessness. She was a very courageous fighter, pulling herself up and down stairs for dinner each day. This was still true five years later at age 92. The therapist was seeing her at that time, although the agitated depression had gone. They seemed unable to give each other up. They would meet approximately once monthly, usually on Saturday afternoon, at which time at her insistence they would have a fine sherry or Madeira together. There were occasions when she would put herself to bed and seem to be failing. However, nothing would be amiss on physical examination and it became clear that these episodes were related to the thought on her part that maybe she was just about to die. In view of her advanced age, this was not such an irrational idea! Then, after several days in bed, she would awaken to the realization that she was neither dead nor dying and would be back up functioning again.

At other times the therapist would simply tell her she was alright, whereupon she would agree and resume life. These episodes were characterized psychologically by great preoccupation with leaving things and with what the recipients would do with the objects of her legacy. It was very important to her that she not be falsely reassured about death but that respectful attention be given to her ideas about dying, death, burial, and the objects of her legacy—religious items, pictures of her parents, old favorite books, etc. Unlike the first patient, she had always had a sound sense of the evolving process of life, the life cycle. But her advancing age—or diseases—narrowed the opportunities in which she could express her personality. Thus she had to rely more and more on verbal or bodily expression of needs (rather than action). She had responsiveness in abundance from her daughter as well as from her therapist. She continued to do quite well.

Rites of passage

Rites of passage are the cultural observances of biological and social changes. Christenings, confirmations or bar mitzvahs, marriages, and burials are the most obvious but there are countless others, all adding structure and meaning to lives. They lend predictability and help to ease the individual's movement from one stage to the next. Such rites help us to "know the score"; offer social supports from time of birth and early development; confirm our religious, sexual, occupational, and social identity; consecrate marriages as well as provide for their dissolution; and offer models for dealing with happiness and fulfillment as well as with failure, grief, loss, and eventual death. However, rites of passage, as with all other cultural institutions, are often out of tune with human needs as history unfolds. It is necessary to understand the nature of the particular life cycle in order to judge the validity of the rites of passage associated with it. Rites of passage undergo constant revision—and, while revising, many humans flounder and suffer from the lack of a meaningful structure. An example in the present is the problem in handling grief, which has resulted from increasing secularization and the loss of religious supports. Older people, and especially their children, often do not know what to do with grief. Should they cry, maintain a stoic front, deny it, become angry, or what? There is no longer a structured and supportive mourning period. Some mourners pretend the loss never happened; others wait silently, hoping grief will go away. Yet we know theoretically what "grief work" is and what could be done to help find the best possible psychological resolution to loss. It remains for such knowledge to become part of popular psychology. People who no longer have a religious belief must learn to do for themselves some of the work they formerly left up to the church or synagogue.

Other parts of the life cycle are changing as a result of alterations in biology and changes in the life-span. Changes occur so quickly that people may be left bewildered. The bewilderment is greatest in those for whom the change is greatest. Small children born today have never experienced anything but accelerating change, and it has been suggested that change itself is an accepted way of life for them. But for the present generation of older people who remember a more slowly moving past the contrast with the present can be horrifying, disconcerting, and disorienting, particularly if the older person feels or is in some way personally victimized by change.

New rites of passage are needed to support new developments. Recent and still growing controls of the events of the life cycle bear comment. Flexibility of classic rites is needed to cope with birth control, liberalized abortion, genetic manipulation, sex prediction before birth—all of which could (and already do) allow considerable control over the occurrence and timing of birth and the quality of children. The arrival of menstruation for girls has moved ahead thirty-six months in the last one hundred years. The rite of marriage (which first became a sacrament in the ninth century A.D., when people seldom lived longer than forty years) is being influenced by trial marriages, the ability to control births, and the notion of divorce by consent. Menopause is being eased by endocrine replacement—even beginning to be considered a treatable disease rather than an inevitable loss of ovarian functioning. The event of death is subject to greater control also. Organ transplants, new thoughts about criteria for death (as a result of medical discoveries), interest in passive and active euthanasia—all produce legal, ethical, and medical considerations that will become part of the evolving rites surrounding death.

One feature of present life—retirement—has almost no formal rites of passage and no precedent historically. The institution of retirement is barely eighty years old and is a consequence of the lengthening of the life-span for vast numbers of people. In the next thirty years, 65 million people will have retired and in the year 2000, about 33 million of these will still be alive. Similar demographic changes are occurring in other countries, some of which are responding more positively than we. Our present lack of structured and meaningful rites for retirement has led to anomic nonparticipation of many people in American life.

Biological control can create social innovation, and vice versa. Thus people can become freer of the previously fixed, unalterable biological states that have long controlled the culturally defined rites of passage. What such freedom means for the future is hard to fathom. What we do know is that present generations of older people need to have a secure place for themselves in a society that makes sense to them. Good mental health is not possible in chaos and meaninglessness.

OBSTACLES TO TREATMENT IN OLD AGE

Ageism and countertransference

We have described the many negative attitudes toward old people under the general term "ageism"—the prejudices and stereotypes that are applied to older people sheerly on the basis of their age.* (Another term, *gerontophobia,* refers to a more rare "unreasonable fear and/or constant hatred of older people whereas ageism is a much more comprehensive and useful concept").† Ageism, like racism and sexism, is a way of pigeonholing people and not allowing them to be individuals with unique ways of living their lives. Prejudice toward the elderly is an attempt by younger generations to shield themselves from the fact of their own eventual aging and death and to avoid having to deal with the social and economic problems of increasing numbers of older people. It provides a rationalization for pushing the elderly out of the job market without spending much thought on what will happen to them when they are no longer allowed to work. Ageism is the sacrifice of older people for the sake of "productivity" and the youth image that the working world feels compelled to project. A terrible awakening comes when these younger people themselves grow old and suddenly find that they are the victims of attitudes they once held against others.

In the mental health field, ageism has become professionalized—often to the point where it is not recognized. Gibson noted in 1970 that psychiatrists were pessimistic about the treatability of older persons. In reviewing the records of 138 patients over 65 who were admitted to a private hospital

*Butler, R. N.: The effects of medical and health progress on the social and economic aspects of the life cycle, Industrial Gerontology 1:1-9, 1969.

†Palmore, Erdman: Gerontophobia versus ageism, The Gerontologist 12:213, 1972.

during a three-year period, it was found that the prognosis was considered poor in 80% of the cases; yet 60% were discharged as improved to their homes within ninety days. Gallagher et al. also found age correlating with therapeutic pessimism.* Of patients between 15 and 29 years of age, 66.7% received psychotherapy; of patients who were 30 to 39, 38.5% did; and of those 40 to 65, only 15.4%. Other mental health professionals are no less pessimistic.

Countertransference in the classic sense occurs when mental health personnel find themselves perceiving and reacting to older persons in ways that are inappropriate and reminiscent of previous patterns of relating to parents, siblings, and other key childhood figures. Love and protectiveness may vie with hate and revenge. Ageism takes this a step further. Staff members not only have to deal with leftover feelings from their personal pasts, which may interfere with their perceptions of an old person; they must also be aware of a multitude of negative cultural attitudes toward the elderly, which pervade social institutions as well as individual psyches.

The GAP report, "The Aged and Community Mental Health," in 1971 listed some of the major reasons for negative staff attitudes toward treating the elderly.†

1. The aged stimulate the therapist's fears about his own old age.
2. They arouse the therapist's conflicts about his relationship with parental figures.
3. The therapist believes he has nothing useful to offer old people because he believes they cannot change their behavior or that their problems are all due to untreatable organic brain diseases.
4. The therapist believes that his psychodynamic skills will be wasted if he works with the aged because they are near death and not really deserving of attention (similar to the triage system of the military, in which the sickest receive the least attention because they are least likely to recover).
5. The patient might die while in treatment, which could challenge the therapist's sense of importance.
6. The therapist's colleagues may be contemptuous of his efforts on behalf of aged patients. (One often hears the remark that gerontologists or geriatric specialists have a morbid preoccupation with death; their interest in the elderly is therefore "sick" or suspect.)

Another factor in ageism is what appears to be a human propensity for hostility toward the handicapped. There is often an unconscious overidentification with old people, especially those who are physically handicapped: they are thought of as "defective," "crippled," "powerless," or "castrated." Excessive sentimentality, sympathy, avoidance, or hostility may result. It is estimated that some 300 million people in the world have highly visible deformities. These cause emotional problems—in part because of the attitudes of society. In primitive cultures such cripples (and, we might add, old people) were often put to death. This "final solution" is not so obvious in present societies but attitudes remain surprisingly similar. In a study done by two German psychologists on attitudes of normal school-age children and adults toward the handicapped, most (63%) thought the victims should be institutionalized (in short, kept out of sight). Many felt "they probably would rather be dead." The younger the children, the less pity they felt and the more aversion. The same thing has been found for differences in skin color. Fear is the basis for the hostility, and ignorance prolongs it. The fear is that this might happen to me, so I must stay away or fight it.

Some people have described the treatment they have received as handicapped patients.

*Gallagher, E. B., Sharaf, M. R., and Levinson, D. J.: The influence of patient and therapist in determining the use of psychotherapy in a hospital setting, Psychiatry 28:297-310, 1965.

†The aged and community mental health: a guide to program development. Formulated by the Committee on Aging, Group for the Advancement of Psychiatry, vol. 8, New York, 1971.

An American writer, Eric Hodgins in his book *Episode: Report on the Accident Inside My Skull** tells of his own doctor, an old friend of many years, who talked to others about him in the hospital room after his stroke as though Hodgins were no longer an aware human being.

Another man, younger and partially blind, has described the confusions he created in a state service for the blind because he had been accepted into a well known university's Ph.D. program and was applying to the state for educational assistance. The counselors, with their bachelor's and master's degrees, did not know how to react to a blind person who was obviously not acting "handicapped." They finally resolved their dismay by allotting the money to the man for three successive years of doctoral training without once calling him in to talk again with a counselor, an apparent collusion aimed at avoiding a confrontation with their own preconceptions.

Publications in the field of mental health are no less innocent when it comes to ageism. One respected clinical psychiatric textbook states:

> A dislike of change, a reduction in ambition and activity, a tendency to become constricted and self-centered in interests, an increased difficulty in comprehension, an increase in time and effort in adapting to new circumstances, a lessened sympathy for new ideas and views and a tendency to reminiscence and repetition are scarcely signs of senile dementia, yet they pass imperceptibly into mental destitution and personality regression. Many elderly people have little capacity to express warm and spontaneous feelings toward others.
>
> . . . The patient resents what he considers as interference by younger persons and may complain that he is being neglected. Some show a hostile but anxious and fearful dependence. Natural affections become blunted and may turn to hatred. A certain tendency to isolation occurs.†

There are half-truths in this statement in the case of persons with senile brain disease. But more obvious is the pessimistic, patronizing view of old age, tempered only slightly by hints that some of the changes might be psychological reactions to loss and stress. The student reading such material is confirmed in his negative attitudes.

Reactions of older persons against treatment

Force, deceit, or any other measure taken by mental health personnel "for the older person's own good," when it is against the wishes of the older person, cannot be justified morally or legally, except in those cases in which the person is a clear and present danger to the life of himself or others. Older people may resist mental health intervention into their lives for many reasons: desire for independence, fear of change, suspiciousness based on past experiences, realistic appraisal of the inadequacies of most "helping" programs for the elderly, clumsy, insensitive, or patronizing intervention techniques on the part of mental health staff, etc. Many times old people will tenaciously hold on to what little they have rather than risk the unknown. They may prefer to live in their own homes despite crime, dilapidation, and isolation. They may resist medical examinations, surgery, and medications. Some have been known to keep guns to use on themselves or others if someone comes to take them to a nursing home—a fate feared by many as worse than death. Pride and desire for self-reliance, as well as depression and mental confusion, must be considered as factors in resistance.

One approaches the resistance of the elderly just as one would the resistances of any age group—by gradual development of trust, provision of information, and a commitment to self-determination and civil rights. Clergymen can often be helpful in talking through problems and decisions, as can family members, neighbors, and friends. The older person must be closely involved in any decision-making about himself. Action, rather than just verbalization by mental health staff, can bring satisfying results. An example is the case of the elderly New York

*New York, 1964, Atheneum Press. This superb account should be required reading for all who work with patients of any age.

†From Noyes, Arthur, and Kolb, Lawrence: Modern clinical psychiatry, Philadelphia, 1958, W. B. Saunders Co., p. 289.

woman with mild intellectual impairment who refused to move out of her condemned apartment. No amount of talking could convince her. Finally a staff member offered to physically help her move and stay with her the first night in the new apartment. The old women accepted. Her fears had met with response.

Another problem affecting treatment is the low self-esteem of some elderly people, who have incorporated the negative cultural view of themselves. This reaction of the victims of discrimination has been called "self-hatred" and takes the form of depression, with passive giving up or active self-denigration. They look at themselves as so many younger people see them and thus do not like what they see. Open discussions about ageism can help such a person reexamine his self-view, particularly if at the same time he begins to experience new acceptance on the part of people around him. Age-integrated group therapy is especially useful in this regard.

Lack of knowledge

We simply do not know much specifically about old age, especially about healthy old age. Most clinical experience and studies have been of the sick and institutionalized aged. Generally speaking, older persons are not admitted to research and training centers. And most experience has been limited over time—to short-term evaluation rather than to treatment.*

One major consequence of this limitation is the loss of the more enduring, intensive relationship of treatment personnel and patients, which can be an important source of data about the older person as well as a check up on one's evaluation of him. Indeed referral for psychiatric (mental health) treatment is not only relatively uncommon in the community, but when it does occur, it is usually late in the course of illness, again affecting our knowledge of evaluation as well as militating against the likelihood of therapeutic success.

Financial and bureaucratic impediments

Mental health care is expensive, especially when private psychiatrists, other psychotherapists, private-duty nurses, and private hospitalization are involved. Such care is far beyond the budget of most older people. Public care is occasionally adequate and at times exemplary, but usually it is a far cry from satisfactory. Old people are one of the last priorities on budgets and the last in line on waiting lists. Medicare has not proved to be the godsend hoped for. Nonetheless, pending adoption of a comprehensive medical insurance plan for all Americans, the major method of obtaining care for the elderly will continue to be the Medicare system. Medicare now covers only 43% of the average elderly person's health expenses. The deductibles (that which the patient pays) are just that—deductions from the care of the elderly. Old people often just do not purchase the excluded items (including dentures, eyeglasses, outpatient drugs, physical examinations) because they cannot afford to. Ironically the out-of-pocket cost of medical care has actually risen for older people since the introduction of Medicare because of increases in physicians' fees, hospital costs, and the general inflationary spiral. There is also no proof that the deductible features of Medicare deter unnecessary use of health services. Instead, the exclusions may actually increase the government's bill by discouraging preventive and early rehabilitative care.

Medicare coverage for psychiatric disorders is unrealistically limited and was inserted as a kind of afterthought. There is a 190-day lifetime limit on treatment in mental hospitals; and the patient must pay 50% of outpatient services from a physician. There is an annual limit of $250 on outpatient care. Social workers, psychologists, and other

*Butler and Sulliman found that 40% of all contact between privately practicing psychiatrists and older people in the greater metropolitan Washington community was for consultation only.

mental health personnel are not appropriately covered on an outpatient basis. The system obviously affords inadequate coverage—and, contrary to sound psychiatric practice, it promotes hospitalization rather than care in the community. Some old people get themselves checked into a hospital just to get a physical examination (basing it on some physical complaint) because this will not be paid for on an outpatient basis.

Nursing homes unfortunately have gotten into the business of providing "care" for psychiatric patients; yet they are not in any sense of the word psychiatric institutions. The conditions for eligibility for extended care under the Medicare program are both inadequate and inadequately applied. As a result, thousands of elderly patients, including those with psychiatric problems, are receiving no more than routine custodial care. Many nursing home facilities are substandard (the frequent occurrence of fires in nursing homes being one example). Too often a nursing home can be defined as a place with few nurses and few of the characteristics of home. Social and restorative services hardly exist, and activity programs usually receive more advertising than implementation. It is very rare for psychiatric or social work services to ever play a part in the nursing home program. In addition, a good deal of nursing home care is not even financed through Medicare; rather it is funded by Medicaid and public assistance, ensuring even more deplorable conditions and lack of standards.

It is necessary to be clear on the financial aspects of psychiatric care for the elderly in order to avoid professional overoptimism and pie-in-the-sky planning. We can speak of ideal community mental health programs and about the facts that more is known than is applied and that our society has not yet made a major commitment to the care of the aged. But we cannot maintain an artificial distinction between care and basic political/financial obstacles. The body politic is not to be underestimated. Mental health personnel should at least acknowledge and deal as creatively as possible with the socioeconomic framework under which research, care, and treatment occur.

Bureaucratic impediments present other obstacles. There is much bureaucratic confusion among services for the elderly. There is a lack of centralized information and referral services. Property and insurance liens prevent some older people from seeking help, since they do not want to sign over all their earthly possessions in return for assistance. The "responsible relative" clause in many jurisdictions, which requires relatives to assume financial responsibility for parents, sisters or brothers, etc., denies public assistance to older persons and forces hardships on families.

The stress and frustration older people must go through to collect Medicare and private health insurance must be experienced to be believed. We present a case which is not atypical in our work with older people:

> We attempted to assist one of our patients who was having trouble collecting payments for psychotherapy. Medicare was sending payments in different amounts for the same service and the same fee and Mrs. K wanted to know why. In addition, her supplementary major medical insurance with Blue Cross–Blue Shield was refusing to pay for psychiatric services even though the insurance agent handling the policy assured us the woman was covered.
>
> In a five-month period we made multiple calls to Medicare (Mrs. K had already talked to eight different people there over the previous six months to no avail), asking for an explanation and a list of allowable charges. We were told that a computer was faulty, and an audit was being done. Five months later Mrs. K received a notice that she had been overpaid $60 and that she must pay it back. There was still no explanation or list of allowable charges. Mrs. K refused to believe anything any longer and decided to ignore the $60, feeling sure another mistake had been made.
>
> During the same five months we were told twice by Blue Cross–Blue Shield that Mrs. K was eligible for psychiatric services and three times that she was not. We were twice asked to resubmit *everything* (previous material had been lost, couldn't be transferred from one part of BC-BS to another, etc.). After five months of work on our part, Mrs. K still had not been paid. Like the carrot on a stick, there was a constant promise of payment—"in a month or six weeks."

We checked with Mrs. K ten months after our first contact. She had finally been paid by BC-BS. She had never paid Medicare the $60 and was never billed for it. She continued to get different payments from them for the same service and said "but I don't question it anymore—as long as I get something back." Medicare never sent a list of allowable charges and BC-BS said they could not furnish her with a list of covered services or allowable charges for people who also had Medicare, because "each case is considered separately." We and she remain to this day in the dark about exactly what is happening, but at least some payments are coming through.

When an elderly person with anxiety, anger, and frustration about public and private health insurance programs comes to the attention of mental health personnel, here are some things to remember before simply deciding that the person is "acting dependent" or that he "can't cope."

1. It is difficult to reach the proper insurance or government official by phone. About half of our calls never reached their target.
2. Phone calls are often not returned, nor are messages received. Materials that are promised may not be sent.
3. Conflicting information is given.
4. Many health insurance employees do not know their own office procedures or the specifics of the programs they serve.
5. Clients are shifted from one person to another and tend to give up before they reach the "right" person.
6. Records seem, routinely, to get lost. Then the client must start all over again.
7. There may be no explanation about payments or inconsistent payments, especially in Medicare.
8. When a mix-up occurs, clients often hear an insurance representative say "It's out of my hands" (in the computer, another office, etc.); there seems to be no way then to retrieve it promptly.
9. Even though insurance or government personnel seem to be pleasant and interested, they give the impression of being "helpless" in straightening out problems efficiently. Thus the older person feels guilty about complaining or causing a fuss.

STAFF CONSIDERATIONS

What kind of people work with the elderly?

It has been suggested that few mental health personnel actively choose to work with older people and that most of them fall into the work by chance. Professionals tend to deny having an original, personal attraction to the field, preferring to say they have responded to a "need" in society or to an intellectual curiosity about aging. Directors of institutions for older people will state that most of their employees developed interests and satisfactions after beginning their work. We submit that these may be subtle denials concealing a reluctance to admit an interest in old age—a reluctance fostered by the societal devaluation of the old and by the often heard professional opinion that an interest in aging represents a morbid preoccupation with decline and death. Naturally chance plays a part in determining one's career opportunities. But conscious or unconscious personal factors are as important in choosing and remaining in the field of aging as they are in any other human decisions. We offer the following as a number of possible emotional motivations for working professionally with older people:

1. Particularly warm relationships in childhood with grandparents, who then leave their grandchildren a legacy of natural sympathy and an interest in old people
2. Early dependence on grandparents (e.g., the "grandmother's children" who were not raised by their own parents) or on older persons (Parents may have been already older than average when they had children; or there may have been a young mother and a much older father.)
3. Death or painful illness of an important older person when a child is

young and extremely impressionable (In studies of physicians, for example, it has been found that a significant number experienced an early death of a loved person. Medicine then became a way of gaining power over death and the helpless feelings of childhood.)

4. Unconscious counterphobic attempt to conquer one's own personal fear of aging and death
5. Conscious attempt to "prepare" for one's own old age, especially if the models of parents or grandparents are unacceptable (A 58-year-old social worker interested in working professionally in the field of aging joined one of our age-integrated therapy groups to prepare, as she said, for old age. She was terrified at seeing herself become more and more like her mother, whom she viewed as a bitter, disillusioned old woman. She felt helpless in the grip of the model her mother presented her.)
6. Personal sense of inferiority that causes one to identify with the elderly, who are culturally defined as inferior
7. Guilt and subsequent reaction formation for feelings of fear and revulsion toward the aged
8. Admiration for and identification with someone working in the field of aging

The importance of determining one's personal motivation is obvious. A mental health specialist must know where he is coming from, emotionally, before he can effectively use himself to help others.

PROFESSIONAL DISCRIMINATION AGAINST THE POOR AND THE OLD

We have touched upon this a number of times but want to keep emphasizing it from different angles because we feel it is so crucial. Psychiatrists must reconsider medical education, psychiatric residency programs, and subsequent postgraduate medical and psychiatric training. The nation's programs, including the National Institutes of Health, still emphasize young patients and acute illnesses. We cannot move blissfully along in our efforts toward meeting the psychiatric problems of the elderly without recognizing the need for far-reaching changes in education and emphasis.* Private psychiatrists see patients who are mostly from a small upper segment of the socioeconomic and intellectual population. For instance, a recent study of private psychiatrists in Boston revealed the following:

> About one-quarter of all Bostonians who are private patients are young women in their twenties and early thirties who live within an area of less than 100 blocks. Most are college educated.†

Another study, done by the American Psychoanalytic Association, showed that of the private patients seen by its members 98% were white and 78% were educated at the college level or above.‡ Other studies, by Hollingshead and Redlich,§ Schaffer and

---

*Despite the leadership of social workers in the field of aging (among them Walter M. Beattie, Jr., Margaret Blenkner, Elaine M. Brody, Helen Turner Burr, James J. Burr, Elias S. Cohen, Theodore Isenstadt, Hobart C. Jackson, Wilma Klein, Virginia Lehmann, Helen Lokshin, Jean M. Maxwell, Helen Padula, William Posner, Ollie A. Randall, Sheldon S. Tobin, and Edna Wasser), their numbers remain a handful—rather like the situation in psychiatry. The Council on Social Work Education has encouraged schools of social work to include study of the middle and later years in the entire curriculum. Certain social agencies have begun placing greater emphasis on work with the elderly; for example, the Family Service Association of America did a four-year study, 1961 to 1965, with Ford Foundation support, to upgrade the content of their casework with older people and their families in the forty Family Services agencies in the United States and Canada. See Wasser, Edna: Creative approaches in casework with the aging, Family Service Association of America, New York, 1966.

†From Ryan, W., editor: Distress in the city, Cleveland, 1969, Press of Case Western Reserve University, pp. 16-17.

‡Hamburg, D. A., et al.: Report of ad hoc committee on central fact-gathering data of the American Psychoanalytic Association, Journal of the American Psychoanalytic Association **15**:841-861, 1967.

§Hollingshead, A. B., and Redlich, F. C.: Social class and mental illness, New York, 1958, John Wiley & Sons, Inc.

Myers,* and Brill and Storrow,† have confirmed these findings. They were summarized by Schofield, who called the selection of private psychiatric patients the YAVIS syndrome—young, attractive, verbal, intelligent, and successful.‡

An article in the *Washington Post* in March of 1972 proclaimed "psychiatric clinic aids non-wealthy," yet a psychiatric resident working in the newly formed clinic stated that he and most of his classmates intended to establish traditional private practices when they finished their training. He said "I find it not very rewarding to see a full day of chronic psychotics—the frustrations are fantastic." This is another case in which the provider's needs predominate over the needs of those to be served.

In large and small ways this attitude appears everywhere. Doctors in nursing homes frequently tell patients and their families "Don't call me directly. I'll deal with your problems through the nurse." The premium prices paid for care do not guarantee personal contact with the physician.

Foreign-born doctors present another problem. Approximately 20% of newly licensed physicians in the United States are foreign-trained. Many of them work in public hospitals and clinics because of the medical discrimination against them in private facilities. Thus the poor and the elderly are especially likely to be treated by foreign-born physicians and psychiatrists, who have language and cultural difficulties. In addition the old and the poor are still the training material in the emergency rooms and the wards. Professor Alonzo Yerby once said that the poor have had to barter bodies and dignity in return for medical treatment. This was to have ended with Medicare but it has not.

*Schaffer, L., and Myers, J.: Psychotherapy and social stratification, Psychiatry 17:83-89, 1954.

†Brill, N. W., and Storrow, H. A.: Social class and psychiatric treatment, Archives of General Psychiatry 3:340-344, 1960.

‡Schofield, W.: Psychotherapy: the purchase of friendship. Englewood Cliffs, N. J., 1964, Prentice-Hall, Inc.

Discrimination that prevents utilization of skills

Physicians will be more and more obliged to reconsider their own roles vis-à-vis those of other mental health personnel. There are not enough physicians available or willing to do the mental health work that is being demanded. The American Psychiatric Association supports the requirement of health insurance carriers that psychotherapy be carried out only by physicians or be supervised by them. Thus social workers and psychologists in private practice must be supervised by psychiatrists—an open form of discrimination when there are no empirical data to suggest that this produces more effective work.* In fact there is increasing evidence that the successfulness of psychotherapy is based more on the personality factors of the therapist than on the kind or length of his training or the acquiring of a medical degree. Recently, by imposing more stringent restrictions, Blue Cross and Blue Shield appear to be having second thoughts about allowing nonphysicians to practice at all.

Because of the realities under which the poor, the blacks, the Spanish-speaking, and the elderly exist, social workers, paraprofessionals, community workers, etc. are in many respects better and more appropriately "trained" to offer therapy and other services than are psychiatrists. This is not said to let psychiatrists off the hook with the poor; it is intended to point to the additional knowledge and skills that physicians have yet to learn.

Seymour Halleck, M.D., in discussing the politics of therapy, has stated:

> It is time to acknowledge what many psychiatrists already know: that it is not necessary to have a medical degree . . . to practice good psychotherapy. Even much of the training involved in obtaining a degree in clinical psychology, counseling, guidance or social work may not be absolutely essential to the making of a good psychotherapist. There are many relatively uneducated but otherwise intelligent and sensitive persons in all strata

*Only the government workers' Aetna Insurance Plan covers psychologists without medical referral.

of our society who could and would make excellent therapists if they were properly trained. There has been more disagreement over how much training is needed to make an intelligent and sensitive person into a good therapist than there has been study of the question, but there are enough data to suggest that it can be done.

I foresee a future in which one of the psychiatrist's major functions will be to train nonprofessional therapists to do psychotherapy. Talented people will have to have ready access to psychiatric educational facilities and to the best psychiatric teachers.

These physicians who would resist any tendency to dilute the medical or professional status of psychotherapy must appreciate that in the short run, at least, there is no other humane choice. In our current climate of need and distrust of professionalism, it seems certain that large numbers of nonprofessionals will start doing psychotherapy with or without training. Thousands of persons with little or no training already are trying to help others with encounter or sensitivity experiences and with counseling, formal and informal. Psychiatrists, if they refuse to commit themselves substantially to the training of lay therapists, will renege on an important obligation to their society.*

We would add that one of the major functions of the "nonprofessional therapists" will be to train psychiatrists in the ways of the varied cultures in which they function.

Paraprofessionals

Paraprofessionals are also known as "new professionals," "nonprofessionals," "lay therapists," "community workers," "community aides," "indigenous workers," and even, condescendingly, "subprofessionals." The abundance of names points to the newness of the concept and the disagreement about roles. We prefer the term "paraprofessional" because its Greek roots mean "along side of" professionals, implying a working together rather than working under other staff members. Paraprofessionals should and will play increasingly more important roles in evaluation and treatment of the elderly. A National Institute of Mental Health study of more than 10,000 mental health paraprofessionals reported in 1969 as follows:

Non-professionals are utilized not simply because professional manpower is unavailable but rather to provide new services in innovative ways. Non-professionals are providing such therapeutic functions as individual counseling, activity group therapy, milieu therapy; they are doing case finding; they are playing screening roles of a non-clerical nature; they are helping people adjust to community life; they are providing special skills such as tutoring; they are promoting client self-help through involving clients in helping others having similar problems.*

Paraprofessionals have certain skills and knowledge often lacking in their colleagues. Some may even not know how to read and write, yet understand infinitely well how to provide assistance to others because of their own personal experiences and personalities. One must caution against overromanticizing the capacities of paraprofessionals; if they can effectively help other people, their skills are real enough and need no embroidery. But there are of course those who are ineffective, just as in every profession, and this too should be honestly acknowledged. Training and supervision are crucial to growth and utilization of inherent skills. Reasonable and uniform standards of performance ensure better treatment capabilities.

A "power" issue occurs in most settings where paraprofessionals begin to function effectively and autonomously. Professionals may become threatened, may feel pushed out and insecure, or insulted and angry. It is difficult to share power and status, let alone giving some of it over completely to a new group. Power must be discussed openly, but it *must* be shared.

We have alluded before to the dangers of developing a two-class system of care, with paraprofessionals caring for the poor and psychiatrists caring for the rich. Obviously

---

*From Halleck, Seymour: Politics of therapy, New York, 1971, Science House.

*From Sobey, Francine: Non-professional personnel in mental health programs, a summary report based on a study of projects supported by the National Institute under contract number PH-43 66-967, National Clearinghouse for Mental Health Information Publication No. 5028, Nov., 1969.

this is unhealthy, undesirable, and unfair. All the professions need to work together to utilize each other's assets and provide optimal care.

In the future, various new careers may evolve—one example, a "personal care worker" who would be trained to absorb a variety of functions now distributed among members of many occupations, from home health aide to homemaker to occupational therapy assistant. This would avoid the jurisdictional disputes that now arise, as shown by the homemaker who will not or cannot change a cancer dressing, the home health aide who will not clean the kitchen, etc.

The changing mental health team concept

The community mental health team is likely to become more comprehensive either by its members' taking on more functions or by its absorption of more occupations (e.g., family physicians, physical and occupational therapists, homemakers, visiting nurses, and home health aides in addition to the more traditional participation of psychiatrists, social workers, psychologists, nurses, and nursing assistants). The leadership of teams is becoming diversified—some centers now being headed by nurses, social workers, and psychologists rather than psychiatrists.* By 1967 one third of all centers were directed by nonphysicians.

The following list shows some characteristics of the elderly, per 150,000 population of an average CMHC catchment area (the area designated to be served by a particular center).

- 15,000 over 65 years of age
  - 14,250 in community (95%)
    - 750 in institutions, nursing homes, state hospitals (5%)
- 4,500 over 75 years of age
- 1,100 black people
- 3,750 below "official" poverty line
- 3,000 living alone
- 130 women to 100 men

*The Federal Register states (June 7, 1969), "The direction of a center may be carried out by a properly qualified worker of any one of the mental health professionals."

In the inner city and rural areas where there are considerable numbers of poor, the black and the elderly, there should be an especially greater active recruitment of paraprofessionals as staff members.

STAFF TRAINING

General therapeutic principles should be applicable in all settings—private offices, community mental health centers, hospital wards, service agencies—where older people are seen in a mental health context. Intrapsychic phenomena, mechanisms of defense, developmental theory, the structure of grief, and the dynamics of dependency are some of the key areas of knowledge. Everyone, including the paraprofessionals, should have a working knowledge of this material. Even difficult concepts can be presented in inservice training in a clear, simplified but accurate manner if the person presenting such material takes the time and thoughtfulness to do so.*

Mental health personnel working as a team can teach each other from their collective backgrounds. Anyone with special training or skills should, ideally, share such knowledge openly rather than retaining it as "secret" prerogatives. Psychiatrists have a particular body of information to teach others, but they need to learn much more about social, economic, and cultural considerations and thus will have to be students as well. Social workers can use increased skills and knowledge in understanding and recognizing medical symptoms and in sharpening diagnostic skills. Paraprofessionals are usually weak on formal knowledge of psychopathology and psychodynamics but strong on information about environmental conditions and cultural factors. A successfully working team will eventually end up sharing a mutual body of knowledge, with the end product being qualitatively more useful than the sum

*For general interviewing principles, presented simply and clearly we recommend Annette Garrett's Interviewing—its principles and methods. Also see Redlich, Fredrick, and Freedman, Daniel: The theory and practice of psychiatry, New York, 1966, Basic Books, chap. 7.

of its parts. Individual disciplines can maintain their individual skills while at the same time gaining from and adding to a larger whole. The result can be a rich blend of similarities and differences stimulating and teaching each other. The danger, of course, lies in the competition and power struggles that seem to arise naturally under such circumstances. These reactions should be anticipated and a plan of action agreed upon before they occur. There is no reason why human beings who have chosen a career of helping others should not be able to help themselves in working peacefully and constructively with their colleagues. Much is theoretically known about group behavior. It remains for us to apply it in our hopefully humane dealings with each other as mental health practitioners.

In working specifically with the elderly, it is safe to assume that all staff members will have some attitudes toward older people that are unclear, untrue, and even prejudicial. A major task in staff training is to clear up uncertainty and misinformation, and to face up to negative countertransference and ageist feelings. Sometimes this can be accomplished by simply providing accurate information. At other times it may require sensitivity training of a sort that brings a staff member's feelings to his awareness and invites and stimulates him to reexamine them. Supervisory sessions, both group and individual, are useful. It is wise to see many kinds of older people in many different settings and circumstances. It is also desirable to work with persons from all age groups and not overspecialize—a life cycle view is helpful.

Inservice training, planning, and problem-solving programs are a way of wrestling with staff conflicts and antagonisms when they arise, providing a forum for resolving countertransference, setting policy and programs, and planning formal and informal learning experiences. Outside teachers and consultants can be used to avoid inbreeding of ideas and outlook. Staff members generally rebel at the thought of extensive outside reading, which should be kept at a minimum and be highly selected for its clarity and direct usefulness.* We have found that one of the best outside reading sources is the daily newspaper; nearly everyone already reads it, and it contains an endlessly fascinating mixture of material regarding health care, welfare, public policy, economic and social conditions, and the like. Special-interest newspapers, including local black or ethnic publications can be pertinent.

Research should be built into any ongoing program. Any unusual observations of the older person or his family, responses to drugs, etc. should be recorded in a special observation book kept available for that purpose, as well as in the person's individual records. Such a practice can result in serendipitous findings that would otherwise be lost and may add to an accumulating body of general knowledge about old people. The material could be available for staff discussion, written research, etc. Another form of research is a routine, periodic reevaluation of the program or service itself. These research methods can both be uncomplicated, do-it-yourself ways of learning more and of revitalizing services. Cooperative and more sophisticated research can be arranged from time to time among various similar institutions or services in an area. Grants can be obtained for applied research studying delivery systems. The Health Service and Mental Health Administration (HSMHA) in Rockville, Maryland, can be contacted for ideas and support.

TREATMENT POINTS TO REMEMBER

What's in a name?

What we call someone often defines how we will treat him or, at least, how we view him. What should an older person be called? Some of the names one hears are aged, elderly, senior citizen, retiree, gramps, granny, old biddy, old fogy, old gal, or just plain old. If the older person comes for mental health care, is he or she a patient? a client? or (an unfortunate but popular term used by medical students) an old crock? In our

---

*See references at end of each chapter as well as lists of films and fiction in Appendix.

experience people prefer the simplest and most dignified title. "Older person" can be used for anyone from a 60-year-old to one of 90 or more years. "Elderly" is accepted in advanced old age—the seventies and eighties. "Aged" to some has implications of decrepitude and is not as favored. We have used the terms "older person" and "elderly" interchangeably and have referred to the older person as "patient" only when it was confusing not to do so. "Patient" implies a limited role in relationship to a doctor or therapist, and we are interesting in presenting the older person as a whole. Viewing someone as a patient encourages his self-evaluation as dependent, inferior.

In contacts with particular older persons it is important to respectfully address them as Mr. or Mrs. unless they specifically asked to be called by their first names. Young students, interns, and trainees are especially tempted to brashly use first names, either through habit or as an attempt to overcome feelings of intimidation from older people. Old people may feel insulted. Black and other minority elderly are even more sensitive and angered or depressed at being called by their first names. The presumptuous use of first names or nicknames implies a careless, thoughtless, even contemptuous attitude toward the feelings of older people who grew up at a time when this was a demeaning and disrespectful gesture. In the case of black people, they have too long been known only as "James," or something similar, while the white person was "Mr. Jones." Hopefully there will be many more black, Chicano and other minority-group professionals who will both act as advocates for patient dignity and set higher standards of care for their white colleagues. The name one is called is only a small part of the problem.

Who decides?

Treatment is a collaboration between the older person, his family, and mental health personnel. Decisions should be mutually agreed upon unless physical or mental incapacity prevents this.

Need for full attention to physical complaints

It is very important emotionally for the older person to feel that medically everything possible is being done, even when there is really little that can be done. To exhaust the limits of the possible is very reassuring. The arthritic pain, the hypertensive flare-up, the constipation, nerves, irritable colon syndrome, unsightly varicose veins, stress incontinence, senile vaginitis, urinary tract infections, dry and itchy skin, gout, parkinsonism, osteoporosis, cold extremities, painful calves, fatigue, edema, irregular pulse, headaches, dizziness, shortness of breath, and confusion are all common complaints that must be treated with seriousness and competence. Sometimes side effects of the treatments must be treated. For instance, magnesium–aluminum hydroxide helps alleviate gastric distress associated with prolonged salicylate therapy for arthritis.

It is extraordinarily painful for a human being to be sold short, to be considered unreachable, beyond help, having received the "maximum benefits" of physical therapy, etc. Imagine the sense of numbing despair. It is equally true, of course, that doing for the sake of doing can be a pointless charade. Necessary is a continuing collaboration, with objective assessment including the person's morale. Treatment should never be discontinued in a vacuum without explanation and some acceptance from the patient. To do so is to risk depression and despair.

Because Medicare does not cover physical work-ups, mental health personnel should become alert to signs of physical illness. For example, early signs of peripheral vascular disease (arteriosclerosis obliterans) such as mild calf pain, loss of hair on toes, slow or unusual toenail growth, cold sensitivity, and shiny skin may be presented as part of an older person's complaint. Early diagnosis obviously means early treatment.

Older people often have a dilemma with regard to their family doctor. Usually one's doctor is older than oneself. As one gets older that is often disadvantageous. It would be ageist to recommend against the older, experienced doctor; but the potential reality of retirement, disability, or death of such a physician must not be overlooked. In some cases this can be overcome by building a parallel relationship with a younger colleague of the doctor. Group practice is another solution.

Psychoanalytic theory as it applies to older people

Psychoanalytic theory provides a valuable means of viewing old age. The ego, id, superego, and ego ideal are useful constructs. In the presence of brain damage, impulses may overrun inhibitions; that is, the id may overpower the superego and the ego, executive functions having been damaged. Incomplete fulfillment of one's ego ideal occupies an important part of the content of the life review in both the brain-damaged and the unaffected. In the person not brain-damaged, considerations pertinent to ego psychology indicate the continuing capacity of the elderly ego to grow and the superego to become more flexible. The notion of the weakening of the id or libido (vitality) with age is reminiscent of Aristotle's observation contained in the *Rhetoric* that the old love and hate less strongly. We do not yet know enough about the outer influences on ego structure or even the id to be certain how intrinsic any observed weakening of the id or ego may be.

The full range of transference possibilities can be seen in the elderly as with any age group. One may see role reversal, with the older person taking the role of parent to the therapist. Coercive, dominating, or patronizing behavior may occur. In older people who manifest helplessness, the therapist may become imbued with magical powers.

How to estimate treatability

When in doubt, treat and see if improvement occurs. This is of course an obvious rule with respect to reversible brain syndromes but should also be applied elsewhere. Improvements can occur in people who are considered hopeless. Overt behavior is too often taken as innate rather than adaptive. On the other hand, patients with apparently positive treatment possibilities may not respond well at all because of hidden, underlying processes. Treatment should be used to both rule in and rule out a diagnosis and should not be separated from evaluation.

Emotional self-treatment

Much mental health treatment is done by older people on their own. One should be alert for this and encourage it. We include an example of Christmas greeting oratory, which hints at self-treatment in progress. A description of catastrophe is followed by the implication of recovery in a vacation resort. The life review search for names in the cemetery shows a self-conscious sense of how this must appear to others. Finally the last stanza proclaims another year of life over, with a sense of stoic realism and a certain air of self-congratulation.

> "Again this year the Christmas spree
> Was held at our house, but no tree.
> The old folks failed to get up steam
> To decorate a tree, 'twould seem.
>
> • • •
>
> "Then finally ———'s luck ran out.
> She'd stretched it far without a doubt.
> She's fallen many times before
> But this time hit the "ice box" door.
> The door won out—broke a rib.
> It hurt a lot, and that's no fib.
>
> "Last fall we took another trip.
> We went by car, not plane or ship.
> New England and New York our goal,
> Back roads, slow speed, we paid no toll.
>
> "——— prowled a cemetery there
> He came away with notes for fair.
> His family tree is growing big,
> But there's a lot more dope to dig
> Before the job is really done.
> It's queer what some folks think is fun.
>
> • • •
>
> "Now Year's end's drawing near again,
> Just like it always does, but then
> Each time it does we're one year older,
> And ev'ry winter seems some colder
> We're both alive and fairly well.
> How we hold up, just time will tell."

Use of nonverbal communication

Because of the greater likelihood of physical impairments, nonverbal communication can facilitate treatment and in some cases become a dominant part of the relationship. Persons who are hard of hearing need to be able to see the lips of the person talking to them, in order to "read" them. (We all do this to some degree, and it is not hard to learn to read lips.) It may be necessary to speak very close to the ear, and it is important to learn if one ear is a "good ear," better than the other. Eye contact also is useful in relating; one can learn to "read" the eyes of a stroke victim or of someone with throat problems or certain forms of aphasia. Older people seem to be very alert and responsive to the tone and inflection of an interviewer's voice—able to judge rather accurately the personality behind the voice. Touch and tactile communication become extremely important. There is often a desire to be literally "in touch" with the person speaking. People who are very sick may respond more to holding their hand than to talking. Shared tears of happiness or sadness on the part of both mental health personnel and older people are common and can be therapeutic. When the older person is physically unable to talk, interviews can be carried out via intuition: the therapist surmises what is on the older person's mind and verbalizes it for him; then the person signals in some way, by a smile, nod, frown, if he is being understood. Affection from an older person should be accepted graciously and warmly—and returned—when appropriate. A kiss on the cheek or pat on the hand for the therapist may become part of the ritual of therapy.

Patience is needed for those struggling to speak. We never shall forget the 75-year-old woman who had had a stroke and was attempting to express her emotional feelings about her suffering. She struggled mightly for a number of minutes but the words just would not come. Finally everything fell momentarily into place and she shouted "Shit" to the heavens, with a triumphant voice and a gleam in her eye—summing up her feelings succinctly. We and she alike considered it a therapeutic victory.

"Listening" as a form of therapy

Listening is an important ingredient in therapy with the elderly.* Some older people have a great need to talk, and their talking should not be dismissed as boring or garrulousness. Reminiscence has meaning for the life review that occurs in nearly all people. Feelings of guilt that result from such reminiscing should not be treated as irrational, to be patched up by cheerful and patronizing reassurance. Guilt is as real in old age as in other any age and must be dealt with therapeutically.

Race and culture—language differences

In Chapter 6 and elsewhere we have emphasized the importance of racial, cultural, and ethnic backgrounds in diagnosis and treatment. We wish to add here the problems of language differences, whether these be regional dialect, slang, or accent differences or use of a totally different language—such as Spanish, Chinese, or German. For example, between 1959 and 1971, some 600,000 Cubans fled from their native land to the United States. By 1971, 40,000 were over 65 and 150,000 were between 45 and 64. Nearly half the exiles settled in Florida. Members of minority groups should be employed in every level of mental health care. Bilingual interpreters having skill in slang or dialect interpretation, as well as actual dual language ability, should be used to train staff, provide direct interpretation, and help older members of minority groups obtain needed services. In addition hospitals and services that hire foreign personnel, including doctors, have a responsibility to adequately train them in English or provide interpretors. Older persons should not have

---

*One might imagine the creation of a National Listeners Corps whose members would function in nursing and old age homes, mental hospitals, etc. One might predict consequent reductions in nursing services, drug use, etc. Older people themselves and high school students would be appropriate listeners.

to bear the burden of treatment personnel's language handicaps.

Myth of termination of treatment

Older persons need the opportunity for continuing support and easy re-availability of services, even when a particular problem has been resolved. Traditional psychiatric and social work thought stresses working through to termination of mental health care, and there is a considerable literature on countertransference and the problem of termination of treatment. With older people it may be necessary to continue the treatment and care, varying it according to changing conditions until a quite different termination—namely, death.

Three directions to move in treatment

Older people need a *restitution capacity,* the ability to compensate for and recover from deeply felt losses. They also need the opportunity for *growth and renewal,* which represent the opposite of obsolescence or stagnation. This can be defined as the effective striving toward discovery and utilization of innate potential. It can mean a rediscovery or even a first discovery of the self. Jung has written of individuation as one of the tasks of late life. Consequent to a successful psychotherapeutic process (or occurring naturally in a private life review) one may see either the emergence of a qualitatively different personality or identity or a renewal.

> I for one have never touched bottom in self, nor even struck against the surface, nor the outline, the boundaries of the self. On the contrary, I feel the self as an energy only which expands and contracts.
>
> BERNARD BERENSON AT 83

And finally they require *perspective,* the ability to see themselves and their lives as wholes rather than fixating on any particular aspect. This is the ability to perceive one's place in the world, free from distortion, and extends to both the outer world and the inner world. It is the sense of "putting one's house in order." Inherent in perspective is a time framework that includes both past and future orientation and that is longitudinal rather than merely situational. The end result is to make acceptable "sense" out of one's life.

We shall be discussing other treatment directions in later chapters: what to do when that which is "possible" becomes limited for older persons; the psychotherapy surrounding death, loss and their emotional trappings; and advocacy—including the therapist as advocate.

RIGHT TO TREATMENT

The right to treatment will hopefully soon be more than a moral obligation—it will be a legal right and requirement. Mental health personnel should not have the unjustified luxury of "deciding" whether to offer services or treatment or of being able to weigh the wisdom of expending resources on the old. (See Chapter 11.) Mental health care is the promotion of human well-being and the alleviation of suffering—from birth to death. If we are serious about this, it must be a right rather than a privilege.

REFERENCES

Aries, P.: Centuries of childhood: a social history of family life, translated by R. Baldick, New York, 1962, Alfred A. Knopf.

Bazelon, D.: Lake vs. Cameron: readings in law and psychiatry. In Allen, R. C., Ferster, E., and Rubin, J. G., editors: Psychiatric hospitalization, Baltimore, 1968, Johns Hopkins Press.

Birnbaum, M.: Some comments on the right to treatment, Archives of General Psychiatry **13**: 33-45, 1965.

Busse, E. W.: Therapeutic implications of basic research with the aged, Strecker Monograph Series No. 4, Philadelphia, 1967, The Institute of Pennsylvania Hospital.

Butler, R. N.: Research and clinical observations on the psychological reactions to physical changes with age. In Proceedings of the Conference on Psychological Reactions to Physical Changes with Age, Rochester, Minn., 1966, Mayo Clinic.

Butler, R. N.: Toward a psychiatry of the life cycle: Implications of socio-psychological studies of the aging process for policy and practice of psychotherapy. In Simon, A., and Epstein, L. J., editors: Aging and modern society—psychosocial and medical aspects, Washington, D. C., 1968, American Psychiatric Association.

Butler, R. N.: The effects of medical and health

progress on the social and economic aspects of the life cycle, Industrial Gerontology **1**:1-9, 1969.

Butler, R. N., and Sulliman, Lillian G.: Psychiatric contact with the community-resident, emotionally disturbed elderly, Journal of Nervous and Mental Diseases **137**:180-186, 1963.

Education and training in gerontology—1970, The Gerontologist **10** (1 & 2):153-164, 1970.

Feldstein, D.: Do we need professions in our society? Professionalism vs. consumerism, Social Work **16**:5-12, Oct., 1971.

Frankl, V.: Man's search for meaning (original, 1959), New York, 1963, Washington Square Press, Inc.

Garrett, Annette: Interviewing—its principles and methods, New York, 1942, Family Service Association of America (16th printing, 1958).

Goldfarb, A. I.: Psychotherapy of aged persons. I. The orientation of staff in a home for the aged, Mental Hygiene **37**:76-83, 1953.

Group for the Advancement of Psychiatry: The aged and community mental health: a guide to program development, vol. 8, series No. 81, Nov., 1971.

Halleck, S.: Politics of therapy, New York, 1971, Science House.

Henry, W. E., Sims, J. H., and Spray, S. L.: The fifth profession, San Francisco, 1971, Jossey-Bass.

Hollingshead, A. B., and Redlich, F. C.: Social class and mental illness, New York, 1958, John Wiley & Sons, Inc.

Noyes, Arthur, and Kolb, Lawrence: Modern clinical psychiatry, Philadelphia, 1958, W. B. Saunders Co.

Office of Research and Statistics, Social Security Administration: Financing mental health care under medicare and medicaid, Research Report No. 37, Washington, D. C., 1971, U. S. Government Printing Office.

Perlin, S., and Butler, R. N.: Physiological-psychological-psychiatric interrelationships. In Birren, J. E., Butler, R. N., Greenhouse, S. W., Sokoloff, L., and Yarrow, Marian R., editors: Human aging: a biological and behavioral study, Public Health Publication No. 986, Washington, D. C., 1963, U. S. Government Printing Office.

Reed, L., Myers, Evelyn, and Scheidemandel, Patricia: Health insurance and psychiatric care: utilization and costs, 1972, Washington, D. C., 1972, American Psychiatric Association.

Ryan, W., editor: Distress in the city, Cleveland, 1969, Press of Case Western Reserve University.

Schaffer, L., and Myers, J.: Psychotherapy and social stratification, Psychiatry **17**:83-89, 1954.

9

DIAGNOSTIC EVALUATION: HOW TO DO A WORK-UP

PURPOSE OF EVALUATION

The mental health evaluation in its simplest sense is a method of looking at the problems of old people, arriving at decisions as to what precisely is wrong, and concluding what can be done to alleviate or eliminate these problems. The older person and the evaluator together try to discover whether the problems are originating from inside (long-term personality factors or personal reactions to situations) or from outside (environmental causes); whether there are physical components; and whether the problems represent a new, first-time experience, an old experience with new implications, or something new superimposed on already existing difficulties. A gathering together and assessment of the many factors that affect the emotional life of an elderly person is the process by which such evaluation is carried out. Evaluators use historical data from the person's past; current medical, psychiatric, and social examinations; and their own personal interactions with the individual to get a many-sided and hopefully coherent picture of what is happening.

On the basis of the evaluation, decisions must be made as to reasonable, reachable treatment goals: can the problem at hand be reversed or merely ameliorated; should treatment be aimed at total recovery, partial restitution, maintaining the status quo, or—of equal importance—supporting the person during some inevitable decline? Is environmental change indicated; would direct medical treatment be useful; or does the individual himself need therapy—whether physical, social or emotional? These are some of the possibilities. It is of course necessary to know what resources are available for treatment purposes: the older person's own emotional and physical capabilities, the assets in his family and social structure, and the kind of services and support available in his community.

An aggravating, ever present factor in working with and planning for older people is the difficulty in obtaining needed services. For example, it is increasingly evident that the elderly make good use of individual psychotherapy; yet it is seldom offered, even when they can afford to pay. In some cases such services are not available for any age group, and the elderly are excluded along with everyone else. However, in many instances, a service may be offered to the general public but old people find themselves put at the bottom of the waiting list or totally denied access to what is theoretically available. This is an example of institutionalized ageism—discrimination on the basis of age. All too many mental health personnel, because of training and background, assume that certain services are not applicable for elderly people and thereby deny treatment possibilities. We hope that Part II of this book will help to overcome the pessimism that has prevailed regarding rehabilitation and treatment in old age.

CONDITIONS FOR A GOOD EVALUATION

Rapport

It is an old mental health principle that the first contact for evaluation is also the first therapeutic treatment hour, the two cannot be separated. Unfortunately for many older people it may be the first and last time they will have a structured opportunity to talk about their problems and feelings. As discussed more fully in Chapter 8, the older person needs to sense certain things in order to feel comfortable about revealing himself: (1) that the interviewer is not turned off or frightened by the physical or mental changes in old age but can accept these changes as a matter of fact and can see through them to the person inside; (2) that the interviewer knows what he is talking about when he deals with old age (the psychological aspect of being old); (3) that the interviewer understands the social problems of old age, having a broad and accurate knowledge of conditions as they exist for the majority of the elderly; (4) that the interviewer himself has the professional skills combined with empathy which will inspire the older person to trust him with his confidence, in the expectation that help will follow.

Confidentiality and privileged communication

Confidentiality is a critical element in gaining an accurate history and in establishing and maintaining rapport. "Privilege" is the legal right of the person to privacy of communication. With the advent of the team concept, using paraprofessionsl and peer review, the legal situation has not yet been clarified. In most states, a patient can sue the medical physician who does not preserve privileged communication, but what about the nurse, the social worker, the nursing assistant, etc.? The increase in insurance forms and computer use complicates the picture. Until clarification, it is essential that practitioners recognize the seriousness of protecting the patient's/client's privacy. For instance, a designing relative may be trying to get an old person's house and attempt to gain significant information from mental health personnel. It is well known that the privacy of the poor who are served in community mental health centers, public clinics, and the like is less protected than that of the privately paying person. Legal suits may curb such practices.

Setting

All persons should be interviewed in dignified, private surroundings—not on the run, in public hallways and open clinic areas.

Time

The old person should be given more time when there is evidence of intellectual retardation (slowing), whether this be due to depression or to organic changes. Interviews and examinations should be unhurried and relaxed. When organicity, severe depression, or paranoid reactions are suspected, there must be several sessions, preferably at different times of day, to take into account variation in general and cerebral circulation. Early-morning confusion—before the older person has shaken off sleep—can be mistaken as chronic, fixed disorientation. There is also a "sundown syndrome"—the increased disorientation and agitation at night resulting from loss of visual orientation when daylight is gone or electric lights are turned off. If this is organically based, it has been called "senile nocturnal agitation."

Clarity of purpose

It is beneficial to clarify with the older person the reason for his seeing a mental health evaluator and what he can expect during and as a result of the evaluation. It is usually wise to make certain the person understands the setting in which he is being seen (a clinic, a counseling agency, etc.) unless this is totally obvious. An older person also has the right to know who is interviewing or examining him (a psychiatrist, mental health specialist, visiting nurse, etc.).

Recognizing the Goldstein catastrophic reaction*

The Goldstein catastrophic reaction describes the tendency of a brain-damaged person to become flooded with anxiety and irritability when confronted with a task he cannot handle. Weinberg's "exclusion of stimuli" may have a similar basis. Any examina-

*Goldstein, K.: Aftereffects of brain injuries in war and their evaluation and treatment, New York, 1942, Grune & Stratton, pp. 71-73, 77-78, 93.

tion may provoke this reaction and thus complicate or delay findings. Careful, skilled use of the interview can alleviate unnecessary stress by being aware of the reaction of the person. (It is also, of course, important to note the presence of this reaction in diagnosing brain damage.)

HOW COMPREHENSIVE SHOULD AN EVALUATION BE?

We recognize the range of opinion regarding the length, style, and content of an evaluation and the methods by which it should be conducted. A number of variations can be justified on the basis of the treatment method and setting under consideration as well as the individual's specific request for help. For example, an elderly person wanting only brief assistance in dealing with feelings about retirement may not require the same work-up as the person needing evaluation for placement in a nursing home. But in general we feel that a comprehensive evaluation has much to recommend it. There is an astounding lack of uniformity about what happens when an old person meets up with mental health practitioners or institutional facilities. Even routine information may not be gathered. An individual may or may not get treatment, which may or may not be based on a solid evaluation and recommendation. Busy agencies and personnel with limited resources plead that their hands are tied. Yet even the shoddiest medical facility or the busiest family doctor would not be able to deal quite as cursorily with patients if they presented physical (rather than emotional) complaints—at least some minimal work-up would be done. Nonprivate mental health specialists have operated, often out of necessity and sometimes out of laxness, in a piecemeal, second-rate manner and then have had to take the blame for their "failures."

Court suits are now being instituted claiming the "right to treatment" for persons requiring care, particularly in the case of the poor. It is hoped that this will result in more meaningful standards of mental health treatment. The old person not only has a right to expect treatment (as opposed to custodial care or no care) but also to expect that it be based on a thorough evaluation.

The following categories of treatment encompass the major services to the elderly in terms of evaluation:

Emergency-crisis intervention
Evaluation for brief service
Evaluation for extended service
Evaluation for referral elsewhere (e.g., a mental health evaluation for referral to a psychiatric hospital or nursing home)
Evaluation for legal purposes (psychiatric commitment, guardianship, etc.)

In all these categories a complete evaluation is indicated for optimal and often time-saving intervention. An emergency, of course, requires attention to the immediate crisis but with older people a crisis often points to underlying problems and requires extended periods of recovery. Thus an evaluation can be begun as soon as the emergency subsides. The evaluation should ideally fulfill a *preventive, screening* function as well as a diagnostic one. As with all ages, the problem first presented by the elderly is often not their major or only difficulty. They may be reluctant to reveal intimate matters or be fearful of appearing demanding and complaining. They sometimes may deny actual problems or be totally unaware of their presence. The value of multiphasic screening (through a routine battery of tests) in mental health care may eventually be recognized. Such screening for prevention and early detection of illness is now becoming a part of physical health treatment in public clinics. Private doctors have been doing this routinely for a long time. When old people do not receive competent mental health care, the twin culprits are usually lack of finances for private care and prejudice against them in both public and private circles because they are old.

WHAT CONSTITUTES A "DIAGNOSIS"?

A diagnosis is not simply a matter of psychiatric nomenclature that an evaluator, by the process of elimination, plucks out of the APA's *Diagnostic and Statistical Manual.* Staffs, particularly in state hospitals and research centers, tend to obsess over a psychiatric diagnosis. The latter is important, but most important is an understanding of the total problem—not just intrapsychic conflicts. One must know the strength of the person psychologically (e.g., his defenses and personality assets); his physical capabilities; and the familial, social, and cultural climate and structure of his life. The direct and immediate environmental influence upon people's lives is finally receiving its due share of importance along with the more traditional emphasis on early developmental and constitutional factors of personality. It is vital also to recognize the vast implications of racism in its institutional and personal forms as they affect the lives of the black, Indian, Mexican, Chinese and other minority and ethnic elderly (Chapters 1 and 6). The serious mental disorders and the emotional reactions seen in old age are multicausal.

A problem may not only have many causes; it may itself be multiple, that is, a combination of many problems. Simon and Cahan have rightly stated that "the doctrine of the single diagnosis, as it occurs in many psychiatric institutions, has probably interfered with a more complete understanding of the individual geriatric patient."* A serious case in point is a diagnosis of senile, arteriosclerotic, or other chronic brain disease, while omitting an additional diagnosis of superimposed, reversible brain syndrome. Another serious and frequent oversight is the failure to recognize the emotional component or overlay to physical illness of the body or brain. An evaluator must search for possible combinations of problems, where some may be less obvious than others but no less damaging.

Diagnosis is best viewed as a continuing, dynamic assessment, particularly in the case of the elderly. Old age, indeed life at any age, is more similar to a motion picture than a still photograph; it is constantly changing. Because of this ongoing, altering process, evaluation too must be continuous, with treatment intervention varied accordingly.

*From Simon, A., and Cahan, R.: The acute brain syndrome in geriatric patients. In Mendel, W. M., and Epstein, L. J., editors: Acute psychotic reaction, Washington, D. C., 1963, Psychiatric Research Report No. 16, p. 10.

A BASIC EVALUATION

The concept of "multiple evaluations" describes the way in which an old person's problems can best be diagnosed. A basic evaluation should include a core collection of material: basic personal information; a psychiatric assessment; a medical assessment; a social-cultural assessment with the older person and, if possible, his relatives; and an on-the-spot evaluation of the home environment where indicated. In addition, any number of special evaluations may be deemed valuable in arriving at a clear understanding of the older person (e.g., special medical tests, nutritional evaluation, etc.) The following outlines list the elements of such an appraisal, as well as some of the special consultants who can be used. Busse has also provided a useful summary of evaluative procedures. It is important that members of consultative specialties be willing to see older people as well as being readily available to people of all incomes. The evaluator may have to act on the older person's behalf in persuading reluctant consultants to participate, particularly if they are being used for the first time. The professional bias against old people remains an interference to collaboration and must be confronted wherever possible.

COMPREHENSIVE BASIC EXAMINATION OF THE ELDERLY PERSON

- Basic background information: Personal, family, economic, social
- Psychiatric assessment
  - Personal and family history
  - Psychiatric examination, including
    - Mental Status Evaluation (or, if time is limited, the Mental Status Questionnaire)
    - Psychiatric Symptoms Checklist
- Medical assessment
  - Medical history, including reports from family doctor
  - Physical examination, including
    - Electroencephalogram (brain wave test)
    - Skull films
    - Electrocardiogram
    - Chest roentgenogram (x-ray film)

- Laboratory tests
  - Complete blood count
  - Hematocrit
  - Urinalysis
  - Fasting blood sugar
  - Blood urea nitrogen
  - Serology
- Hearing test: Audiometry
- Vision examination
  - Refraction
  - Glaucoma check
  - Retinal examination
  - Visual fields examination (peripherals; centrals)
- Dental examination

Sociocultural assessment
- Intimates: Family and friends
- Financial status/work
- Housing/transportation
- Social status and participation

On-the-spot home evaluation (where indicated)

SPECIAL EVALUATIONS

Additional evaluation of the elderly person
- Psychological tests
  - Bender Visual-Motor Gestalt Test
  - Wechsler Adult Intelligence Scale (WAIS)
  - Kent E-G-Y Test
  - Raven Progressive Matrices
- Medical tests
  - Lumbar puncture (for pressure, cells, protein, serology)
  - Brain scan
  - Pneumoencephalogram
  - Angiogram
- Other specialties to consider
  - Internal medicine
  - Neurology
  - Ophthalomology
  - Otorhinolaryngology (ENT)
  - Physiatry/Rehabilitation
  - Dermatology
  - Radiology
  - Podiatry
  - Physical therapy
  - Occupational therapy
  - Pharmacology
  - Homemakers–Home health aides
  - Visiting nurses
  - Recreation
  - Education
  - Employment opportunities
  - Home economics
  - Nutrition/Dietetics
  - Transportation
  - Legal services
  - Shopping services
  - Meals-on-Wheels
  - Visitation services
  - Telephone reassurance service

Basic background information

The question of how to collect background information or "histories" for use in mental health evaluations has always been a controversial and confused one. This is largely because mental health as we define it today encompasses every aspect of a person's life, and the task of collecting so much information boggles the mind. Add to this the need to take a longitudinal life cycle view, as in the evaluations of older people, and the problem grows. Medical doctors can limit themselves to the body and its ills, traditional psychiatrists to "inner" problems, social service workers to "outer" difficulties, and ministers to spiritual life—but mental health personnel must familiarize themselves with the whole picture in order to prescribe and carry out sound treatment.

Collection of basic background information should be done in a manner that ensures comprehensiveness without being rigid. The goal is a high quality evaluation, whether it takes place in a private hospital, a public clinic, a doctor's office, or a nursing home. The following elements are important considerations in planning data or "history" collection:

1. The method of obtaining the mass of data desired must be flexible in terms of how it is collected and who can collect it. Some psychiatric facilities may provide only one interview for this purpose while others can offer a more leisurely accumulation of the data during actual course of treatment. Anyone, from psychiatrists to paraprofessionals, should be able to do initial interviewing. At times, the older person's relatives or even the older person himself may be the most appropriate person to collect the data, independent of outside assistance. Certain material—name, addresses, reason for needing help, etc.—naturally must be available shortly after the first contact; but other background material should be collected in a way that is compatible with the needs and personality of the older person, the realistic working conditions faced by mental health staffs, and the setting in which service is being given. We stress, however,

that the end result should be a broad and thorough review of the person's history and current life situation.

2. Data should be in a transferable form, able to be passed from one staff member to another, and from one treatment setting to another, with the patient's permission. This is particularly true with older people because numerous personnel may participate in their care and the elderly frequently move from one setting or agency to another as their conditions change. Sharing information is timesaving and protects patients from repeating themselves—the confidentiality being maintained by sharing appropriately.

3. Data collection ideally serves an organizing function for experienced evaluators (by organizing their manner of thinking about a person) and a teaching function for less experienced personnel (by guiding them in what to look for and what to consider important).

4. The life history is organizing for the patient. Using the opportunity to review one's life—to take an inventory and to evaluate the meaning(s) of one's life—should be encouraged. The sense of approaching death is believed to be related to the life review. Reactions to one's death—equanimity, fear, or denial—should be appraised. The life history becomes both diagnostic and therapeutic. We consider the concept of the life review in several contexts in this book (Chapters 3 and 12).

5. Research potential should be built into any data collection system. There are still tremendous gaps in our knowledge about old age, and direct treatment contact is, of course, a rich source of information about the elderly.

As a result of our own work experiences in various hospitals, welfare departments, community mental health clinics, nursing homes, research, and private practice, we have devised a method of collecting data, which combines for us an adaptable format with a thorough content. (See the Personal Mental Health Data Form for Older Persons, pp. 149 to 163.) It can be compiled either piecemeal or all at once, and at any time during contact with a patient. For example, when seeing a person in crisis, one must deal with the immediate situation and may not be able to obtain much background data until the crisis subsides. When we know we will be seeing the person over a period of time, we generally fill out the form ourselves in an unhurried manner as the data accumulate. However, in a period of crisis or shortage of time, a relative may complete the form, either at home or in the office. (Material of course is not as rich as when the patient is directly involved.) In other cases it is appropriate and even highly therapeutic for the patient to fill out the form alone. Patients report that it is a life review process, which is organizing to them in evaluating themselves and planning for their future. We would generally not recommend this for patients having obvious severe organic brain syndrome, poor eyesight, or severe hand tremors or for those who would become frustrated without help. It can on the other hand be extremely useful for the hard-of-hearing patient (with whom interviewing is difficult) and for those who pride themselves on their independence. We also use the form this way for patients who are entering group therapy and may be seen in only one individual, pregroup session.

A completed personal data form is like a baseline electrocardiogram. It indicates the person's present situation and provides a standard against which to measure changes in the future. It is often not accurate to think in terms of eventual "discharge from treatment" for the old in the same way as for the young. Many will need various kinds of service the rest of their lives, thus it will save time to collect proper information right from the start. Mental health personnel need to review their own thinking and attitudes about the quality of evaluation given to older people. A sloppy, haphazard approach cannot be rationalized as time-saving nor as humane care.

Psychiatric assessment

The traditional psychiatric interview derives from the medical model; it can be an

Text continued on p. 163.

PERSONAL MENTAL HEALTH DATA FORM FOR OLDER PEOPLE

1. Basic background information Date: ____________

A. Patient/client's full name: ____________

Age: ______ Complete birth date: ____________

Birthplace: ____________

Social Security No.: ____________ Medicare No.: ____________

Medicaid No.: ____________ Public Assistance No.: ____________

Where spent childhood to age 21: ____________

Present addresses: Residence: ____________
(Street)

____
(City) (State) (ZIP)

Work: ____________
(Street)

____
(City) (State) (ZIP)

Telephone numbers: Residence: ____________

Work: ____________

Data source:

Name of person supplying data: ____________

Name of person recording data: ____________

Date first seen: ____________

Referred by: ____________

In case of emergency: Current doctor(s)

Name: ____________

Address: ____________

Phone: ____________ Specialty: ____________

In case of emergency: Nearest relatives and/or friends

Name: ____________

Address: ____________ Phone: ____________

Name: ____________

Address: ____________ Phone: ____________

Continued.

PERSONAL MENTAL HEALTH DATA FORM FOR OLDER PEOPLE—cont'd

B. Religion

Of family of origin: ______

Present affiliation, if any: ______

Active? ______

Any internal religious conflict? ______

C. Ethnic, racial, or cultural background: ______

Year of immigration to U. S.: ______

From: ______

D. Family status

Present marital status: Single: ______ Separated: ______ Widowed: ______

Married: ______ Divorced: ______

Marriage, most current: Full name of spouse: ______

Age difference: ______ (years older) ______ (years younger)

Religion: ______

Place of birth: ______

Courtship duration: ______

Date of marriage (month, day, year): ______

Closest anniversary attained: ______

Date of separation, divorce, or widowhood (month, day, year): ______

(Specify which): ______

Marriage, previous: Full name of spouse: ______

Age difference: ______ (years older) ______ (years younger)

Religion: ______

Place of birth: ______

Courtship duration: ______

Date of marriage (month, day, year): ______

Closest anniversary attained: ______

Date of separation, divorce, or widowhood (month, day, year): ______

(Specify which): ______

Other marriages (describe): ______

Children:	Name	Sex	Age	Address	Date and cause of death?
1. ______					
2. ______					
3. ______					
4. ______					

(Use additional space for children if needed; include miscarriages, stillbirths, etc.)

Your age when last child left home: ______

Grandchildren:	Name	Sex	Age	Address	Date and cause of death?
1. ______					
2. ______					
3. ______					
4. ______					

(Use additional space for grandchildren if needed.)

Your age at birth of first grandchild: ______

Members of current household (Include everyone who lives with you.)

	Name	Sex	Age	Relationship to you
1. ______				
2. ______				
3. ______				

E. Education (years of schooling): ______

Description of schools:	Name of school	Year of graduation	Degree
Grammar: ______			
High school: ______			
College: ______			
Graduate or professional school: ______			
Later courses; other education: ______			

Continued.

PERSONAL MENTAL HEALTH DATA FORM FOR OLDER PEOPLE—cont'd

Self-rating, as a student (check) Above average: ______

Average: ______

Below average: ______

Any honors, awards, scholarships: ______

F. Work

Preretirement

Occupation or profession: ______

Second occupation or profession: ______

(Describe): ______

Last three positions and the durations of employment:

1. ______
2. ______
3. ______

Occupation of spouse: ______

Major work interests: ______

Military service: ______

Did you experience age discrimination at work? ______

(Describe): ______

Postretirement

Did you work after retirement? ______

If so, describe employment: ______

How many hours per week? ______

Employed or self-employed? ______

Did you experience age discrimination at work? ______

(Describe): ______

Are you currently employed? ______

G. Retirement

Date of retirement: ______

Was it voluntary? ______ Welcomed? ______

Was it compulsory through company or union? ______

Was it forced because of illness? ______

Did you have preretirement preparation (seminars, etc.)? ______

______

Did you have postretirement counseling? ______

H. Economic status

Indicate sources of income

Employment: ______

Social Security: ______

Veterans benefits: ______

Railroad Retirement: ______

Private pension plan: ______

Public assistance: ______

Insurance payments: ______

Annuities: ______

Investments: ______

Savings: ______

Assistance from family: ______

Other: ______

Do you have financial problems? ______

(Describe): ______

Indicate sources of health coverage

Medicare: Part A? ______ Part B? ______

Blue Cross–Blue Shield: ______

Group health: ______

Aetna: ______

Champus: ______

Medicaid: ______

Other: ______

Have you given over power of attorney? ______ To whom? ______

Guardianship? ______

Conservatorship? ______

I. Residence (state which)

House or apartment: ______

Continued.

PERSONAL MENTAL HEALTH DATA FORM FOR OLDER PEOPLE—cont'd

Owned or rented: ______

If owned, is there a mortgage? ______ Amount per month: ______

Number of years left to pay: ______

Nursing home: ______

Home for aged: ______

Mental hospital: ______

Chronic disease hospital: ______

Personal care home: ______

Foster care: ______

Public housing: ______

Hotel: ______

Rooming house: ______

Boarding house: ______

No regular residence: ______

Other: ______

Total monthly cost of housing: ______

Any problems with living situation (describe): ______

Any problems in neighborhood (describe): ______

If you are not in your own home, is someone caring for your possessions? ______

Your pets? ______

Your plants? ______

J. Transportation and mobility

Do you drive a car? ______ Own one? ______ Have access to one? ______

How do you usually get around? ______

Is public transportation available? ______ Do you use it? ______

Any physical disabilities that affect your mobility (describe): ______

______

Do you feel safe going out during day? ______

Do you feel safe going out during night? ______

Do you have a telephone? ______

K. Interests (describe)

Avocations or hobbies: ______

Sports and exercise: ______

Commercial recreation (movies, nightclubs, etc.): ______

Music: ______

Languages: ______

Travel (places and years): ______

Vacation habits (frequency; what do you do?): ______

Gardening: ______

Collect anything: ______

Pet(s): ______

Use community centers, senior centers, etc.: ______

L. Community involvements (describe)

Memberships—organizations, clubs, etc. ______

Retiree or "senior citizens" groups: ______

Veterans organization: ______

Political activity: ______

Voluntary work: ______

Church work: ______

M. Family history

Parents

Father's full name: ______

Occupation: ______

Year of birth: ______ Birthplace: ______

If dead: Year of death: ______ Age at death: ______

Cause of death: ______

Your age at his death: ______

Brief description of his personality: ______

Mother's full name: ______

Occupation: ______

Year of birth: ______ Birthplace: ______

Continued.

PERSONAL MENTAL HEALTH DATA FORM FOR OLDER PEOPLE—cont'd

If dead: Year of death: ______________ Age at death: ______________

Cause of death: ______________

Your age at her death: ______________

Brief description of her personality: ______________

During childhood, who lived in your home other than immediate family? ______

____

(Include relatives, nurses, maids, boarders, etc.)

Did anyone other than your parents help care for you? ________

(Describe): ______________

Siblings:	**Name**	**Sex**	**Age**	**Address**	**Date and cause of death**
1.					
2.					
3.					
4.					

(Use additional space for siblings if needed.)

Grandparents: Amount and quality of contact

Paternal: ______________

Maternal: ______________

Socioeconomic conditions during childhood

Poor? ______________

Average? ______________

Wealthy? ______________

N. Friendship patterns

Who are the three closest living persons in your life?

	Name	**Number of contacts per week** (In person, by phone, by letter)
1.		
2.		
3.		

Do you have someone to depend on in an emergency? ____________

If so, who? ____________

Are you lonely? ____________

Is there someone you can talk to whenever you feel like it? ____________

If so, who? ____________

Describe contacts (List names, frequency of contact, and nature of contact; is the relationship a good one for you?)

1. Children: ____________
2. Grandchildren: ____________
3. Siblings: ____________
4. Other relations: ____________
5. Friends: ____________
6. Neighbors: ____________

(Use other side of page for these descriptions.)

O. Prejudice (directed against you?) (describe)

Age? ____________

Sex (male or female)? ____________

Race? ____________

Ethnic origin? ____________

Religion? ____________

2. Medical information

(List the doctors or medical specialists you see now or saw in the recent past)

	Name	Address	Phone	Problem
1.				
2.				
3.				

Date of your last medical checkup: ____________

How do you rate your general medical health?

Excellent ____________ Fair ____________

Good ____________ Poor ____________

Continued.

PERSONAL MENTAL HEALTH DATA FORM FOR OLDER PEOPLE—cont'd

History: Any health problems

When born: ______

When growing up: ______

List any illnesses that seem to run in family: ______

Have you ever had the following? (List dates)

1. Accidents, injuries, and falls

   Fracture: ______

   Hip injury: ______

   Head trauma: ______

   Other: ______

   Any operation as a result: ______

2. Circulatory disorders

   Heart disease: ______

   High blood pressure: ______

   Stroke: ______ Any residual: ______

   Leg cramps: ______

3. Operations: Prostatectomy, cataract extraction, others: ______

   ______

4. Arthritis: ______
5. Heart attack: ______
6. Lung conditions (bronchitis, emphysema): ______
7. Diverticulitis: ______
8. Bladder problems: ______
9. Prostate problems (men): ______
10. "Change of life" problems (women): ______
11. Allergies: ______
12. Other symptoms

    Nervousness, tension: ______

    Frequent, severe headaches: ______

    Difficulty in breathing (dyspnea): ______

Dizziness: ____________________

Fainting spells: ____________________

Fever: ____________________

Ringing or buzzing in ears: ____________________

13. Psychosomatic disorders

Asthma: ____________________

Peptic ulcer: ____________________

Essential hypertension: ____________________

Ulcerative colitis: ____________________

Ileitis: ____________________

Other: ____________________

Do you have any physical limitations?

Hearing loss? __________ Do you wear a hearing aid? __________

Vision loss? __________ Do you wear glasses? __________

Cataracts? __________

Glaucoma? __________

Memory loss? ____________________

Are you ambulatory? ______ Bedridden? ______ Some of each? ______

Incontinent? ____________________

Do you wear dentures? Partial? __________ Complete? __________

Can you dress, bathe, and generally care for self? __________

Daily living habits

Alcohol consumption per day: ______ Before dinner: ______ Before bed: ______

Water consumption: __________ glasses per day

Coffee and tea consumption per day: __________ Coffee __________ Tea

Do you smoke? ______ How many per day? ______ How long have you smoked? __________

Are you on a special diet? (describe)? ____________________

Is diet medically prescribed or self-prescribed? ____________________

Do you take vitamins? ______ What kind? __________

Current weight? __________ Has there been recent loss? __________

Have you ever had weight problem? ______ Maximum weight? ______

Continued.

PERSONAL MENTAL HEALTH DATA FORM FOR OLDER PEOPLE—cont'd

Sleep

Any difficulty falling asleep? ____________________

Any difficulty staying asleep? ____________________

Average number hours of sleep a day? ____________________

Take naps? ____________________

Do you take sleeping pills? ________ Kind: ____________________

Drug usage (dates drugs were taken and amount of dosage)

Sedatives: ____________________

Tranquilizers: ____________________

Stimulants: ____________________

Laxatives: ____________________

Diuretics: ____________________

Digitalis: ____________________

Hormones: ____________________

Nitroglycerin: ____________________

Others: ____________________

Sexual activity:

Do you experience a desire for sexual activity? ____________________

Has there been a recent change in your sexual desire? ____________________

(Describe): ____________________

Do you currently have sexual outlets? ____________________

(Describe): ____________________

How frequently? ____________________

Are there any problems—emotional, physical, social—as far as you are concerned regarding sex? ____________________

(Describe): ____________________

Males: Any problems with potency? ____________________

Females: Any vaginal pain or irritation? ____________________

How important is sexual activity in your life?

Very important: ____________________

Moderately important: ______________________

Unimportant: ______________________

3. Psychiatric information

A. General

What brought you here (complaints, concerns, symptoms? ______________________

____

Have you recently felt

Depressed? ______________________

Anxious? ______________________

Lonely? ______________________

Guilty? ______________________

Fearful? ______________________

Have you had recent losses of any kind (health, loved ones, job, etc)? ______________________

____

Previous psychiatric contact? With whom (psychiatrist, psychologist, social worker, others): ______________________

____

When? ______________________

Describe treatment form (individual or group therapy, other): ______________________

____

How long? ______________________

Drugs? ______________________

Electroshock? ______________________

Hospitalization? ______________________

Outcome of treatment in your opinion: ______________________

Has spouse had psychiatric problems? ______________________

Anyone in your family with psychiatric problems? ______________________

B. Attitudes toward aging and death

First experience with death (describe): ______________________

____

Continued.

PERSONAL MENTAL HEALTH DATA FORM FOR OLDER PEOPLE—cont'd

Losses of loved ones (include relatives, friends, describe person and date)

When you were a child (up to 10 years of age): ____________________

From 10 to 21 years: ____________________

From 21 to 60 years: ____________________

After age 60: ____________________

What are your feelings about old age? ____________________

What are your feelings about death? ____________________

Do you worry much about illness? ____________________

Do you worry much about your own death? ____________________

Do you worry much about death of others? ____________________

Have you made arrangements concerning your death? ____________________

Whom to contact? ____________________

Insurance? ____________________

Plans for funeral or memorial services? ____________________

Burial arrangements? ____________________

A will? ____________________

Describe the old age of your parents: ____________________

Describe the old age of your grandparents: ____________________

Have you modeled your own later life after that of anyone else? ____________________

If so, who? ____________________

C. Self-view (use extra space as needed)

Describe yourself (appearance, personality, personal assets and liabilities): ____________________

____

How do you feel about your present status in life? ____________________

Do you feel you have much control over your own life? ____________________

Do you feel you have much influence on others? ____________________

Are you or have you been an independent person? ____________________

Describe persons or things that have most influenced your life (friends, family, teachers, books, etc.): ____________________

Do you tend to reminisce? ______

Subject matter? ______

What are your earliest memories? ______

Do you dream? ______

Much? ______

Little? ______

Describe recurrent or significant dreams: ______

Nightmares? ______

Have you composed a diary? ______

Photograph album? ______

Autobiography? ______

Saved letters, mementoes, souvenirs? ______

Conclusion

What have been your reactions to this review of your life?

unimaginative, tedious, rigid procedure of limited usefulness in mental health care unless attention is given also to psychodynamics* and socioeconomics. A completed personal data form such as we have described can provide background and direction for the psychiatric interview. But we also urge caution in the opposite direction. In the interest of dealing with the crises of the moment, or at any time concerning oneself only with the immediate environmental context, the value of the psychiatric view can be overlooked completely. A psychiatric diagnosis, perhaps more for the elderly than any other age group, is immensely important. One must be ever alert to the possible presence of reversible brain syndromes and functional disorders, both of which can be treated if properly diagnosed. A psychiatric look at the everyday crises of living, too, can be valuable. Much that is swept under the rug as "senility," or even viewed as reaction to environmental stress, may have a psychiatric component that rightly deserves clarification and treatment.

In conducting a psychiatric examination, it is obviously not wise to be bound to a cookbook routine. Rather one must continue to build upon one's skill in observation, perception, and intuition (for hypothesis-making), while at the same time taking a comprehensive approach. The degree of comprehensiveness—the width and depth—of the study will vary according to time pressures, purposes, motivation, and (sadly) the economic status of the patient and his ability to pay.

We will not discuss the general techniques of psychiatric examination, since these have

*The systematized knowledge of theory of human behavior and its motivation, the study of which depends largely upon the functional significance of emotion. Psychodynamics stresses the role of unconscious motivation.

been well described elsewhere.* Instead, those components of the examination which are found to be especially pertinent to old people will be stressed. The appearance and general behavior of the person can offer significant clues: Does she walk like an "old" person, or does her walk belie her age? Does he dye his hair and pretend to be youthful? Is there a peculiar gait (for instance, the distinctive parkinsonian "march," the marche à petits pas with its characteristic short shuffling steps, the patient leaning forward so that the gait is propulsive, the arms not swinging)? Does she look blank-faced (indicating organicity? depression?)? An ironed-out masklike facies may point to parkinsonism. Is he slow moving in speech and action, distractable, flighty, incoherent, or irrelevant? Does she speak sotto voce, quietly, while looking about suspiciously (possible paranoid feature)? Is the appearance one of premature age and debilitation (there may be a basic physical process or illness underlying the psychiatric symptomatology)? One must also be aware of behavior that might be inappropriate for younger people but is "normal" in old age—a good example being the fact that an old person may arrive an hour or more early for an interview. This is because old people often are highly time-conscious and want to compensate for any unavoidable delays along the way that may be hard for them to cope with; thus they tend to overcompensate by starting very early.

At the beginning of an interview, it must be made clear to the older person what the purpose of the interview is. Many people still see attention from psychiatrists and other psychiatric staff as indications that they are "crazy," and they need reassurance that the examination is taking place to help to discover what is causing discomfort, pain, or anguish for them—that it is a way to get to know them better. Some need to be told this directly, others will assume it from the general manner of the examiner, and still others arrive already convinced. One generally starts off the examination by asking the person what brought him for treatment—what is his chief problem or complaint. The history of the problem in the person's own words is next. Family and chronological life histories follow. Careful questioning is necessary to discover how the old person feels about his family: does he see himself as a burden, is he angry at them, do they indicate annoyance with him? At every step, care must be taken to watch the nonverbal communications and revelations of the unconscious. One should try to record important aspects of the person's descriptions in his own exact words, not only for any later medical-legal reasons but also for later reflection upon psychodynamics.

A psychiatric checklist such as the accompanying is a useful device for ascertaining symptoms upon admission and for comparison with follow-up impressions.

The examiner must also be especially alert for "new" and "peculiar" behavior—keeping in mind the immediacy of the life situation as well as the life history. Immediate precipitants are crucial in old age where change, loss, and deprivation are so powerful in their effects.

Certain symptoms in old age practically guarantee medical and/or psychiatric problems. Persons with organic brain disorders and severe depressions may survive—even well—in the community, and then suddenly a change in their lot makes the pathology visible. Wandering at night, evident confusion, and incontinence are examples of problems that are usually organic in nature—all of which can, however, be functional. Wandering, for instance, may have as its psychogenic root the need to escape. Incontinence may be an expression of anger.

The alert facade or appearance and normal-looking social habits can be deceptive, masking the presence of severe brain damage. Korsakoff's syndrome, presbyophrenia, and the presenile dementias are conditions in which an observer can be misled by first impressions:

*For example, see Lewis, N. D. C.: Outline for psychiatric examinations, ed. 3, New York, 1943, New York State Department of Mental Hygiene.

PSYCHIATRIC SYMPTOMS CHECKLIST*

	At time of admission	At time of follow-up
1. Conversion symptoms		
2. Hypochondriacal ideas		
3. Somatic delusions		
4. Suspiciousness		
5. Persecutory trend		
6. Idea of unreality		
7. Depersonalization		
8. Nihilistic ideas		
9. Depressive trend		
10. Suicidal attempts		
11. Elation		
12. Grandiose ideas		
13. Hallucinatory experiences:		
a. Auditory		
b. Visual		
c. Tactile		
d. Gustatory		
e. Olfactory		
14. Illusions		
15. Misinterpretations		
16. Obsessions (including death)		
17. Compulsions		
18. Phobias		
19. Anxiety; fear (including death)		
20. Nightmares; dreams		
21. Sexual adaptation (homosexuality or other)		
22. Psychosomatic symptoms		
23. Psychogenic exacerbation of somatic pathology		

*From Perlin, S., and Butler, R. N.: Psychiatric aspects of adaptation to the aging process. In Birren, J. E., Butler, R. N., Greenhouse, S. W., Sokoloff, L., and Yarrow, Marian R., editors: Human aging, a biological and behavioral study, Washington, D. C., 1963, U. S. Government Printing Office.

Two sisters were admitted to the National Institute of Neurological Diseases and Blindness in 1960 for studies of familial essential hypercholesterolemia and general research studies. One was 57, the other 55. They were anxious, depressed, fearful, restless, and perplexed. Verbal productivity was somewhat increased. There was slurring of speech, as well as delay in responses and little spontaneity of thinking. They had difficulty finding words; they were distractable. There was perseveration of ideas but in these cases not of words.

They appeared outwardly intact. Their personal habits and conduct were fine. The successful social facade, however, fell away drastically when tested in the mental status examination. They knew all the "right things" to say. They just didn't know such simple facts as what day it was.

Intellectual deficiency, memory loss, acalculia, inability to abstract proverbs, and impaired judgment were present. Both began to show signs of illness in their early fifties. Their courses were insidious and progressive. There was a family history of Alzheimer's disease, one of the presenile dementias. Four of five siblings showed signs. Brain biopsies confirmed our studies, which showed reduced cerebral blood flow and oxygen consumption.

Concentration, memory retention and immediate recall, mental grasp and comprehension, counting and calculation, and judgment must be appraised with delicacy. Although there have been advances in recent years in psychiatric techniques for rating or measuring the psychological functioning, mental status, and symptoms of the elderly, much

MENTAL STATUS EVALUATION*

1. Retention

Say to the patient: "I am going to tell you an address which I want you to remember. I will ask for it at a later time."

This is the address:	(Alternate)
Apartment C	Room 7
Arbor Estates	Carrier Hotel

Then say, "Repeat that for me now." This is essential to be certain the address has been registered in the memory. Then continue with the examination, 2. Remote memory (time interval: 5 minutes).

Then, "Do you remember the address I gave you a few minutes ago?"

Raw score: (-1, 0, 1, 2, 3, or 4). ______

2. Remote memory

Write out subject's response. Score 1 point for each correct answer.

Score

1. Where were you born?

   ______ ______

2. Where did you go to school?

   ______ ______

3. Highest grade completed?

   ______ ______

4. How old were you when you finished school?

   ______ ______

5. How old were you when you began work?

   ______ ______

6. Name of first employer?

   ______ ______

7. Address of first employer?

   ______ ______

8. Mother's maiden name?

   ______ ______

9. Who was President of the United States when you began your first job (in this country when foreign born)?

   ______ ______

Remote memory score: Sum of correct answers.† ______

*From Perlin, S., and Butler, R. N.: Psychiatric aspects of adaptation to the aging process. In Birren, J. E., Butler, R. N., Greenhouse, S. W., Sokoloff, L., and Yarrow, Marian R., editors: Human aging, a biological and behavioral study, Washington, D. C., 1963, U. S. Government Printing Office.

†Authentication of the correctness of answers should be based, where possible, on information obtained from family members, records, etc.

3. Orientation

(Rate 1, 2, or 3 for A, B, and C) **Score**

A. Time: ______________________ ________

What is the date today?

What year (month, day) is it? What season is it?

1. No awareness of correct time (e.g., does not know month, season, or year).
2. Disturbed orientation, but some degree of awareness (e.g., knows season or year, etc.).
3. Knows exact time (month, approximate day, year, and season).

B. Place: ______________________ ________

What is the name of this place?

Where is it?

1. No awareness of location.
2. Disturbed orientation, but can give an approximation that is reasonably accurate.
3. Knows exact location.

C. Person: ______________________ ________

What is my job? (Other members of the staff?)

1. No knowledge of above.
2. Some knowledge of above.
3. Knows exactly who and what they are.

Orientation score: Sum of A, B, and C. ________

4. Recent memory

(Check when you are certain he is correct; otherwise write in subject's response. Leave blank if incorrect. One point for each correct response.)

1. Where do you live? ______________________ ________
2. How long have you lived there? ______________________ ________
3. How long have you been here? ______________________ ________
4. Where were you a week ago? ______________________ ________
5. How many meals have you had today? ______________________ ________

____

Continued.

MENTAL STATUS EVALUATION—cont'd

6. What did you have for breakfast?* ________________ ______

________________ ______

7. What is my name? ________________ ______
8. When did you see me for the first time? ________________
9. Have you been in this room before? ________________ ______

________________ ______

Recent memory score: Sum of correct answers.

________________ ______

5. Reading (logical memory)†:

"I am going to read you a story. Listen carefully." Then, "Now tell me what I read. Begin at the beginning and tell me everything that you can remember . . . and what else?"

(21 possible memories. Check every memory. Leave spaces beside wrongly remembered or omitted facts blank. When in doubt write out response. One point for each memory.)

Logical memory score: Sum of memories.

________________ ______

*The evaluator should check beforehand where possible to uncover confabulation, that is, some patients with organic problems cover up their memory loss.

†From Terman, L. M., and Merrill, M. A.: Measuring intelligence, Boston, 1937, Houghton-Mifflin Co., pp. 255-256.

work remains to be done. The clarification and differentiation of age-relevant behavior from lifelong behavior (as well as disease-determined, culture-deprived, and other behavior) is an unsettled problem. There have been efforts toward the development of quantified forms for mental status examination, covering memory, orientation, judgment, etc., but none have been generally accepted for standard use. The Mental Status Questionnaire of Kahn, Goldfarb et al. (included here) is probably the most widely used, but it is no substitute for a full mental status examination. The Mental Status Questionnaire is correctly used when a quick mental appraisal is required for screening and

MENTAL STATUS QUESTIONNAIRE*

Where are we now?
Where is this place located?
What month is it?
What day of the month is it?
What year is it?
How old are you?
What is your birthday?
Where were you born?
Who is the president of the U. S.?
Who was president before him?

*From Kahn, R. L., Goldfarb, A. I., Pollack, M., and Peck, A.: Brief objective measures for the determination of mental status of the aged, American Journal of Psychiatry 117:326-328, 1960.

cursory diagnostic purposes. We prefer the more comprehensive Mental Status Evaluation (pp. 166 to 168), derived from the National Institute of Mental Health's human aging studies, comparing state hospital and healthy community populations.

A note should be made here with respect to two special features in evaluation, which are of interest to us: observation of handwriting and interviewing in front of a mirror. Parkinsonian patients typically write in small script (micrographia); thus attention to handwriting can be diagnostic. Mirror-interviewing also has diagnostic value in revealing a patient's self-image. It is not a routine procedure but can be quite helpful for in-depth evaluations. A fuller description will follow later.

We wish to point out also that psychiatrists are by no means the only people qualified to do "psychiatric" evaluations. In community mental health centers, psychiatric hospitals, and elsewhere, a team of persons from many disciplines may arrive at a joint evaluation. In addition, well-trained paraprofessionals can learn to assess the psychiatric condition of patients. With inadequate psychiatric coverage in most public and many private facilities, such skills can and should be learned by others.* Responsible supervision and competent training can ensure quality care, regardless of the primary discipline.

Medical assessment

A thorough physical exam is mandatory, in addition to a medical history (we use the medical section of a patient's completed personal data form to provide some beginning background information) and recent reports from the patient's family doctor or other involved physicians. The latter reports are often obtained verbally by phone but should be summarized in written form in the patient's record. It must be known what drugs are being taken, for what condition, for how long, and what, if any, have been the side effects, especially adverse reactions. A routine physical exam includes the laboratory tests listed in the outline on p. 147, supplemented by any further tests suggested by the patient's symptomatology. Electroencephalography (brain wave test) is the process or method of making a graphic record of the electrical activity of the brain. Healthy aged persons have essentially the same records as younger people with the exception of the observation of Busse and Silverman of left temporal foci, the meaning of which remains unclear. Thus evidences of diffuse or other focal changes are significant indications of organic brain disorders.

Tests measuring the cerebral blood flow and oxygen consumption by the brain would be invaluable diagnostically, but the present methods including the original nitrous oxide method of Kety and Schmidt (1948) are too dangerous for routine clinical use, requiring the skills of highly trained medical personnel. It is hoped that a simple and safe test will be developed so that it can be part of the basic examination.

Hearing tests, a visual examination with a check of eyeglasses, and a dental exam are obviously important for elderly people. Nutrition and sleeping habits must be noted. Because of widespread poverty among the elderly, combined with the physical incapacity of some to care for themselves, many suffer from malnutrition in subtle or gross forms.* Malnutrition and dehydration therefore are among the major medical problems to recognize.

The medical evaluation should be comprehensive, multiphasic, continued at regular intervals, and if possible, computerized. Hopefully there will soon be a baseline body of quality data available through automated

*There is a danger that must be avoided, wherein psychiatrists will care for the well-to-do and paraprofessionals care for the poor.

*One should not overlook the possibility of pellagra in the diagnostic work-up. The complete syndrome of this vitamin deficiency disease may not be present. One can look for redness of the mouth and tongue (more obvious in acute cases), skin changes, and—of special interest to mental health personnel—evidence of intellectual changes in a chronic brain disorder.

technology and telemetry (to send information quickly, long distance) to aid in diagnosis. Heart disease, diabetes, glaucoma, emphysema, and cancer are particular foci. Indeed, after age 45 there should be annual medical checkups for the healthy, and more frequent ones for the ill. Unfortunately Medicare does not cover routine checkups, making it difficult for the elderly to take advantage of the early detection and prevention possible through regular physical examinations.

Another difficulty for old people is lack of knowledge about health, medicine, and their own bodies. For obvious reasons they know less than later generations will know. Physicians have not been the major source of health education that they could be for old people. Often they are reluctant to impart information—saying it takes too much time, there is no good purpose to it, etc.—while the elderly remain unenlightened as to what is being done to them. Many, for example, are given medication without knowing what it is for or what the side effects may be. Numerous other examples could be given of medical care administered in a manner that produces needless anxiety and emotional anguish.

Besides the usual diagnostic benefits, medical evaluation has two particularly important functions for the elderly patient. First the examination is essential for the detection and early treatment of the reversible brain syndromes. These syndromes must be diagnosed early or they can become complicated, losing their reversibility. The medical exam also helps to "rule in" the functional disorders by clarifying those situations in which no physical basis can be found. Thus an evaluator is clued into the possibility of a functional disorder (paranoid states, depression, etc.) and is more inclined to explore psychogenic processes.

Socioeconomic assessment

The immediate social environment has substantial influence upon the older person's psychological behavior and attitudes, and this has been investigated in studies at NIMH and elsewhere. "As the environment showed qualities of deprivation or displacement of the person (in loss of intimate persons, loss of income, in cultural displacement), the attitudes and behaviors of the aged showed more deteriorative qualities. Losses of significant persons were especially associated with deteriorative functioning,"* and further, "findings of this study lead to the suspicion that psychological reactions to the loss of friends and other environmental supports may amplify if not initiate changes in the older nervous system and thereby the rest of the organism."†

Having intimate friends in whom one can confide is very important. It must be recognized, however, that social isolation per se is not causative of emotional and mental reactions in old age. Persons who have lived isolated lives throughout the years—"loners"—are not necessarily more liable to the occurrence of late-life psychopathology.

A socioeconomic evaluation should include general background information concerning details of family structure, housing, work or retirement, friendship patterns, economics, social roles, activities, and interests. (See example of personal mental health data form—pp. 149 to 163.) Interviews with the older person and members of his family can provide valuable insight into the contribution of social factors to the patient's problem and into potential assets that can aid and support treatment. The evaluation of the family itself is crucial, since the genesis, precipitation, and maintenance of disorders may derive from a family context. The older person may be expressing what is really a family-wide pathology in which he or she is the scapegoat or the victim of ancient angers. Sometimes the "problem" of the old person is the means by which a son or daughter seeks treatment but is unable to ask for it directly. A skilled evaluator is

*From Birren, J. E., Butler, R. N., Greenhouse, S. W., Sokoloff, L., and Yarrow, Marian R., editors: Human aging, Washington, D. C., 1963, U. S. Government Printing Office, p. 314.

†Ibid., p. 316.

able to detect this phenomenon and help the younger family members to obtain treatment themselves. In other situations, the older person may exploit the family; an example is the domineering parent who becomes even more tyrannical in old age by playing on guilt feelings of children toward the aging and decline of a parent. A prideful overemphasis on independence and a manipulation of others through passivity are other patterns of behavior in the elderly that can cause family conflict. Old people must not routinely be judged helpless or fragile. Indeed, a fair number of them wield substantial influence over family and friends.

In working with the total family, it is imperative to share evaluation findings as openly as possible, guided by judgment as to the effects of such sharing on the older person. Family therapy involving the old person may be indicated—couples' therapy with the patient and spouse can be beneficial even in marriages that have been difficult for years and/or have deteriorated. At times, the family approach is used as a rationale to exclude the elderly patient (usually the result of countertransference problems on the part of treatment personnel):

> There is no point seeing the patient—you know his memory is gone. He feels rejected—I find it more useful to see the son and daughter-in-law.

One must recognize the vast implications of race as well as racism in the lives of the black elderly, Mexicans, Indians, Chinese, and other groups. A knowledge of cultural patterns and traditions and knowing the discriminatory practices and prejudices experienced in a lifetime are fundamental parts of a thorough evaluation. This applies also to ethnic origins, since so many of the elderly are immigrants. However, a note of caution is warranted here: at times, race or ethnic origin may be used to rationalize another form of prejudice. The elderly black person can be denied psychiatric care because his problems are viewed as social or racial while intrapsychic problems remain unnoticed. People in every culture develop internalized emotional difficulties that require treatment beyond changes in the social condition.

Treatment should ideally be planned to coincide, insofar as possible, with those cultural elements which are familiar and valued by the old person. An elderly black man in a nursing home might prefer "soul food," whereas a Norwegian immigrant could long for "lutefisk." Patient comfort, satisfaction, and dignity are important in a positive treatment program.

Not least among the steps in an adequate evaluation is determining the patient's health care coverage and economic circumstances. Pending the introduction of a truly comprehensive national health insurance, it is usually necessary to appraise the patient's "ability to pay" for treatment, although this notion of personal financial responsibility is generally obsolete, given the realities of escalating costs and, for the elderly, the denial of adequate income programs and job opportunities. Third-party medical payments include Medicare, Medicaid (see p. 172), and sometimes insurance supplementary to Medicare. A routine check should be made to determine whether the older person is a member of one of the national organizations for the elderly, which sell such supplementary insurance. The National Council of Senior Citizens and the American Association of Retired Persons offer policies, as do the so-called nonprofit Blue Cross–Blue Shield plans and the commercial insurance carriers. One must be on the lookout for fly-by-night, fraudulent Medicare supplements that have been sold to old people. A check of the additional income resources listed on a personal mental health data form (pp. 153 and 154) and information about average living expenses will complete the economic assessment. Old people, like others, may be sensitive to questions about economics, fearing that they will be billed unjustly for treatment or simply resenting an intrusion into their privacy. Some are ashamed to admit their meagre incomes and out of pride may refuse to accept financial benefits to which they are entitled. Every effort should be made to help them exploit all possible out-

HEALTH INSURANCE FOR THE AGED—HOSPITAL INSURANCE
(Popular name: Medicare)

This program provides hospital insurance protection for covered services to any person 65 or over who is entitled to Social Security or Railroad Retirement benefits. A dependent spouse 65 or over is also entitled to Medicare based on the worker's record. The covered protection in each benefit period includes hospital inpatient care, posthospital extended care, and home health visits by nurses or other health workers from a participating home health agency. It does not include doctors' services.

Under Social Security, workers, their employers, and self-employed people pay a contribution based on earnings during their working years. At age 65, the portion of their contribution that has gone into a special Hospital Insurance Trust Fund guarantees that workers will have help in paying hospital bills.

HEALTH INSURANCE FOR THE AGED—SUPPLEMENTARY MEDICAL INSURANCE
(Popular name: Medicare)

Social Security's medical insurance program helps pay for doctor bills, outpatient hospital services, medical supplies and services, home health services, outpatient physical therapy, and other health care services.

Medical insurance is not financed through payroll deductions and is not based on earnings or period of work. As a voluntary supplemental extension of Medicare's hospital insurance protection, it helps pay for many of the costs of illness not covered by hospital insurance.

MEDICAL ASSISTANCE PROGRAM
(Popular name: Medicaid Title XIX)

This program provides grants to states to administer medical assistance programs that benefit: (1) the needy—all public assistance recipients in the federally aided categories (the aged, blind, disabled, and families with dependent children) and those who would qualify for that assistance under federal regulations; (2) at a state's option, the medically needy—people in the four groups mentioned above who have enough income or resources for daily needs but not for medical expenses; and (3) all children under 21 whose parents cannot afford medical care.

State plans must include at least five basic services for the needy, and a similar or less extensive program for the medically needy. Family planning services may be included in both.

side resources in order to protect their own incomes during treatment.

Medicare coverage may be expanded and will probably be incorporated within a national health insurance plan. In the meantime, actual coverage is limited (43% of the health bill of the elderly in 1970). There are many exclusions—outpatient drugs, eye glasses, dentures, blood transfusions, routine physical examinations—all of particular importance to the elderly. No third-party payment covers the medical problem of malnutrition due to inadequate income or difficulty in obtaining food. Referral for public assistance, food stamps, and Meals-on-Wheels programs are among some available resources.

On-the-spot home evaluation

To see how old people of all socioeconomic classes live is a first-rate diagnostic tool.

> An old man lived in an unpainted, roach-infested, windowless closet, sleeping on a urine-smelling mattress that could not be fully extended because of the small size of the closet.

With 95% of the elderly residing in the community, a home evaluation is a logical way to get a sense of the day-to-day existence of the patient. One looks for pets (companionship), calendar (to what month is it turned?), clock (is it running and set properly?), odors (gas leaks, spoiled food, signs of incontinence), food supply (is the person eating regularly and adequately?), mementoes (what does the old person consider important?), family pictures. The safety and security of the home, the ability of the older person to get around the house, and the presence of others can be assayed. (It is not uncommon to find an old person caring for someone who may be even sicker than he.) A realistic evaluation of the fear of crime, and financial and physical limitations to transportation can be made.

Such outreach services as home visiting are still rare in the United States. Some cities (e.g., Baltimore) have health aides who work for the city health department's bureau of special home services. These workers collect data about the elderly in their homes and are a useful adjunct to the mental health specialist. The physician, psychiatrist, psychologist, social worker, nurse, or paraprofessional all should make use of home visiting to keep in touch with the realities of the urban, suburban, or rural life of the elderly from various walks of life.

PSYCHOLOGICAL TESTS

Except for special research purposes, we do not necessarily feel that psychological tests must be done in every case. However, when there is uncertainty around the differential diagnosis of organic brain damage versus depression, such tests can be very useful; but one should not forget that the patient with an organic problem can still be depressed. A patient with chronic organic brain syndrome generally produces lower test scores than one with the reversible brain disorder; however, at the height of the acute reversible crisis (e.g., delirium), the patient is likely to be untestable.

The Bender Visual-Motor Gestalt* is the most useful measure of organic change. The person is presented with a series of cards, one at a time, with a simple geometric figure on each. His task is to copy each figure on a sheet of paper. The first card shows a circle flanked by a diamond, with one corner of the diamond touching the circle. The second card shows a series of dots in a straight line. The person must be able to retain his spatial orientation. The patient having organic difficulty may rotate the figures, misplace them, or perseverate (e.g., be unable to stop making the series of dots).

The Wechsler Adult Intelligence Scale† is a standardized test of intelligence, for which national figures are available. Moreover, there are standardized figures for old people, taking education into account to

---

*Bender, Lauretta: A visual-motor Gestalt test and its clinical use, Research Monograph No. 3, New York, 1938, American Orthopsychiatric Association.

†Wechsler, D.: WAIS manual: Wechsler Adult Intelligence Scale, New York, 1955, The Psychological Corporation.

some extent. However, a cultural bias is present against foreign immigrees, blacks, and other racial minorities. The WAIS can be given in abbreviated form by asking the odd-numbered items—1, 3, 5, and so forth —of Information, Comprehension, Calculations, Similarities, Vocabulary. The verbal subtest—Similarities—is an excellent measure of the ability to abstract; patients with organic disorders will tend to be concrete on this test. The Raven Progressive Matrices, utilizing geometric figures, is presumably culture-free but there is some question of this.

Another popular test is the Kent E-G-Y,* a ten-item, quick-screening test for intelligence. Some people, such as Goldfarb, find M. Bender's Double Simultaneous Tactual Stimulation (Face-Hand) Test† of value in the important differential diagnosis between organicity and depression.

DIAGNOSTIC USE OF MIRROR AND SELF-DRAWINGS

Any technique that is useful in eliciting rich, spontaneous information and response from older people can become part of one's diagnostic repertoire. Such techniques may be discovered quite by accident. Clinical experiences (by R. N. Butler) of observing certain elderly people communicating with their mirror images led to investigation of self and body concepts through the experimental use of the mirror and self-drawings. These techniques were introduced as cues for a collaborative self-exploration *with* the older person as an active participant—how does he view himself now, how did he in the past, and what does he see in his future?

Mirror

To help illustrate the psychological significance of one's mirror image, let us quote from a Tolstoi short story, *The Death of Ivan Ilych* (1886):

> . . . and Ivan Ilych began to wash. With pauses for rest, he washed his hands and then his face, cleaned his teeth, brushed his hair, and looked in the glass. He was terrified by what he saw, especially the limp way in which his hair clung to his pallid forehead. While his shirt was being changed he knew that he would be still more frightened at the sight of his body, so he avoided looking at it.

Asking an old person to look into a mirror and tell about what he sees is an exceptionally excellent way of acquiring data about body image and reactions to changes with age. The mirror is a powerful trigger or cue to thoughts and observations about one's self and one's changes. One often obtains much richer data in less time than by way of elaborate verbal questioning about physical, personality, and other changes. The range of reactions may be accounted for by (1) reality factors in appearance, (2) personality factors, whether lifelong or in reaction to old age, and (3) organic factors. (See following outline.)

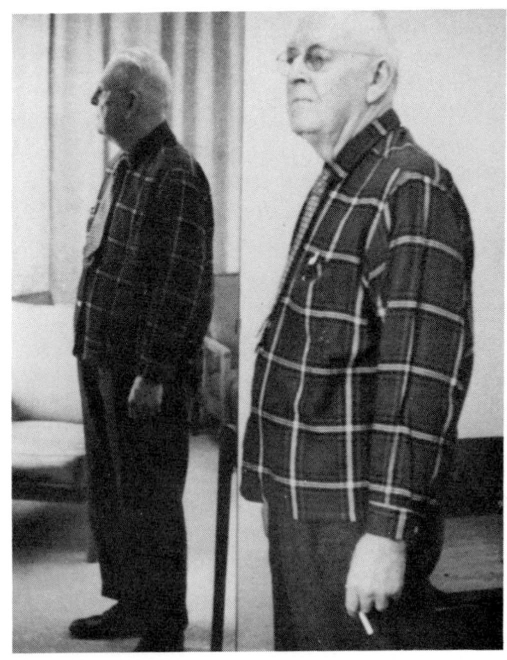

Diagnostic use of the mirror.

From Butler, R. N.: Geriatrics **18**:220-232, 1963.

*Kent, Grace H.: Kent E-G-Y test: series of emergency scales, manual, New York, 1946, The Psychological Corporation. See Delp, H. A.: Correlations between the Kent E-G-Y and the Wechsler batteries, Journal of Clinical Psychology **9**:73-75, 1953.

†Bender, M. B., Fink, M., and Green, M.: Patterns in perception in simultaneous tests of the face and hand, Archives of Neurology and Psychiatry **66**: 355-362, 1951.

1. *Reality factors in appearance*
   a. Skin-wrinkling; pigmentation; flabbiness; leathering
   b. Bodily movements—slowing
      Physical impairments
         Arthritis
         Palsies—tremors
   c. Facial changes—palsies; wrinkling
   d. Hair—balding; graying
   e. Eyes—opacities of the lens
   f. Teeth—absence; discoloration
   g. Cartilage growth—ears; nose
   h. Chest—increase diameter; breathing rate
   i. Abdomen—protuberance
   j. Weight—loss; shrunken
2. *Personality factors*
   a. Lifelong
      Focal emphasis (cathexis) Parts vs. Whole —e.g., nose; profile vs. frontal view; sexual organ
      Character—narcissism, self-hate, etc.
      Identity—crisis
      Mood—depression, hypomania, etc.
   b. Old age
      Fear—shudder—tension—aging and death
      Denial of aging changes; reparative vs. depression
3. *Organic factors*
   a. Perceptual factors
      Vision affected (can be defensive; cf. exclusion of stimuli—Weinberg)
   b. Organic factors
      Organic brain damage: "Not me"
      Disorientation for person

As is known, cartilage continues to grow in old age, so the ears and nose may consequently become more prominent, but these changes are not mentioned as much by people as wrinkling, sagging around the eyes, hair loss, and general appearance of "oldness." On the other hand most healthy older people find it difficult to see themselves as having essentially changed. Of course, much turns upon the term "essentially." It appears that they are in effect recognizable to themselves, and in their own minds they have not drastically altered in their character and nature in the course of time; their identity has remained solid. A sudden and rapid deterioration and change of appearance can cause an identity crisis or reaction, even in otherwise healthy people. Adjustment and acceptance are much easier when physical change comes slowly. A clue to shaky identity or difficulty in adapting to changes can be seen in people who reject their mirror image.

A middle-aged woman who expressed a profound fear of aging could not accept her mirror image as herself. She regarded the image as something foreign and experienced her "real" self as being on the inside of her body, feeling and reacting, while people responded to her "foreign" outside image in a way that was unacceptable to her.

Personality factors before the mirror can be strikingly obvious. People exhibiting defensive preoccupation with themselves (narcissism) are pleased and attracted by their image, whereas those who are ashamed and guilty shun the mirror, reject their images, become anxious. A focal emphasis upon or cathexis of a particular body part (e.g., the nose) is observed and provides diagnostic clues. Usually a part rather than the whole is seen by the older person. Other common reactions are fear, shudders, suddenly occurring thoughts about aging and approaching death or, conversely, a denial of aging changes and denial of fear of death.

Organic factors can affect the mirror reaction. Persons with organic brain damage may insist the image is "not me" or illustrate vividly a "disorientation for person" by not recognizing the person in the mirror. Perceptual impairments of vision can be actual or defensive in nature, the latter recalling Weinberg's concept of exclusion of stimuli, in which the person blocks out images that are too painful.

Self-drawings

Some classic examples of the emotion-laden quality of self-drawings are the variety of self-portraits done by well-known artists (many using their mirror image). A 1972 museum exhibit displayed such portraits with expressions ranging from pleased and serene to displeased and tortured. Goya made his self-portrait defiantly ugly and troubled, not bothering to idealize himself or impress his audience. Cezanne dressed himself in overalls and a lumpy, battered hat, beneath which he seemed to be shy and retiring. The self-portrait of Dürer was exquisitely and lovingly drawn.

Self-drawings by patients are revealing, whether done in front of the mirror or by themselves. The technique is to focus the person directly upon himself. Self-drawings of the elderly with and without the mirror often suggest a self-view of dissolution, sometimes bizarre; they do not appear as some have said, similar to the drawing of children. The accompanying figure shows examples of self-drawings of normal elderly men.

Barring severe hand tremors or profound visual problems that would affect expression, drawing provides other clues to the feelings of old people. Things to look for in drawings are the size of the image and placement of figures on the page, amount and kind of detail, underemphasis or overemphasis of a body part, omissions, facial expressions, activity or inactivity of the figure, and the general emotional quality of the picture.

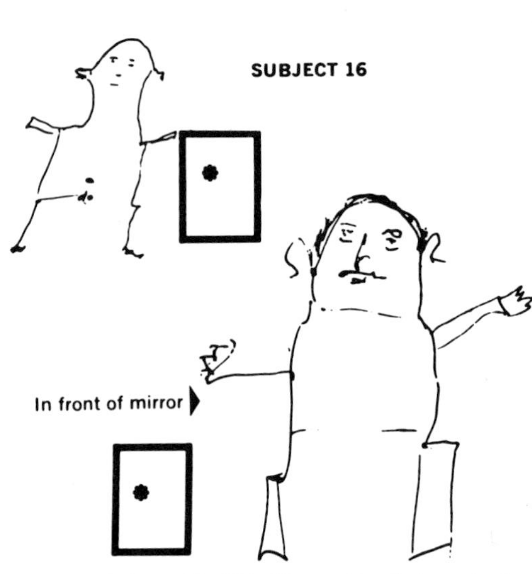

A

Subject 16. *This 76-year-old retired merchant's counterphobic activity helped him to ward off depressive symptoms. Although emphasizing his physical well-being, his self-drawing suggests incompleteness. Character trait disorder.* Subject 20. *This 78-year-old retired clerk has recurrent nightmares related to death. He describes himself as a "silent worrier." No psychiatric diagnosis.*

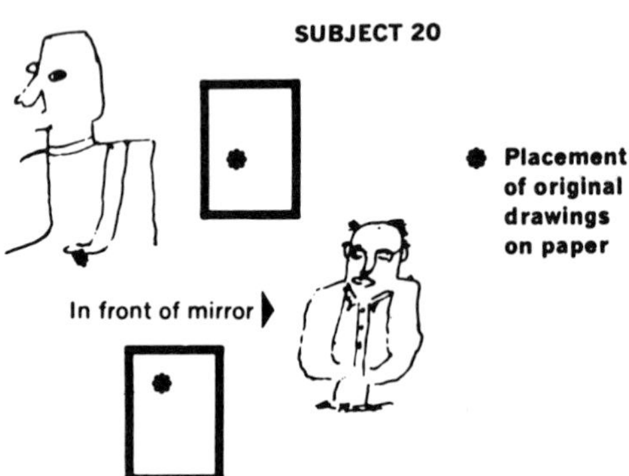

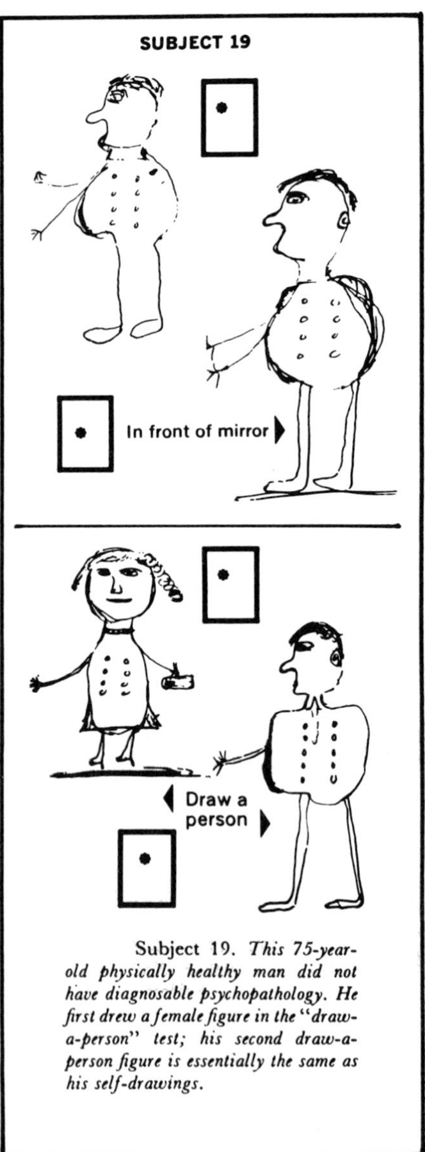

Subject 19. *This 75-year-old physically healthy man did not have diagnosable psychopathology. He first drew a female figure in the "draw-a-person" test; his second draw-a-person figure is essentially the same as his self-drawings.*

Self-drawings of normal elderly men.

From Butler, R. N.: Geriatrics 18:220-232, 1963.

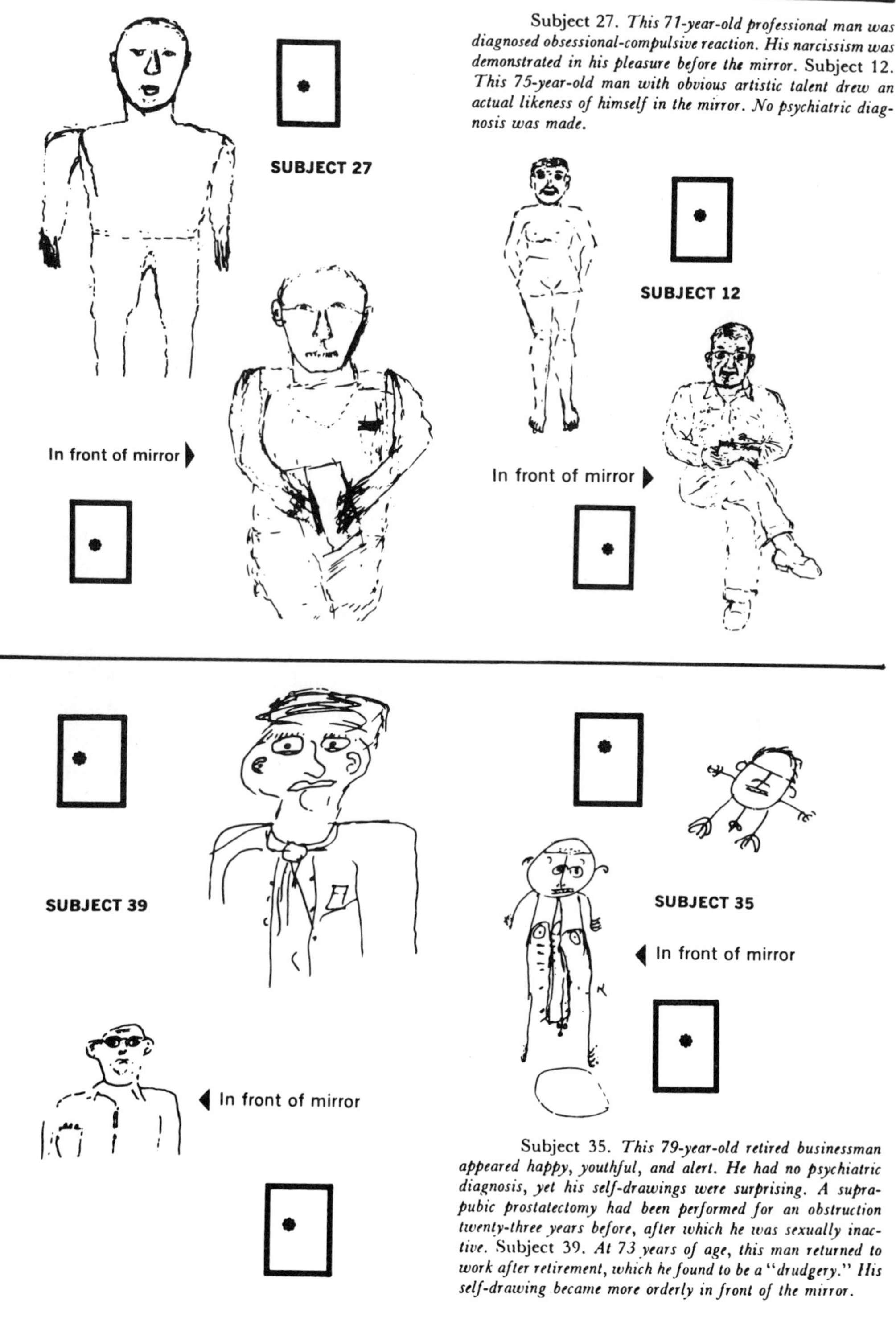

Subject 27. *This 71-year-old professional man was diagnosed obsessional-compulsive reaction. His narcissism was demonstrated in his pleasure before the mirror.* Subject 12. *This 75-year-old man with obvious artistic talent drew an actual likeness of himself in the mirror. No psychiatric diagnosis was made.*

Subject 35. *This 79-year-old retired businessman appeared happy, youthful, and alert. He had no psychiatric diagnosis, yet his self-drawings were surprising. A suprapubic prostatectomy had been performed for an obstruction twenty-three years before, after which he was sexually inactive.* Subject 39. *At 73 years of age, this man returned to work after retirement, which he found to be a "drudgery." His self-drawing became more orderly in front of the mirror.*

"Draw your insides"

This device is an interesting one because of the preoccupation of so many elderly people with their bodily ailments and changes. One can get clues about the emotional impact of such changes by observing the older person's response in this kind of drawing. Shown here is the figure provided for the male subject. A female figure should be provided for women.

Items most commonly drawn are intestines, heart, lungs, and stomach. Placement and size of these organs in the drawing can give indications of their meaning emotionally. In experimental tests, 20% of inner body parts were drawn as protruding out from the body or as completely outside, suggesting possible mental confusion and organicity.

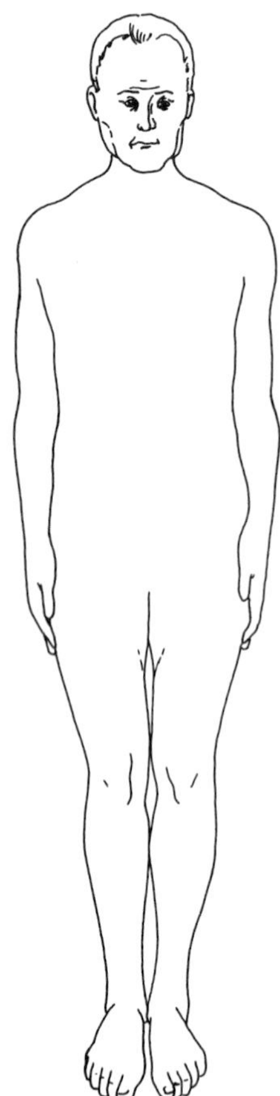

Figure given to patient when he is asked to draw his insides.

Since comparative data for other age groups or various diagnostic entities are not available, no concise inferences can be drawn from findings; indeed anatomical knowledge may be quite limited in the elderly population, which did not receive as much educational emphasis on biology, health, etc., as more recent generations have. But the draw-your-insides procedure, along with mirror reactions and self-drawing, produces rich emotional data without unduly threatening the older person. In the same way, reviews of family photo albums and scrapbooks can provide stimulation and diagnostic clues, while often giving immense pleasure to the elderly person in the process.

COMMUNITY ASPECTS OF AN EVALUATION

The older person's community should be included in the evaluative process, both to determine what the community has to offer and to engage community services in ongoing evaluations of patients. A homemaker working in a patient's home may be able to furnish a picture of the person's day-to-day life. Visiting nurses, workers in Meals-on-Wheels programs, occupational therapists, and others can offer their particular viewpoints.

STUDIES OF COMMUNITY-RESIDENT "HEALTHY" ELDERLY

Quests for a psychological baseline against which to measure "illness"

Busse's group and the NIMH group are among those which have evaluated the community elderly, who make up 10% of the total population. In the NIMH studies, begun in 1955, physical and emotional health was a criterion in selection for study. Part of the purpose in such work was to obtain, for evaluating old people, a baseline consisting of a composite of the statistical norm (the average) and the healthy (the ideal). A longitudinal view of the life cycle has begun to receive attention. Senescence as a developmental stage or process in the course of the life cycle has a psychology of its own, which thus far has only been crudely delineated.

Evaluation of the effects of lifelong personality

The list given here indicates the contribution of some aspects of lifelong personality to the psychological nature of old people.

1. Adaptive qualities
   Candor, ease of relationships, independence, affirmation, positive self-concept, sense of usefulness
   Defense mechanisms: insight, denial, use of activity
2. Maladaptive qualities
   Paranoid isolation
3. Maladaptive in early life—adaptive in late life
   Obsessive-compulsive features
   Schizoid mechanisms
   Dependent personality

Both adaptive and maladaptive features are brought by the person into old age. We must caution observers, however, that only through a careful knowledge of life history can differentiation be made between those qualities possessed by the individual throughout his life and those which first came into being in old age through a reorganization of personality. The Swedish film "Wild Strawberries" reflects the potential of an old man, set in his ways, to make rather basic changes in his personality late in life.

Lifelong personality traits that have been found useful in old age are a sense of self-esteem, candor, ability to relate easily with others, independence and self-motivation, and a sense of usefulness. Measures of the "ego strength" (the ego's function as the moderating and reality-testing component of the personality) enable judgments to be made regarding the capacity to cope and adjust. Some defense mechanisms (by which the ego copes) are more useful than others. Naturally, insight is a valuable aid in alleviating anxiety and guilt by realistically appraising the changed circumstances of life and body. Denial can be beneficial if it does not interfere with needed medical or emotional care and if it facilitates relationships and activities. Old people who use appropriate activity, ranging from the creative to merely "keeping busy" in order to counteract fear or depression, also have a defense that is an asset. Less adaptive are the counterphobic defenses, wherein some old people undertake excessive activities, which are dangerous to life and limb, in order to prove their continued prowess, youthfulness, and fearlessness.

In judging the adaptations of the elderly it is vital to remember that the old commonly deal with more stresses (in actual number, frequency, and profundity) than any other age group. Thus evaluation of restitutive attempts must be viewed with this in mind. Sometimes maintenance of the status quo may be all that is possible; indeed, this may be a triumph under the circumstances. A pride in present accomplishments, no matter how small, is appropriate.

Paranoid personality features have a particular maladaptiveness in old age, since so much happens to reinforce the notion that the problems are all "out there." In addition, hearing and other sensory losses increase the inability to deal with threatening forces and compound the isolation of the person with paranoid tendencies. A defensive use of perceptual loss, such as "hearing what one wants to hear," may be present. Tendencies to use age, disease, or impairment as a defense (by acting more helpless than is warranted) are common problems. Personality characteristics of rigidity, despair, depression, and the whole range of psychopathological reactions can further hamper adaptation to old age.

As we stated in Chapter 4, certain psychopathology can become increasingly adaptive as people age. Obsessional maneuvers fill the emptiness of retirement; schizoid detachment apparently insulates against loss; dependency can result in a welcoming of greater care and help from others.

Diagnostic attention to the inner experience of old age

Aside from the complex of reality factors and the influences of the individual personality, there are inner reactions to old age, which seem to be part of the developmental work of late life. One of these inner processes, the life review, appears to be of universal occurrence. (See Chapters 2 and 3.) It takes place through reminiscence accompanied by feelings of nostalgia, regret, pleasure. Complications that can occur are extreme pain, despair, guilt, obsessive rumination, panic, and suicide. A resolution or working through of the life review may bring atonement, serenity, constructive reorganization, and creativity.

PROBLEMS COMMONLY MISDIAGNOSED OR OVERLOOKED

Some conditions that require special diagnostic care are named in the following outline. These conditions, commonly overlooked, are recoverable and treatable. Look for:

1. Reversible brain syndromes
   a. Alone
   b. Superimposed on chronic brain syndrome
2. Depressive reactions simulating organic brain disorders
3. Paranoid states without organic brain disease
   a. Generalized
   b. Circumscribed
   c. Chronic paranoid state with superimposed, reversible crises
4. Subdural hematomas
5. Drug reactions

The list below contains key diagnostic concepts.

1. Insight and depression may be present in early phase of cerebral arteriosclerosis.
2. Depression may mask itself as organic confusion.
3. Reversible (acute) brain syndromes are often misdiagnosed as chronic brain syndrome.
4. Acute and chronic brain syndromes may coexist.
5. Depression and brain syndromes may coexist.
6. Retinal arteriosclerosis is *not* diagnostic of cerebral arteriosclerosis.
7. Suicide is frequent in old men.
8. Paradoxical excitatory drug reactions to barbiturate sedatives may occur.
9. Tranquilizer-induced ("iatrogenic") brain syndromes occur.
10. Tranquilizer-induced depressions are not uncommon.

Reversible (acute) brain syndrome

As Simon and Cahan state, "We found a large proportion (over half) of geriatric patients admitted for mental illness to be suffering from acute brain disorder and in urgent need of psychiatrically oriented medical care. A gratifying proportion of them improved sufficiently or recovered to return to society."*

The reversible brain syndromes are extremely important to diagnose early so treatment can be given before further illness complicates the picture. Such disorders have been called acute, but the salient fact is that they are reversible. Abruptness of onset, brevity of the illness, and obviousness of the symptoms are not so clear in the elderly as they may be in younger people and, therefore, require heightened diagnostic awareness.

The physiological disturbances responsible for onset are varied and include malnutrition, occult (hidden) cardiac failure, febrile illnesses, dehydration, cerebrovascular accidents, trauma, alcoholism, and drugs. The signal importance of a comprehensive examination is clearly demonstrated by the diagnostic work-up of the reversible brain syndrome. For instance, the hematocrit level may reveal dehydration or blood urea nitrogen may be elevated—both would be picked up in a routine examination.

One is more likely to observe the reversible brain syndrome in patients who are younger on the average than those with chronic brain syndromes. Most cases come to medical attention within a month of onset; but when malnutrition is the cause, the duration of illness before diagnosis is frequently longer. There also seems to be a social element present in this disorder. Simon and Cahan reported that patients with reversible brain syndromes were likely to have fewer family ties (often being divorced and living alone) and that retirement tended to occur before age 65.

---

*From Simon, Alexander, and Cahan, Robert B.: The acute brain syndrome in geriatric patients. In Mendel, W. M., and Epstein, L. J., editors: Acute psychotic reaction, Washington, D. C., 1963, Psychiatric Research Report No. 16, p. 8.

Psychometric tests are generally lower in the presence of chronic brain syndromes, as compared to reversible syndromes—the more chronic the syndrome, the lower the score. But testing results are of uneven reliability in diagnosing the reversible syndromes because of fluctuating levels of awareness.

Judging from the work of Simon and Cahan and that of others, perhaps 10% to 20% of older patients have reversible brain syndromes *only* and another 30% have mixed acute/chronic disorders. Thus as many as 50% of all older patients may have treatable organically based conditions and can be expected to improve if treated promptly. Treatment itself is part of the diagnostic work-up. *One often cannot know if a condition is reversible until it has been reversed.*

Depression versus organicity

It is imperative to diagnose depression that may be masked as organic states. Observe the content of thought and capitalize upon the sense of interpersonal responsiveness. The depressed are prone to express a sense of worthlessness. The patient with an organic disorder is likely to be perceived as presenting a "biological," rather than an "emotional," problem. Depressive episodes are self-limited; organic states are not. Identify the specific events or stimuli that precipitated the feelings of depression. Many depressive episodes are realistic responses to loss. Some are influenced by the unconscious or the past history but, because they cannot be readily explained by the present, they are referred to as "exogenous" rather than "reactive." There is a relief of symptoms when actual loss or threat is relieved, compensated for, or replaced; not so with organic disorders. Depression may look similar to the organic disorders, but careful evaluation can differentiate the two. (See Chapter 5.) Here psychological tests, the Goldstein catastrophic reaction, EEG, and other components of the comprehensive examination are most helpful. It must not be forgotten, however, that depression and organic brain disorder can coexist. In depressions one may also see a paranoid trend.

Paranoid states without organic brain disease

Look for ideas of ruin and for delusions of noxious fumes, delusions of marital infidelity, and the like. Note isolated evidences of projection as well as comprehensive delusional systems. Be aware of cases of folie à deux.* Check for hearing loss, which is associated with suspiciousness and paranoid states.

Subdural hematomas

Falls and fractures are common in old age. Persons over 65 account for 72% of all fatal falls and 30% of all pedestrian fatalities. Subdural hematomas are collections of blood between the dura mater (the hard outer membrane over the brain) and the skull. They may be clinically silent. Again, a careful history may elicit a story of head injury, concussion, perhaps coma, delirium, or a syndrome (Korsakoff's) marked by fabrication and confabulation. Subdural hematomas, as well as brain tumors, hypertension, and extracerebral vascular occlusion or narrowing, can often be successfully treated—provided they are discovered.

Drug reactions

The prevalent wide use of drugs, from tranquilizers to antidepressants, has produced a number of negative drug reactions. Although they are useful when properly prescribed and controlled, drugs are also overused and misused. A striking illustration is the use of chemical straightjackets (heavy doses of quieting drugs) to handle patients in nursing homes. Drugs may make a differential diagnosis between functional and organic disorders exceedingly difficult, and discontinuation of the medications during an evaluation period may be required.

*Folie à deux is a form of psychosis in which symptoms, especially paranoid delusions, are shared by two people—most often mother and daughter, two sisters, or husband and wife.

SUICIDE INDICATIONS

Suicide in old age was discussed in Chapter 4. We wish to list here (not necessarily in order of frequency or importance) some of the major diagnostic clues for suicide in old age.

Depression
Withdrawal
Bereavement (especially within year)
Isolation: widowed; single
Expectation of death from some cause
Less organization and complexity of behavior
Induced helplessness
Institutionalization
Physical illness
Desire and rational decision to protect survivors from financial disaster
Philosophical decision: no more pleasure or purpose
Meaninglessness of life
Decreased self-regard
Organic mental deterioration
Changes in sleep patterns: nightmares
Male
Note: A threat to commit suicide is relatively uncommon in this age group. Old people tend to simply kill themselves.

One must be alert for statements from people about killing themselves and be aware of any previous suicide attempts. Self-destruction can be abrupt or be drawn out over long periods of time (not eating, not taking one's medicines, alcoholism, delay in seeking treatment, excessive risk taking). Old people account for one fourth of all reported suicides. Therefore, a mental health evaluation should give serious consideration to behavior that might indicate self-destructive tendencies.

THE LEGAL EXAMINATION

Medical doctors, especially psychiatrists, may be called upon to evaluate an older person's need for involuntary commitment to an institution or to ascertain aspects of competency (contractual or testamentary capacity). Human beings have a fundamental right to make their own decisions, enter into contracts, vote, make a will, and refuse medical or psychiatric treatment. Each of these decisions represents one's control over one's own life, with the understanding that the consequences may be unfortunate as well as fortunate, folly as well as wisdom. Limitations of such rights or freedom ideally come about only when illnesses invalidate the capacity to make choices or, in the case of legal commitment, when the older person is a danger to himself or to others, physically, or is in clear and present need of immediate care or treatment. Old people also need protection when they are vulnerable to exploitation by others.

In examining an older person for forensic (legal) purposes, the examiner should spell out in detail that fact. The person needs to know that he can be represented by an attorney and that his statements to the examiner will *not* be protected either by privilege (the legal concept) or by confidentiality (the relationship). The examination should be thorough, and we again suggest use of the personal mental health data form on p. 149.

What is the test of incompetency? "Understanding" is the crucial criterion: the person must have sufficient mental capacity to *understand* the nature and effect of the *particular* transaction in question. The psychiatric diagnosis is not considered, in courts of law, to be as important as judgment.*

Contractual capacity (the ability to make contracts) is related to the degree of judgment required—selling a major business is a complex situation that may require a greater degree of judgment than selling a car. One problem sometimes emerging in contractual cases is that in which an older person's judgment may indeed be adversely affected by mental or physical disorders but this fact is unknown to the other party in the contract.

A 69-year-old woman was profoundly depressed but outwardly cheerful. She sold her $75,000 home for $55,000. It was a bona fide sale, so there was no later recourse.

The concept of the "lucid interval" is a vague and difficult one, implying the capacity to exercise sound judgment at one time and and not another. The multicausal aspects of

*Commitment to a mental hospital is *not* the equivalent of incompetency.

the emotional and mental disorders of old age indicate the possibility of such intervals. For example, a person with cerebral vascular insufficiency may do well until severe emotional stress (e.g., widowhood) compromises his equilibrium; after a period of time he or she may again stabilize and be considered "lucid." An evaluator must be extremely thorough in examining the older person for such a possibility.

Testamentary capacity (the ability to make a will) requires that the testator (person who makes the will) be "of sound mind and memory," knowing the condition of his estate, his obligations, and the import of the provisions of his will. The psychiatric examiner must consider whether the older person is unduly suggestible or under "undue influence" from others. Severe depression and paranoid states, as well as organic brain disorders, may affect the capacity to write a will; however, diagnosis of psychosis, adjudication of guardianship, or commitment per se does not invalidate a will. "Extreme age, mental sluggishness, and defective memory do not render a testator incapable of making a will if he is able to recall to mind his property and the natural objects of his bounty." Alcoholism, addictions, and unusual beliefs (e.g., spiritualism) do not by themselves invalidate wills. When there is any doubt of testamentary capacity or when a contesting of the will is anticipated, it is wise of the testator to arrange for a comprehensive medical and psychiatric evaluation while he is alive, with a careful and complete report filed until his death. By so doing he can prevent further grief and turmoil for his family.

An 87-year-old man married his nurse and rewrote his will. Other members of the family challenged his mental soundness and pushed for a postmortem examination of his brain, resulting in bitterness and anguish for everyone concerned.

Guardianship or the appointment of a committee for a person or his estate should be solely for his benefit and protection. The test is whether the person can or cannot protect himself or arrange his own affairs. Emotional disability, as well as intellectual impairment, is important. (Guilt or feelings of worthlessness may lead a person to give everything away.) Injudicious management and improvidence are difficult to evaluate and are not precisely correlated with intellectual debility. Laws are unclear on many points, and there is a quality of all-or-none, whereas a continuum or scale of impairment would be more appropriate. Certain disabilities are not considered at all by the law—visual and auditory impairments, loss of speech, etc. Poor people are disadvantaged because of the legal costs of conservatorships; since few states provide for public guardianship (the poor man's conservatorship), estates are easily eroded. The poorly educated and the uninformed are not protected, and the Roman injunction "caveat emptor" (let the buyer beware) holds sway to a greater degree in old age than ever before.

Involuntary commitment will be examined more thoroughly in Chapter 11, but we wish to discuss here the question of court cases for mental patients and old people in general. In what passes for kindness it is often argued that court appearances are too disturbing for the elderly patient. Even when a hospitalized person decides to call for a jury trial, the hospital psychiatrist may back away and discharge the patient first. We believe there are serious faults with these attitudes. They conceal from the public, from the person involved, and from the psychiatrist and mental health personnel the realities of legal processes and of property and personal rights. Patients often learn from the painful court proceedings; it becomes clear what the situation really is, and the process can have therapeutic effects. Our traditional overestimation of the fragility of patients and, indeed, our paternalism and infantilization can deny people their rights and the opportunity for self-expression.

Court appearances may also assist mental health personnel in sharpening up their diagnostic thinking. A few embarrassing moments under cross-examination in a court of law can be a humbling experience and worth hours of postgraduate training or review. Psychiatrists and other staff who complain of wasting time in court might be well advised to keep eyes and ears open, taking the occasion to learn something more of the human condition as it unfolds in a courtroom.

The adversary system does have its cruelties, and one might argue for dispassionate commissions wherein commitment, competency, and contractual and testamentary capacities are evaluated. We would support the use of independent commissions (comprised of physicians, mental health personnel, and lawyers) but subject to administrative and judicial reviews. Hearings must include patients, well represented by counsel. The amount of time provided must be adequate and not just a token. In Washington, D. C., it was found that the mental health commission operative at St. Elizabeths Hospital often made judgments within minutes. We also feel, along with others, that the various capacities under consideration (contractual, testamentary, etc.) should be considered separately and in their special contexts, rather than under a global concept called "competence."

REFERENCES

Allen, E. B., and Clow, H. E.: Paranoid reactions in the aging, Geriatrics **5**:66-73, 1950.

Birren, James E.: A factorial analysis of the Wechsler-Bellevue Scale to an elderly population, Journal of Consulting Psychology **16**:399, 1952.

Busse, E. W.: Treatment of the non-hospitalized, emotionally disturbed, elderly person, Geriatrics **11**:173-179, 1956.

Butler, R. N.: The facade of chronological age, American Journal of Psychiatry **119**:721-728, 1963.

Butler, R. N.: The life review: an interpretation of reminiscence in the aged, Psychiatry **26**:65-76, 1963.

Butler, R. N.: Psychiatric evaluation of the aged, Geriatrics **18**:220-232, 1963.

Butler, R. N., and Perlin, S.: Physiological-psychological-psychiatric interdisciplinary findings. In Human aging: a biological and behavioral study, Washington, D. C., 1963, U. S. Government Printing Office. Reprinted Publication No. (HSM) 71-9051, 1971.

Butler, R. N., and Sulliman, Lillian G.: Psychiatric contact with community-resident emotionally disturbed elderly, Journal of Nervous and Mental Diseases **137**:108-186, 1963.

Cowdry, E. V., and Steinberg, F. U., editors: The care of the geriatric patient, ed. 4, St. Louis, 1971, The C. V. Mosby Co.

Diagnostic and statistical manual of mental disorders, ed. 2, (DSM-II) Washington, D. C., 1968, American Psychiatric Association.

Ehrentheil, O. F.: Differential diagnosis of organic dementias and affective disorders in aged patients, Geriatrics **12**:426, 1957.

Gaitz, C. M.: Functional assessment of the suspected mentally ill aged, Journal of the American Geriatrics Society **17**:541-548, 1969.

Goldstein, K., and Scheerer, M.: Abstract and concrete behavior, Psychological Monograph **53**(2): 239, 1941.

Grier, William, and Cobbs, Price: Black rage, New York, 1968, Basic Books, Inc.

Hollender, M. H.: Role of the psychiatrist in homes for the aged, Geriatrics **6**:243-250, 1951.

Kahn, R. L., Goldfarb, A. I., Pollack, M., and Peck, A.: Brief objective measures for the determination of mental status in the aged, American Journal of Psychiatry **117**:326-328, 1960.

Kety, S. S., and Schmidt, C. F.: The nitrous oxide method for the quantitative determination of cerebral blood flow in men: theory, procedure, and normal values, Journal of Clinical Investigation **27**:476-483, 1948.

Lawton, M. P.: The functional assessment of elderly people, Journal of the American Geriatrics Society **19**:465-481, 1971.

Menninger, K. A.: A manual for psychiatric case study, New York, 1952, Grune & Stratton, Inc.

Norris, Vera, and Post, F.: Treatment of elderly psychiatric patients: use of diagnostic classification, British Medical Journal **1**:675-679, 1754.

Perlin, S.: Psychiatric screening in a home for the aged. I. A follow-up study, Geriatrics **13**:747-751, 1958.

Perlin, S., and Butler, R. N.: Psychiatric aspects of adaptation to the aging experience. In Birren, J. E., Butler, R. N., Greenhouse, S. W., Sokoloff, L., and Yarrow, Marian R., editors: Human aging: a biological and behavioral study, Washington, D. C., 1963, U. S. Government Printing Office, Reprinted Publication No. (HSM) 71-9051, 1971.

Redlich, F. C., and Freedman, D. X.: The psychiatric interview and examination. In Redlich, F. C., and Freedman, D. X, editors: The theory and practice of psychiatry, New York, 1966, Basic Books, Inc.,

Rossman, I., editor: Clinical geriatrics, Philadelphia, 1971, J. B. Lippincott Co.

Roth, M.: Natural history of mental disorder in old age, Journal of Mental Science **101**:281-301, 1955.

Rypins, R. F., and Clark, M. C.: A screening project for the geriatric mentally ill, California Medicine **109**:273-278, 1968.

Simon, Alexander, and Cahan, Robert B.: The

acute brain syndrome in geriatric patients. In Mendel, W. M., and Epstein, L. J., editors: Acute psychotic reaction, Washington, D. C., 1963, Psychiatric Research Report No. 16.

Sullivan, H. S.: The psychiatric interview, New York, 1954, W. W. Norton & Co., Inc.

Werner, Martha M., Perlin, S., Butler, R. N., and Pollin, W.: Self-perceived changes in community-resident aged: "aging image" and adaptation, Archives of General Psychiatry 4:501-508, 1961.

10

HOW TO KEEP PEOPLE AT HOME

Do older people who are ill really prefer staying home if they can get the help they need? Would the rest of us? Knowing what we all know about hospitals and other institutions: the high-priced, impersonal, medically oriented concepts of care and the grim reputations of most institutions for the elderly, it seems clear that some alternatives would be eagerly and even desperately welcomed. Institutions seldom feel like home to people who were raised from infancy in family units, and little is done to make them feel homey. Still worse, little is done to make them therapeutic or even livable. A tour of many state hospital geriatric wards, nursing homes, and other treatment and custodial settings designed "especially" for the old is enough to frighten brave men and turn steady stomachs. We shall be discussing institutional care in Chapter 11. Here we wish to examine the care of people in their own homes with the aid of a variety of services.

HOW IMPORTANT IS "HOME"?

Home is extraordinarily significant to many older persons. It is part of their identity, a place where things are familiar and relatively unchanging, and a place to maintain a sense of autonomy and control. Some insist upon remaining at home "at all costs" to their emotional and physical health and personal security. Such tenaciousness can be laid to a desire for freedom and independence; a fear of loss of contact with familiar and loved people, places, and things; a fear of dying, because of the reputation of hospitals and nursing homes as "houses of death" from which there is no return; and a trepidation about change and the unknown, which frightens people of all ages. In this nation of homeowners where 67% of older people own their homes the idea of a personal house is deeply ingrained; and communal living is viewed as a loss of personal liberty and dignity.* The notion of home can refer primarily to the four walls surrounding one, to the neighborhood in which one is located, or to the possessions that make one feel at home. Home may mean certain other individuals living with one or it may mean neighbors, pets, and plants. It can either be a place where one has lived a good part of one's life or be a new place, as when older people move into a retirement community or leave the farm for a home in town. Thus home is whatever the "concept of home" means to each person.

Home can be a euphemism. In our eagerness to recognize the importance of a feeling of home we must not overlook those older people who dislike their living conditions, who have never felt "at home" where they are, and who are eager to move somewhere else—even to an institution. They may live in a crummy rooming house, having a bare room with a lone light bulb suspended from the ceiling, in a boarding house with skimpy meals, in a cheap "retirement hotel" where the bath is shared with junkies, alcoholics, or street drifters. Some old people are themselves drifters with no regular

*With changing life styles and living arrangements, the importance of "place" and the definition of "home" may be quite different in the future. Present-day communal dwellers and apartment renters may be prepared for a different kind of old-age living arrangement.

residence, no fixed address. They sleep on park benches or in subways, bus and train stations, bowery missions, doorways.

Home may be fine physically but miserable emotionally because of family circumstances. The in-law problem is classic, where an older person moves in with a son or daughter. Everyone may end up bitterly unhappy.

One 69-year-old woman was living with her son and daughter-in-law. The mother and daughter-in-law had never gotten along and couldn't tolerate talking to each other. The mother was discouraged from participating in housework. She therefore would remain in her pajamas all day, watching television. When the son was due home, she would dress, put on her makeup, and become warm and friendly. She and her daughter-in-law vied for his attentions. The mother complained that she was not invited to help the family and was considered a burden. The daughter-in-law stated that mother expected total care. The son, caught in the middle between the two women in his life, finally asked mother to leave.

Many situations with an older parent in the home fortunately work out much more satisfactorily. But one must avoid falling prey to one's own slogans, such as "keep people in their own homes," when this may be totally inappropriate and even cruel. The other battlecry of reformers, "return institutional patients to the community," needs to be looked at with the same careful skepticism. What kind of community? What kind of home will be involved? Successful adjustment and adaptation is no more ensured in the community than anywhere else. Each new generation of reformers and each new change in political administration tend to grab that easy problem-solving device known to bureaucrats as "reorganizing"—to give the impression of progress (change names and titles, shift personnel, start new programs, abandon old ones, move patients around: into institutions, back to communities, into nursing and foster homes, or back to institutions with new names). Actual provision of care is rarely improved by all this shuffling. In fact the complaints about nursing homes heard in the latest back-to-the-community trend* sound amazingly like the previous complaints about mental institutions, citing poor food, understaffing, fire hazards, and unsanitary conditions. Each decision concerning home care versus institutional care must be based on the older person's needs, but both alternatives should be as attractive and as therapeutic as it is possible to make them. In general we believe that home care offers the best treatment location except when people are physically dangerous or require inpatient medical treatment. But it is beneficial only when the home is an adequate place to begin with or can be made adequate by selected interventions.

ADVANTAGES OF HOME CARE

Of course one of the obvious advantages of home care is that most older people prefer it. Care at home offers better morale and security as long as proper services are given to provide comfort, support, and direct treatment of physical and emotional ills. Relatives and service personnel such as homemakers and home health aides can often give more individualized care than nursing staffs in institutions. Families tend to become intimately involved in treatment. Familiar surroundings are reassuring and the older person does not have to be separated from family members, friends, possessions, pets. Earlier intervention is possible, since it is not necessary to wait until hospitalization to begin treatment. Hospital beds can be saved for those who are more critically ill. Older people who may be very ill or not ambulatory are not forced to leave home and travel to get treatment. Physicians, nurses, social workers, and members of all other disciplines involved can become more familiar with community resources and be able to use them more fully as well as point up the need for services not presently available. Older people and their families can receive not only medical and psychiatric care but also social and economic help. And, finally, the older person

*We consider nursing homes to be institutions rather than homes. Thus we do not consider them to be "community" facilities any more than hospitals are.

and the people in his life receive a different view of illness and treatment. Instead of being whisked off to the hospital or an institution, people remain where their care can be observed and participated in. It becomes evident that mental or physical illness can be lived with. Life does not have to stop or become totally disrupted, and rehabilitation and recovery may be seen occurring even in the very old and sick. It is clear that removal from home for treatment or long-term care is perceived by many older people as a "punishment" for getting sick. They fear the isolation, the loneliness, and the separation from familiar patterns and people, not to mention the boredom. The thought of "dying alone" becomes a frightening preoccupation. Older people should not have to "serve time" in an institution just because they become ill unless such care is an absolute necessity or their own personal preference.

It should also be mentioned that home care is a potential consumer market, which could create many new jobs and a whole new service industry. It could open up the mental health professions to an influx of new personnel and new ideas. There are some excellent nursing homes, but all too many are inadequate and seem to be run exclusively for profit. Some day nursing homes and home services may be operated as social or public utilities, well regulated and run in the public interest. New professions may well evolve, having a broader base of skills than is now seen.

USE OF THE HOME FOR SCREENING AND EVALUATION

Keeping older people at home can begin at the beginning when a request or referral for mental health services is received. Part or all of the evaluation can be done at home, except for technical (usually medical) examinations that require a specific setting. Even when most of an evaluation must be carried out elsewhere, it is important that a direct evaluation of the person's home situation be made. In addition to telling much that is useful about people's lives, such evaluations make it possible to bring services to those older persons who cannot or will not leave their homes to come to a clinic, hospital, or agency.

Referral requests for mental health care come from older people themselves, their families, agencies, the police, and other sources, as shown in the list below.

Self-referral
Family
Friends and neighbors
Clergymen
Doctors—often internists
Visiting nurse service
Welfare department
Community agencies
Police

The more isolated the older person, the more likely that his or her difficulties will remain unnoticed until an emergency occurs and the police are called. Health inspectors, shopkeepers, and service workers such as postmen, meter readers, hotel and apartment clerks may be the link that connects the isolated older person with the police after something begins to obviously go wrong.

After an evaluation of the specific nature of the person's problem has been completed (Chapter 9), a mutually agreeable decision must be made among family members, the older person, and mental health personnel as to the nature and location of treatment to be given. Is home care always preferable to institutional care? Does mental health care include such diverse services as provision of adequate income, homemakers, or even podiatry (foot treatment)? Our view is that a comprehensive, broad concept of care includes whatever has to be done. We are interested in preserving and rebuilding any aspects of the older person's life that contribute to his physical and emotional well-being. Rather than offering the rather narrow specialty skills most of us learned during professional and vocational training, we advocate learning the additional skills necessary to meet the variety of needs older people present. This is both good mental health treatment and good preventive care as well as sound education for mental health personnel.

SOME FACTORS TO CONSIDER REGARDING HOME CARE

The decision to provide treatment in the home is influenced by what the older person needs and/or wants, the family situation, and the services and choices of care available in a community. In terms of the individual, one must know if he or she is physically and mentally capable of self-care, either alone or with assistance. The list below gives the most important of the skills needed for living at home, particularly if one is alone part or all of the time.

Orientation to time, place, person
Cooking and feeding oneself
Bathing
Dressing
Grooming
Toileting
Continence
Transferring from bed to chair
Standing and walking
Climbing stairs
Fire and accident security
Shopping
Money management
Ability to follow instructions (e.g., medication)
Ability to seek assistance when needed
Social participation

Other considerations are adequate transportation, socializing opportunities, quick availability of emergency medical care, financial circumstances, and the neighborhood crime conditions. Can the rent or mortgage be paid—and the utilities, repair costs, and property taxes? Does the older person have the inner resources to manage on his own? Are there interests and activities? Personal relationships? Sexual outlets? Religious and spiritual supports?

One must also consider those people whom the older person will be living with or relying on heavily. Does home include other family members, roomers, or companions? Is it possible to be at home in someone else's home, perhaps with sons or daughters. Can sharing and communal living work in the average family? Or would the older person be more content in a communal arrangement with elderly persons or mixed with other age groups? Relatives or friends with whom an elderly person lives may not be willing or able to care for the older person at home any longer. Sometimes there are no comfortable or easy solutions as the needs of the older person clash with those who are younger. In most situations families will make every sacrifice to keep an older person and may need help in reconsidering whether this is the wisest course of action. In other cases they need support and opportunity for respite if they do decide on home care.

The essential consideration in opting for home care is the kind of services one can expect to be available to the older person. Often these will ultimately determine whether it is possible for him to stay at home. In this chapter we will be going further than in any other in describing care that should and may exist but probably does not. Medicare and the insurance programs for older people encourage hospitalization rather than outpatient care in their coverage. The very poor may be able to get some home services through welfare, but self-supporting people tend not to be able to afford them. Free care or care based on the ability to pay is sporadically available through charitable agencies and United Fund organizations. The federal government, through Medicare, has weakly sponsored provisions for home health aides, cutting back funds in the 1970s. Food stamps are always perilously close to discontinuance as politicians wax and wane on the issues of feasibility and "moral efficacy."*

*One wonders why old people have to be reexamined and recertified for food stamps on a regular basis to determine whether their incomes have changed; it hardly seems likely that fixed incomes will miraculously expand. We have seen old people waiting in food stamp lines at 6 o'clock in the morning and being told three hours later to come back the next day because an office could process only a certain number of applicants. This kind of harassment causes many older people to refuse to apply for the stamps or any of the other services that require systematic humiliation and endless red tape.

HOME CARE—WHAT *REALLY* EXISTS AND WHAT *IDEALLY* SHOULD EXIST

Any truly serious national effort to keep people in their own homes requires provision for direct home delivery of health services. The middle class as well as the poor suffer from the unavailability of such care. Home care should be available to the chronically ill, to those recuperating from hospitalization, to those who may be acutely ill but can be treated outside a hospital, and finally to all those older people who simply need some help here and there to fill in the gaps left by various losses or declining functions. We will be describing the services we feel are essential if home care is to be a comprehensive approach to the treatment and prevention of mental illness. Evaluations, treatment plans, and coordination of care by some responsible person or group are of course essential. It is usually not difficult to figure out who the responsible coordinating person should be because there are precious few agencies and individuals, professional or otherwise, who work directly in the community despite much rhetoric to the contrary. In the past the family doctor took care of physical problems (using the house call, long since placed on the endangered list of extinct medical practices) and clergymen attended to spiritual and/or emotional matters, buttressed by neighbors and nearby family members.* However, doctors and clergymen began spending more time in their offices, crime frightened away many of those who might have preferred direct community work, and only two major groups now routinely make house calls: public health nurses and social workers. Much to their credit members of these professions—usually female—continue working unarmed and often alone in high crime areas where the poor and many of the urban elderly reside. Some medical doctors, psychiatrists, and related professionals are becoming reinterested and involved in community work, particularly through community mental health centers and outreach programs. Paraprofessionals of all kinds are beginning to do mental health work. But the faithful standbys are still the nurses and the social workers. Thus for the time being, they are likely to be the central coordinating figures in any plans for provision of home care.

The outline here summarizes the range of services that should be part of the repertoire of home care.

- Mental health intake, screening and evaluation
- Mental health care
- Physician's services
- Nursing services
- Homemaker–home health aides
- Physical therapy
- Occupational therapy
- Speech therapy
- Dental care
- Nutrition service (Meals-on-Wheels, group dining, food distribution programs)
- Social services
  - Information and referral
  - Financial support
  - Personal needs (transportation, telephone reassurance, grooming, shopping, companions, pets)
  - Family "respite" services
  - Home safety
  - Recreation (community center, senior center)
  - Employment and volunteer work (VISTA, Senior Aides, SCORE, Peace Corps, Foster Grandparents, Green Thumb, etc.)
  - Education (home library service, academic courses)
- Religious support (clerical counseling, "practical" ecumenism)
- Outpatient care in clinics, community mental health center, day hospitals, day care centers
- Multipurpose senior centers
- Protective services
- Screening before hospital admission

We repeat that many communities will not have all or even most of these resources. Some can be created at little or no cost by volunteer groups. Others can be lobbied for in state legislatures. Pressure can be put on professional groups and voluntary agencies to make their services available or create new services. Research studies have already examined the fiscal, psychological, and med-

*As can be seen, home care is not a radical new idea but a return to some of the sound principles of the past, strengthened by newer medical and psychiatric understanding and techniques.

ical results of home care as compared to results with institutionalization or with no care at all.*

Old people themselves should voice their opinions about the kind of mental health care they want in old age.

In planning a program of home care, one must be clear about the objectives, whether rehabilitation, maintenance of the status quo, or support through decline and eventual death. Change is the most constant factor in the treatment of the elderly. Treatment must be constantly evaluated for its appropriateness and be altered whenever circumstances change in the direction of either improved functioning or greater illness. It can be as harmful to over-treat someone who is trying to get better as to under-treat. Dependency and loss of functioning can result if people of any age are overprotected and coddled when they do not need it. Conscientious mental health practitioners tend to err in this direction.

HOME DELIVERY OF SERVICES

Mental health services

All the services mentioned in this chapter are considered by us as part of mental health care. In addition, the specific services of psychiatrists, social workers, and all other members of mental health teams should be routinely available in people's homes. The two major types of psychiatric outreach care are emergency care (usually for persons making suicide threats and attempts or for those wandering in the streets as a result of brain damage or functional psychosis) and ongoing therapy for those who find it difficult to leave home. Evaluations for mental health services as well as screening for institutional admissions can be done in homes.* Screening should of course emphasize keeping people out of institutions, when appropriate, by use of home care. Mental health services will be discussed more fully in Chapter 12. With outreach services one sees many people who would never appear at clinics and would only be seen in hospitals as a result of an emergency.

Physicians' services

Physicians should be on call for emergency home visits on a 24-hour basis and for ongoing medical evaluation and management of patients. Contact may vary from brief intensive care to weekly or monthly medical supervision and treatment. Laboratory services can also be provided. Specimens—blood, urine, feces, etc.—can be obtained from the person at home and analyzed in the laboratory. Electrocardiograms and other selected studies can be made in the home.

There are two major problems standing in the way of home medical care: doctors' reluctance to make house calls and a lack of financial resources that might make it possible to tempt them from their offices. Government figures document the decline in house calls. In 1957-1958 doctors made about 45.7 million calls; in 1966-1967 only 27.3 million were made although the population had risen. In 1972 less than half the doctors in the country still made house calls, and most of these practice in rural areas. In most cases doctors feel they can treat a patient better in an office or in a hospital emergency room and that the house calls take too much time. "It is rare that a house call is justified" is a common viewpoint. The hospital emergency room has become the place

*Special Committee on Aging, U. S. Senate: Alternatives to nursing home care: a proposal, prepared by staff specialists at the Levinson Gerontological Policy Institute, Brandeis University, Waltham, Mass. (Dr. Robert Morris, Director), Washington, D. C., 1971, U. S. Government Printing Office. Also Special Committee on Aging, U. S. Senate: Home health services in the United States, prepared by Brahna Trager, Home Health Consultant, 1972.

*Arne Querido's famous Amsterdam psychiatric emergency service sent teams to the homes of persons in crises. The San Francisco Geriatrics Screening Project ably coordinated by Mary Lou Clark, ACSW, and the Baltimore City Health Department Geriatric Evaluation Service directed by Mary Guth, MSW, are illustrative of the better screening programs in the United States that stress home visits.

where patients go who might otherwise have been served by house calls.

Profit-making house call organizations have been established but so far only in a few large cities. The oldest is Health Delivery Systems, Inc., of New York City. Next is the Bridge Medical Associates of New York. Los Angeles has Health Systems, Inc. Some local medical societies offer emergency services. Residents in teaching hospitals, older semiretired doctors, newly licensed doctors, and moonlighting military and government doctors make up the bulk of manpower for these organizations. Armed guards are sometimes available to accompany doctors into "hazardous neighborhoods." Radio equipment vans are used by the Los Angeles organization. The patient's own doctor receives a report from the house call doctors. Fees range from $20 to $25. Medicare will cover 80% of what is determined to be the customary and prevailing fee for a particular area.

Doctors who make house calls catch emergency situations such as heart attacks and appendicitis in early stages as well as providing relief from relatively minor but extremely painful ailments such as ear infections. They can determine if hospitalization is called for or if other services are needed. And they provide an enormous sense of security to the older person who may be worried about health or unable to leave home for care of aggravating but noncritical illnesses.

Mrs. H, a black woman of 85 years, lives in a public housing project with her daughter's family. She is confined to her second-floor room because of arthritis and a disabled hip. She seldom sees a doctor because her son-in-law has a heart condition that prohibits him from carrying her down the stairs. In addition, her daughter must take off a day's work to transport her in the family car. Mrs. H. does not want to put an extra burden on them so she seldom mentions her aches and pains. She wept with disbelief at the sight of the physician from the neighborhood community mental health service who came to see her in her room.

Doctors are poorly distributed geographically. Some areas—the urban poor and the rural—typically have few doctors and other health personnel.

In Washington, D. C., 90% of doctors are located west of Rock Creek Park, which essentially divides white (west) from black Washington, where some 60% of the population live.

The National Health Service Corps is the unit within HSMHA, U. S. Public Health Service, charged with carrying out the Emergency Health Personnel Act of 1970 (P.L. 91-623). This Act authorizes the assignment of commissioned officers and civil service personnel of the Service to areas in the United States where health services are inadequate because of critical shortages of health personnel. This program is not meant to solve the problem of the overall shortage of physicians and other health personnel in the nation but is aimed at alleviating some of the more acute problems stemming from the maldistribution of health manpower in this country.

The United States has only one physician for every 650 people, compared to 580 in Italy and 400 in the U.S.S.R. The 1970 report of the Carnegie Commission on Higher education prescribed a shortened program for medical schools and residency programs. Women and minority group members, who now make up only 7% of doctors, should be vigorously encouraged. One state, California, has passed a law permitting physicians' assistants to work under doctors' supervision, doing much of the medical work. At present some 35,000 highly trained medical corpsmen are discharged annually from the military services. The Vietnam veteran has a knowledge of emergency medicine that is often far superior to the experience of doctors in civilian life. By 1970 some forty schools in the United States had training programs for assistant physicians who are known as paramedics, clinical associates, and health practitioners. Nurses also are taking over certain functions of the physician and are called "nurse practitioners."

Area of specialization is another handicap for older people. Of 85,000 new physicians produced annually, less than 3% enter general practice, which has become a dying profession. Old people will look in vain for a "family doctor." Recent congressional legislation aims at encouraging doctors to enter family practice. Geriatric medicine has not been recognized as a speciality in the United States, although 40% of the average internist's patients are older people with whom he spends 60% of his time.

Nursing services*

The services included under home nursing care are those of *registered nurses* (RNs), whose two specialties pertinent to the elderly are public health nursing and psychiatric nursing; *licensed practical nurses* (LPNs); and *home health aides*. The latter two groups are supervised by registered nurses.

We shall attempt to clarify the work of each of these groups as they care for the elderly. *Public health nursing* refers to registered nurses and sometimes licensed practical nurses who work for tax-supported city or county health departments. They visit families in their homes, provide direct nursing care, give health guidance, participate in communicable disease control programs, and staff public health clinics. They may give emergency care as well as care for acute and chronic illness. They can instruct people in the use of community health and social resources and make authorized investigations of convalescent homes, nursing homes, and other institutions. Referrals usually come from public health clinics or city and county hospitals as well as other public agencies. There is a heavy concentration of poor and inner-city people as clientele. Services are free of charge to those eligible.

Another group of nurses works with the *Visiting Nurse Association* (VNA),† a voluntary organization supported by local united givers' funds, endowments, gifts, patients' fees, and contracts with health and welfare departments, the American Cancer Society, the Multiple Sclerosis Assocation, the local Heart Association, the Veterans Administration, Medicare, and others. These nurses provide approximately the same services as public health nurses* but tend to have smaller caseloads and can devote more time to individual patients. Public health nurses may each have several hundred patients as well as responsibilities in clinics and schools. Both groups wear similar blue uniforms. Community familiarity with these uniforms gives them protection as they work in high crime neighborhoods. Visiting nurses do more direct home nursing, while public health nurses carry an added responsibility for preventive and community work. Referrals to visiting nurses come from private doctors and private hospitals, in the form of patient and family self-referrals, and from overloaded public health nurses. Visiting nurses care for both poor and middle-class patients. Elderly people are required to pay a fee adjustable to their income or may be eligible for free service through one of the organizations contracting with VNA and the third-party payments of Medicare and Medicaid.

Licensed practical nurses (LPNs) work under the supervision of registered nurses and perform many of the same nursing skills. *Home health aides* also provide simple nursing care, to be discussed later. For those who can afford very expensive services, a number of agencies supply *private duty RNs, LPNs,* and *nurses aides* for anywhere up to 24-hour total nursing care.

Home nursing service enables older people to leave hospitals sooner as well as keeping them at home longer before institutionalization. Some of the common ailments for which persons are treated are strokes, cerebral vascular accidents, arthritis, cancer, hip fractures, paraplegia, and minimal to moderate chronic brain syndromes. Teaching is another function; an example is the self-administration of insulin for diabetes. Family members can be taught to do a variety of tasks, including physical therapy. Problems with incontinence, bedsores, personal care of teeth

*Nursing education has not given adequate coverage to geriatric care (Moses and Lake, 1968).

†Other services provided by the VNA include homemaker–home health aides, physical and speech therapies, medical social work, and psychiatrically trained nurses.

*In some communities visiting nurses and public health nurses have merged their staffs and functions, while in others they work separately.

and mouth, bed baths, skin care, grooming, and feeding are tasks of the nursing personnel. They are also trained to look at the patient's family from a life cycle perspective: if there are children, are they immunized? is the mother receiving prenatal care? what can be done about the father's chest pains? All these are in addition to the original reason for the visit, which was to serve the older patient.

There has not been an increase in nursing personnel to meet the growing numbers of older people in the community. Federal and state funding programs have not recognized the need for care other than for short-term intervention linked to acute illness. Only 15,152 professional nurses and 1,409 licensed practical nurses were employed in home health agencies as of July, 1969. Many agencies are now cutting back on nursing staff because of restrictive Medicare regulations, curtailment of Medicaid benefits, and reduced voluntary support.

Homemaker–home health aide services*

The term "homemaker–home health aide" refers to one and the same person although in some parts of the nation these functions are distributed among several persons; for example, a housekeeper, nurses aide, etc. "Homemaker" describes the full range of homemaking activities available to people with either short-term or long-term physical and emotional illness or disability. "Home health aide" is a title found in Medicare regulations and describes a somewhat narrower definition of care, somewhat like a nursing assistant or nurses aide in a hospital who complements RNs and LPNs by performing simple medical procedures as well as "personal care." They may take the patient's vital signs, apply simple dressings, give massages, baths, grooming assistance, and physical therapy. Anything directly connected with an individual's care is part of their work: light cooking, cleaning the patient's room, and washing clothes for the patient. Strictly speaking they are not allowed to provide the broader, family-wide care of the home, which is the realm of the homemaker. Training and supervision emphasize both aspects of the homemaker–home health aide: the performance of household tasks and the nursing care that is medically prescribed.

Homemaker–home health aides are always employed by an agency, organization, or administrative unit that selects, trains, and supervises them. They can be obtained through the recommendations of physicians, nurses, social workers, and health institutions as well as on a self-referred basis. Services may be free (for those eligible for welfare assistance) or paid for by third-party payments. In some cases fees are charged, according to ability to pay or on a straight fee basis. The Upjohn Homemakers, Inc., is an example of a private pharmaceutical company's offering a wide range of home care services, from nurses to homemakers and live-in companions, in fifty metropolitan areas.

Many communities across the nation are without homemaker–home health aide services according to the National Council of Homemaker Services (NCHS).* There are an estimated 30,000 homemaker–home health aides available, compared to an estimated need for 300,000.† In January of 1972 there were 2,850 agencies providing services. England, with nearly 50 million population (one quarter of the United States population), has 60,000 persons serving as home helpers. Sweden, with 8 million population,

*Home health aide services are covered by Medicare, whereas homemaker services are not. As of 1972, Part A of Medicare allowed 100 free home health visits during one year after discharge from a hospital. Part B allows an additional 100 visits a year but the patient pays the first $50 and 20% of the bill thereafter.

*National Council of Homemaker Services, 1740 Broadway, New York, N. Y. 10019. One can obtain a "Directory of Homemaker Services" from the Superintendent of Documents, U. S. Government Printing Office, Washington, D. C. 20402.

†Special Committee on Aging, U. S. Senate: Home health services in the United States, Washington, D. C., 1972, U. S. Government Printing Office.

has 35,000 homemakers (called "samaritans").

Homemaker–home health aide services in the United States began fifty years ago and were first funded voluntarily. Later they were included on a limited basis in public welfare programs but financing for the most part still comes chiefly from voluntary sources such as United Community Funds. Federal funds are usually small and available only for pilot programs to establish services or innovative features in an ongoing program.* Medicare and Medicaid provide limited coverage, and federal matching funds have helped finance services in a few areas under public welfare auspices. As of April 1, 1974, the Department of Health, Education, and Welfare will be required by the Social Security Act to set up homemaker services for the needy, aged, blind, and disabled on a national basis.

Quality homemaker–home health aide services that meet national professional standards will not be purchased cheaply, yet the cost is a small fraction of the expense of supporting an infirm or disabled person in a public or private institution. This is illustrated by the estimate of the Department of Health, Education, and Welfare that shortening each hospital stay by a single day would reduce the present astronomical cost of hospital care in the United States by $1 billion a year.

The 1971 White House Conference on Aging delegates urged provision of broadened services in the home and other alternatives to nursing home care, as a public service, without out-of-pocket payments required under Medicare. The National Council of Senior Citizens has long urged homemaker and home health services as an alternative to nursing home care. A resolution adopted by the 1971 National Council convention reads as follows:

> A nationwide program of comprehensive long term care is urgently needed and should be developed without further delay. The deficiencies of long term care, so evident in existing health services, are becoming more and more acute.
>
> Programs of long term care, sought by delegates to the National Council's tenth annual convention, should recognize the potentials of such innovations as day care hospitals and neighborhood health services so as to obviate need for expensive nursing home care and provide a more pleasant environment for those requiring long term care.

Physical, occupational, and speech therapies

These therapies, especially physical and speech therapy, are partly reimbursable under Medicare but severe restrictions limit their use. Thus patients may receive a great deal of rehabilitative work in hospitals following bone and joint diseases and strokes, but the investment is lost because home care follow-up is not given.*

A word should be mentioned about occupational therapy (O.T.), which is often stereotyped as "arts and crafts." At its best O.T. is geared toward helping the individual improve his functioning in any way possible, as defined by the person, his family, and the therapist. This can be done through any form of therapeutic activity that encourages self-expression and use of those resources available to the individual.

The physical therapist should be responsible for any necessary equipment and appliances necessary for rehabilitation, in addition to the actual provision of therapy.

Dental services

"Visiting dentists" are available in some areas and should be provided for all older

---

*For example, the Office of Economic Opportunity funded a pilot training program for "family health workers," recruiting trainees with a minimum fifth grade education from welfare rolls.

*The Curative Work Shop in Milwaukee is an example of an outstanding rehabilitation agency. This comprehensive community outpatient center offers among its components an adult rehabilitation program and home services program. It is a voluntary agency, begun fifty years ago, and is certified under Medicare and Medicaid.

people who find it difficult to leave their homes. Dentistry is not covered by Medicare even though it is a critical element of nutrition and general health.

Nutrition services

Food stamps, governmental supplemental food programs, Meals-on-Wheels, group dining, and homemaker–home health aides who shop for and prepare food are some of the techniques to combat the hunger and malnutrition found in so many older people. The best medical prescription for countless elderly persons would be a prescription for food rather than drugs. Reversible (and ultimately irreversible) brain syndromes can result from malnutrition. It is imperative to examine for evidences of malnutrition and hypovitaminosis even in the affluent, whose eating habits may be poor. Low-income elderly must scrimp on food. Psychological conditions—loneliness, depression, apathy, confusion—can induce malnutrition, which in turn furthers these symptoms. Physical disabilities can keep people from shopping and cooking.

Congress passed legislation in 1972 for a national program for one nutritiously planned hot meal a day, five days a week, to people over 60 years of age. They are served in the form of group dining in schools, churches, synagogues, and community centers and are also delivered to people's homes.* The sum of $250 million was authorized for two years beginning July 1,1972, to provide 90% matching money, with state and local governments or private nonprofit organizations providing the remaining 10%. Although the measure emphasized that the projects be located in low-income areas, this is not a requirement and there is no eligibility test. Anyone over 60 can eat the meals. This is particularly important in our opinion because "means tests" or special low-income programs for the poor lead to angry public feelings toward the poor and humiliation for the recipients of such programs.

The Department of Agriculture has a Commodities Distribution or Donable Foods Program that dates back to the Depression. Five hundred thousand elderly used it in 1971 but it is not available to everyone. For example, the District of Columbia distributes this food through the D. C. Department of Public Health under the title "Supplemental Foods Program," but people over 65 are not eligible. (Only children and pregnant women or new mothers are eligible.) The food in the program consists of evaporated milk, canned meats, scrambled egg mix, canned juices and vegetables, farina, and other staples.

The Food Stamp Act was passed by Congress in 1964 to provide immediate food for needy families. The program is part of the Department of Agriculture. Low-income people purchase stamps at less than face value and redeem them for food in standard food stores. Of the 9.5 million registered in 1971, 1.5 million (or 11%) were 65 and older. Food stamps can also be used for Meals-on-Wheels but not for group dining.

In some areas nutritionists are available to consult with patients and families about food needs and food preparation.*

Social services

We are referring here to all the services that are not strictly medical or psychiatric but instead represent economic and social supports. In the past, social service has been synonymous with social work but this is no longer true. Many other professions have become involved: clergymen, policemen, nurses, government officials, volunteers, paraprofessionals, and physicians who are actively working in the community. In home care, however, it is still most often the social worker who works together with nursing personnel to coordinate a program designed for

*There have been scattered programs in the past to bring food to people's homes (Meals-on-Wheels), sponsored by voluntary groups. However, in 1971 only 12,000 people were being fed through these methods.

*It is still uncertain, but 1972 legislation may have ended the food stamp program for most needy elderly.

an individual. Many homemaker–home health aide services are administered and/or supervised by professional social workers. However, only 20% of certified home health agencies offer social services.

Information and referral

How does the older person find out about services? Some cities have information and referral services especially for the elderly. If not, local or state commissions or advisory committees on aging may be helpful. Social services, human resources, or welfare departments (the names vary in municipalities and states) usually have information numbers to call. The same is true of local health and welfare councils and local mental health associations. The 889 Social Security district and branch offices can provide information. Family Service agencies are another resource. There are over 200 of these in the United States. For information one can write to the Family Service Association of America, 44 East 23rd Street, New York, N. Y. 10010.

Some of the agencies and institutions furnishing direct service to older people are welfare offices, voluntary agencies (the Hearing Aid Society, Societies for the Blind, etc.), public health departments, including community mental health centers, hospitals (both medical and psychiatric), visiting nurse services, nursing homes, employment offices, departments of vocational rehabilitation, religious organizations, and the police.

Financial support

Regardless of potential benefits of home care one must be realistic about whether a person can survive economically. All sources for financial support must be explored for the elderly person at home, including free or low-cost services and any pensions or financial assistance for which he might be eligible. It is not unusual to find older people who do not know they are eligible for Medicare, Medicaid, Old Age Assistance,* Veterans benefits, and even Social Security and income tax benefits. Federal tax laws allow a double exemption for people over 65 years of age and two double exemptions for a married couple. For the blind, still another exemption is allowable. It is hoped that in the future there will be money available for families to keep older people at home—direct payments, monies for construction of home additions or renovations, etc.

For homeowners it is important to understand the upkeep and property tax situation. Many elderly homeowners face financial crises and may be forced to sell their homes. Between 1964 and 1969 property taxes spiralled 28%. Elderly renters experienced substantial rent rises, partly necessitated by property tax increases.

For the very poor the welfare worker is usually the last resort. Old Age Assistance from the welfare departments is not enough for decent subsistence but at least promotes a slower rate of starvation than would occur without it. Money for food must often be sacrificed for medical care and medical supplies as well as other crucial living expenses. Clothing is not a part of many welfare budgets, nor are household articles and furniture. Free emergency food and clothing can be gotten from a variety of agencies, most of which are unadvertised to avoid being swamped with requests. In this respect some seasoned social service workers have their own private sources for help, depending on their ingeniousness and initiative. They can get food, furniture, jobs, clothing, etc. when no one else can. Their lucky clients can depend on them to come up with the things they need, but most clients must go without because such workers are rare and do not divulge their methods for fear of administrative reprimand or inundation of their sources. In our experience good social service workers know how to keep their wits about them and their mouths shut and know how far to go in enabling people to survive, without endangering themselves or their clients. Inadequate welfare policies make "humane collusion" inevitable on the part of anyone touched by human suffering.

*Replaced in the 1972 legislative sessions by a federal program of a guaranteed annual income floor, effective January, 1974.

Personal needs (companions, pets, telephones, shopping, transportation, grooming, etc.)

Older persons may need live-in or part-time companions, help with shopping and transportation,* instructions or direct help with grooming (home visits from beauticians and barbers do wonders for mental health), and appliances and aides to support or compensate for various disabilities (special handles near toilet and tub, wheelchairs, wide doorframes, etc.).

A telephone can mean a longer life. The National Innovations Center of London, England, reported in 1972 that people without a phone had a significantly higher mortality rate. In increasing numbers of urban, suburban, and rural areas, telephone reassurance services have been established under the auspices of private and public agencies. Volunteers often man the phones and check to see if older people living alone are all right.† Special telephones are available for the hard-of-hearing.

Given the state of loneliness and isolation affecting significant numbers of old people, pets can be directly supportive of mental well-being. Dogs and cats are the most favored pets in that order. For the older person a dog has the added advantage of providing some protection. Size, the need for exercise, and economy are three key points in selection. A large dog requires a daily walk and eats a great deal. On the other hand, a small dog like a poodle is expensive to maintain because of necessary grooming every six weeks to avoid skin problems, sore feet, and eye problems. Poodles and certain other dogs have the advantage of not shedding, helpful to allergic persons and to housekeeping. One can acquire a free dog from the Humane Society or an animal shelter. A female dog is usually more tractable. Big dogs may bark less than little dogs, and the bark of a little dog may fend off an intruder. In England one can get house insurance at lower premiums if one owns a dog, and in the United States a dog is tax deductible if you obtain one *after* a robbery. Older people may enjoy participating in dog shows.

Cats are easier to train than dogs and cost less to maintain. Birds bring pleasure to many older people. Canaries, finches, and parakeets are especially popular. Perhaps the easiest, least expensive, and least time-consuming pets to care for are fish. Plants are "pets" to many older people.

Family "respite" services

Although home care may be the treatment of choice for most older persons, it can place such a strain on family members who live with them that care is undermined and the family's own mental health is compromised. Any program of care must therefore consider regular social supports to the families themselves.

"Respite" services (more available in England than here) are a great relief to families and can make it possible for the generations to live together under even stressful circumstances. Such respite includes sending someone to care for the older person at home so the family can take holidays, weekends, and vacations by themselves. At times of particular stress or when the older person needs more attention, it should be possible to admit them briefly to an institution to give the family a chance to rest and recover. This also helps to acquaint the older person with institutional life and reduces the symbolic and real associations of institutions as places of no return. Day and night sitters should be available when the family wants to go out

*An interdisciplinary workshop conducted by the Adminstration on Aging and the Departments of Transportation and Housing and Urban Development has provided a multifaceted depiction of the interrelationships of transportation and aging. (Cantilli, E. J., and Shmelzer, June L., editors: Transportation and aging: selected issues, Washington, D. C., 1970, U. S. Government Printing Office.) An especially valuable description of older people's medical and physiological characteristics was included. (Libow, L. S.: Older people's medical and physiological characteristics: some implications for transportation, ibid. pp. 14-18.)

†Guidelines for a telephone reassurance service. Superintendent of Documents, U. S. Government Printing Office, Washington, D. C., 1972. (Booklet gives a description of the service along with instructions on how to initiate such a service.)

or when the older person requires inordinate attention at night, exhausting family members. Home appliances and aids—wheelchairs, special handles and bars to assist walking, or anything else that alleviates undue dependency or physical stress on the family—can make care easier. The availability of psychiatric, medical, and social assistance on an emergency or routine basis can provide significant relief to a family.

Home safety

Accidents both in and out of the home are an area of legitimate concern. Among people 65 and older, accidents are the third leading cause of death, claiming some 30,000 victims yearly and disabling 800,000 more.* Although older people make up only 10% of the population, 26% of all accidental deaths and 17% of all accidental injuries happen to people over 65. Accidents that do not result in death can cause permanent emotional reactions and may end the older person's independence of movement.

Falls lead as the cause of accidental injuries and deaths. Most of them occur in the home. Losses in muscle strength and coordination, sense of balance, and speed of reaction are factors. Reduced blood flow and oxygen to the brain can result in dizziness and faintness. Older people should beware of sharp moves of the head because of changes in the balancing mechanism of the inner ear. Some people suffer "drop attacks"—sudden and unexpected falls without loss of consciousness but with loss of muscle power of body and legs. Drugs, especially sedatives and tranquilizers, may confuse and slow response. The home should be made as safe as possible. Staircases are especially dangerous at the top and bottom steps. Steps should be highly visible and have good illumination, nonskid treads, and handrails. Slippery floor coverings should be eliminated. Linoleum, small mats, and sliding rugs are offenders. Nonskid floor waxes, wall-to-wall rugs or rubber-backed rugs, and tacking are wise. Corrugated shoe soles help. Nonskid mats and grab rails should be used in bathtubs and near toilets and beds. One must also be alert to the disorientation that can follow a move to a new residence:

> A 73-year-old carpenter moved to Florida after living in his home for thirty-six years. He was accustomed to turning to the left from his bedroom door to enter the bathroom. Suffering from nocturia, he had to get up several times a night. In his new home a stairway was to the left. Several nights after moving, he fell down the stairs and fractured his hip.

Burns, cuts, and poisonings are other hazards. Especially dangerous practices like smoking in bed should be stopped. Room heaters and heating pads must be carefully controlled. Fires can occur when one is cooking while wearing long sleeves or bed clothes. Medicine bottles must be read with caution; it is recommended that they be read *twice* before medicine is taken and *once* afterward.

Loss of one's driver's license can be a blow to self-esteem as well as mobility. But losses of visual and auditory acuity, slower reflexes, poor night vision, and arthritic limitations on neck movements can affect the ability to drive a car. Only 14% of old people have licenses to drive, a reflection of the fact that many older people have never driven at all. Interestingly, studies show that older drivers have lower accident rates than younger drivers.*

Recreation, education, and employment

The world must be brought inside to the bedridden and the homebound. There are friendly visitors programs through which visits are made to isolated individuals. Fre-

*A useful booklet called "Handle Yourself With Care" has been prepared by the Administration on Aging and the National Safety Council. It is for sale (price 30 cents) by Superintendent of Documents, U. S. Government Printing Office, Washington, D. C. 20402.

*Finesilver, S. G.: The older driver: a statistical evaluation of licensing and accident involvement in 30 states and the District of Columbia, College of Law, University of Denver, January, 1969.

quent contacts with family, friends, and neighbors help keep emotions and minds interested and responsive. Television, radio, phonographs, and newspapers can be rich sources of enjoyment. Older people have been known to sacrifice food to pay for television repairs because it is so important to them. Some people leave their television on all day ("like a friend in the house") or sleep with it on at night. Large screens are a visual help, and volume can be adjusted for hearing difficulties. Television and radio offer recreation, education, and even religious services on Sunday morning. One man described watching television as rather like sitting on the park bench and watching the world go by, a continuous nonstop show. Another spoke of the sense of having world events at his fingertips; he had two sets, one on top of the other, which he watched simultaneously. People call or write to broadcasting stations, avidly follow their favorite newscasters and M.C.s, and participate in "audience talk shows."

For those who can move outside their homes, senior centers and community centers may offier a variety of possibilities. There are increasing numbers of senior centers* and also a National Institute of Senior Centers (a program of the National Council on the Aging).† Their primary aim is recreation and they may have activities a few hours each week or may be open all day five days each week. Shows, parties, music, beauty salons, handicrafts, candle-making, cooking, flower-arranging, trips, discussion groups (also group therapy), games, television, walks, group shopping trips, and special programs for the blind are some of the activities in a well-functioning center.

Continuing their education is an interest expressed by many of the elderly. Some communities offer home library service. Inexpensive or free mail order courses should be offered by high schools and colleges, and older people could be encouraged to enroll in regular academic classes if scholarships and low fees were possible. Elementary and junior and senior high schools located right in communities where elderly people live could remain open after the regular class day and provide recreation, education, and food service. Colleges could work up curricula especially designed for older people.

Employment and volunteer work allow the elderly to supplement their incomes and involve them in absorbing activities that benefit themselves and the community. In Bethesda, Maryland, the Over-60 Counseling and Employment Service of the Montgomery County Federation of Women's Clubs, Inc. developed a program that provides job opportunities for elderly women—acting as companions for other elderly persons as well as caring for children. There have been other scattered programs to train unskilled older persons as family aides. In 1966 an experimental project in New Jersey, known as Operation BOLD (Blot Out Long-term Dependency), financed under Title V of the Economic Opportunity Act of 1964, taught homemaking skills and home care of the sick to aides. VISTA, Senior Aides, SCORE, the Peace Corps, Foster Grandparent programs, Green Thumb, Mature-Temps, and other employment and volunteer activities are designed especially to accommodate the elderly.

Religious support

Clergymen of all faiths are involved in the care of older people. Some concentrate only upon spiritual aspects while increasing numbers of others become directly involved in social services, counseling, and other "secular" activities. Many older people are deeply religious and their clergymen can become an integral part in planning and providing for their care. Clergymen have traditionally formed one of the few professional disciplines whose members are trained to care directly for dying people. Home visiting with the sick and infirm is also common

---

*Three to four thousand senior centers are operated in the United States, sponsored by churches, synagogues, clubs, and nonprofit corporations. Financial support derives from private donations and from local, state, and federal governments.

†National Council on the Aging, 1818 L Street, NW, Washington, D. C. 20036.

practice, and clergymen therefore are an important source of referral for medical and psychiatric problems.

Religious groups have for centuries given special attention to older poeple. Some of the better, as well as the worst, examples of homes for the aged and old age–oriented community activities can be found under their auspices. But the need to maintain doctrinal differences has led to fragmentation of services. Each denomination builds its own little island of concern, isolated from everything else. A "practical ecumenism" could allow churches and synagogues to protect their identities yet pool their resources in a planned effort to help the old.* For example, buying necessary supplies together for old age homes could sharply cut costs. Pooling skilled manpower would increase the range of services each home could give. Cooperative planning of vital community programs such as Meals-on-Wheels, friendly visitors, etc. could reach many more people with the churches of all denominations acting as neighborhood bases for all the elderly, regardless of denomination. A national church program including all denominations could register all eligible older people for health programs, coordinate food programs, provide friendly visitors and telephone reassurance, set up information and referral services nationally, help coordinate home care programs, and much more. Clergymen could receive special training for work with the elderly. Religious groups should use their power and influence for improvement of old people's economic and social conditions.

OUTPATIENT CARE

Outpatient services (sometimes called "ambulatory care") refer to care given to people who live in the community rather than in institutions. This care is provided by hospital outpatient clinics, neighborhood health centers, family agencies, day hospitals, and day care centers. Outpatient service may be given in or outside of the home, either bringing the person to the service or taking the service to the person. We have already described home care; therefore, this section will emphasize the facilities where people can go for outpatient care rather than having it brought to them.

Hospital emergency rooms are the major 24-hour facilities available for medical and psychiatric emergencies. In addition, hospitals generally offer *outpatient medical clinic care;* some have *outpatient psychiatric clinics* as well. Currently only 2% of patients in outpatient psychiatric clinics are over 60 years of age. Few of the clinics offer the services necessary for older people, especially psychotherapy.

Community mental health centers are another potential but thus far unrealized resource for the elderly. In 1961, proposals regarding the establishment of community mental health centers were made and published by the Joint Commission on Mental Illness and Health in "Action for Mental Health," resulting in the emergence of such centers in 1963. This first publication was very hopeful and stands in contrast to such later books as "The Community Mental Health Center: An Interim Appraisal," by the Joint Information Service of the American Psychiatric Association and the National Association for Mental Health (Glasscote et al., 1969).

The Federal Community Mental Health Centers program was enacted by Congress in 1963 and amended in 1965 and 1967. If nothing else, it has certainly focused attention upon the fact that the system of delivery of mental health services is woefully inadequate. The community mental health center is required to offer a minimum of five services, four of which are direct clinical activities: inpatient care, outpatient care, partial hospitalization (such as day care), and around-the-clock emergency service. The fifth required program element is community education and consultation services oriented toward prevention. Community mental

*Butler, R. N.: Toward practical ecumenism, Bulletin of the American Protestant Hospital Association 34:6-12, 1970. See also Hospital progress, Journal of the Catholic Hospital Association, July, 1970.

health centers are responsible for specific catchment areas, but certain of the center programs (such as those for children, the elderly, and drug addicts) may serve several catchment areas.

Both public and private agencies have participated in the establishment of centers. Among federal grantee agencies, 45% are incorporated as private, nonprofit corporations, and 55% operate under public auspices—state, county, and municipal agencies. It should be pointed out also that, whatever the nature of its sponsorship, the typical community mental health center is supported through a combination of public and private funds. Public monies meet 75% of the total operating costs of typical centers during the first year of operation. Private funds derived from varying combinations of patient payments, third-party payments made in behalf of patients, and voluntary contributions meet the remaining 25%.

As of June, 1969, a total of 350 centers had been funded; 175 received construction grants only; 81 received staffing grants only, and 75 received both. As of June, 1970, federal construction and staffing grants had been made to 420 centers; 245 were in operation. On the basis of an average of 155,000 persons to be served per center, about a fourth of the country's population are included in the catchment areas of the funded centers. It is estimated that the nation needs between 1,800 and 2,000 such centers. They may be absorbed within health maintenance organizations.

The community mental health centers have been criticized. The facts are that they have never been adequately funded, housed, and staffed. There are no standards. Inservice training and personnel development have lagged. Racism and stereotypes about "the poor" have been negative influences. As is usual when some ideal hope does not work out to eminent satisfaction, there are those who are ready to do away with these ventures, not realizing (or in fact realizing very well) that the reasons they failed are related to inadequate support and the fact that they have not been validly tested.

The Glasscote study explores the many reasons why the community centers have not fulfilled the key purpose of federal funding, which is to appreciably diminish the flow of mentally ill patients of all ages to state hospitals. The Glasscote work also points out the slowness of progress toward meeting the problems of the indigent mentally ill, who make up a large share of the state hospital-bound patients. Many explanations can be given for this slowness, including insufficient and ill-timed appropriations, rigid geographical guidelines, inadequate psychiatric training and experience of operating personnel, and lack of consensus as to the purpose of the center. The work of Hollingshead and Redlich (1958) is pertinent to the problems of middle-class mental health professionals attempting to serve the poor of varied ages and races. Old people make up only 4% to 5% of community mental health center clientele.

Day hospitals for patients with psychiatric problems enable persons to come to the hospital for any indicated treatment during the day and return home at night. This provides a degree of care intermediate between outpatient therapy and total institutional care. It is particularly useful for former mental hospital patients and persons with significant organic mental impairment. In this way families obtain substantial support in keeping an older person at home. Nursing and old age homes should offer similar partial care. One of the greatest problems with day hospital programs is the need for transportation, particularly in rural areas. In England ambulances are used to transport people. Taxis (paid for by Medicaid in some states), volunteers' cars, and staff cars may be used. An ideal day hospital service should offer medical care, individual and group psychotherapy, drug therapy, occcupational and physical therapy, entertainment, education, a library, a store, a beauty and barber shop, free lunches, baths, some form of patient government, and plenty of opportunity for congenial socializing. Day hospitals can ease the return of former mental hospital patients to community life and monitor the physical condition and reactions to medications of all patients. Relatives, friends, and community volunteers should have free access and play vital roles.

Day care centers offer day care in a nonhospital setting but provide many of the same social and recreational services. The first recreational day center for the aged, the William Hodson Community, was set up in 1944 as part of New York City's Department of Public Welfare.* This center emphasized self-government, poetry, music, dramatics, woodwork, painting, birthday parties, discussion groups, counseling, and an added fillip in the form of country vacations.

Various other groups now offer similar programs, of which the following is an example:

Levindale Hebrew Geriatric Center in Baltimore, Maryland, provides day care and a community orientation. A bus picks up twenty to thirty mentally or physically handicapped old people daily at their own homes and takes them to Levindale for a schedule of activities, including meals.

MULTIPURPOSE SENIOR CENTERS

Congressman John Brademas (D-Ind.) introduced legislation in December, 1971, to authorize construction of multipurpose senior citizen community centers. A revolving fund would be established to insure mortgages for such centers. The senior center movement illustrates the continuing debate over the development of comprehensive versus categorical programs: whether the services needed by old people should be assured within comprehensive programs for all people of all ages or be provided in specialized ways. Philosophically, socially, and psychologically, integration of services is the more desirable. Experience demonstrates, however, that old people get lost in the shuffle, fall through the cracks. Until there is a finely honed change in the cultural sensibility so that the elderly do not get lost, it is necessary to press for special, highly visible programs.

*Kubie, Susan H., and Landau, Gertrude: Group work with the aged, New York, 1953, International Universities Press, Inc.

Multipurpose senior centers can provide a range of services beyond the walls of their facilities. Social workers and aides (paraprofesssionals, who are sometimes called "geriatric aides") and friendly visitors may visit the homes of clients. Residential homes may be organized. Group shopping trips by bus, for check-cashing as well as shopping, may be chaperoned. Little House in Menlo Park, California, has been a pioneer example of a multipurpose senior center since 1949.

PROTECTIVE SERVICES

Protective services is the name for a group of services given to a person who is so mentally deteriorated or disturbed as to be unable to manage his affairs in his own best interest and who has no relative or friend able and willing to act on his behalf. Social work, legal, medical, psychiatric, nursing, homemaking, and home health aide services may be provided. Small amounts of cash may be available for use in certan situations.

Federal legislation* has been enacted that will permit local welfare offices to set up protective service programs for which the federal government will provide 75% of the cost.

Protective service clients often need assistance because of some mental condition such as paranoid ideas, organic brain syndrome, overwhelming anxiety, or severe personality disorder. Most of these clients are best helped by social workers and nurses who are generalists in the sense that they manage their cases with the support of medical, legal, and psychiatric consultations and can call on homemakers, visiting nurses, and paraprofessionals for help. A typical case illustrates the importance of such services to mental health.

A mildly confused old woman developed paranoid ideas about the gas company, which resulted in her not paying her bills for several months. She

*1962 Public Welfare Amendment to the Social Security Act. Among pioneering books on protective services is that of Virginia Lehmann and Geneva Mathiasen, editors: Guardianship and protective services for older people, Albany, N. Y., 1963, National Council on Aging Press.

was threatened with having the gas turned off, which would leave her without heat in mid-winter. Had she been without help, her gas probably would have been turned off; after a while police and medical help would have been called for, and her eventual transfer (probably in a very deteriorated condition) to an inpatient psychiatric ward would have been necessary. With protective services, the crisis with the gas company was averted. A casework aide, under the supervision of a social worker, was able to gain the woman's confidence enough to convince her to pay the gas bill. Since she had no money for an immediate payment, protective services made a partial payment of the bill and arranged with the gas company for the woman to pay the rest later. Continuing contact with the protective service worker enabled the lady to continue living in her own home. A homemaker was also provided for a few hours a week. All of these helpers used psychiatric consultants to help them react appropriately to the client's psychiatric condition.

The protective service and the community mental health approaches are closely related in that both provide a variety of services to meet a person's needs while the person remains in his home, thus utilizing less-than-total-care institutions whenever it is in the patient's best interest. The patient is seen not just as having a certain illness but in the context of his psychological, social, physical, and economic conditions. Also, his psychiatric needs may be met without requiring him to accept the idea that he is a "mental patient."

Historically, legal concern for the elderly centered on the protection of property holdings against dissipation and exploitation. In recent times there has been more emphasis on protection of the person.

In 1962 the Social Secuirty Administration made a grant to the Benjamin Rose Institute of Cleveland, one of the few agencies providing extensive protective services to old people, for a research and demonstration project. Margaret Blenkner,* director of this research, has contributed to our understanding the problem of protective services.

It has not been established how many people need protection. The number who have mental impairment is substantial and applies in institutions as well as in the community. Studies show that about 50% of institutionalized populations have mental impairment.*

Other studies suggest that one sixth of the noninstitutionalized population—3 million old people—have some degree of mental impairment. Even if these figures include unrecognized or simulated depression, for practical purposes this describes a vulnerable population. Some of the earliest studies concerning "certifiable" persons in the community† estimated 5% in need of protection. Less stringent studies by Blenkner, Goldfarb, Lowenthal, and others have estimated closer to 16%. (None of these studies are strictly comparable because of varied criteria.)

Burr cites data indicating that 10% of the adult caseload of public welfare agencies (largely Old Age Assistance) are in need of protective services.‡ However, most welfare departments still do not supply them.

In 1967 the Administration on Aging of the Social and Rehabilitation Service (HEW) began its National Protective Services Project in three rural Colorado counties and

*Blenkner, Margaret, Bloom, M., Wasser, Edna, and Nielsen, Margaret: Protective services for old people: findings from the Benjamin Rose Institute study, Social Casework **52**:483-522, 1971.

*Goldfarb, A. I.: Prevalence of psychiatric disorders in metropolitan old age and nursing homes, Journal American Geriatric Society **10**:78-84, 1962. See also U. S. Department of Health, Education, and Welfare, National Center for Health Statistics: Characteristics of residents in institutions for the aged and chronically ill, United States, April-June, 1963, Public Health Service Publication No. 100, Series 12, No. 2, Washington, D. C., 1965, U. S. Government Printing Office.

†New York State Department of Mental Hygiene, Mental Health Research Unit: A mental health survey of older people, 1960, New York State Hospitals Press.

‡Burr, J. J.: Program goals and the specialist's function in public welfare. In: Planning welfare services for older people. Paper presented at the Training Institute for Public Welfare Specialists on Aging, Cleveland, Ohio, June 13-24, 1965, Washington, D. C., 1966, U. S. Department of Health, Education, and Welfare, pp. 5-12.

Washington, D. C.* Referrals for protective services came from county welfare departments, OAA, Social Security offices, housing authorities, health programs, social agencies, counseling, referral and information services, and probate courts. Some of the referred older people were rootless, isolated, "loners," reflecting a multigenerational chain of psychopathology. Some had chronic brain syndromes, others were severely depressed or neurotic, a few were mentally retarded. Physical disease was common. Most were poor, with less than grammar school education.

In Blenkner's approach social casework was the core service and the directive was "do, or get others to do, whatever is necessary to meet the needs of the situation." Rapport, trust, mutual respect are necessary. In our Washington work we found gradualism (nonprecipitous, careful intervention) a guiding concept; we did not accept the idea that it was crucial to think in terms of completing a case, except as nature dictated through death. Needs included, of course, medical, financial, home health aide, homemaker, nursing care, psychiatry, and legal services. The following are some principles crucial to protective services:

1. Client or patient must have decision-making power.
2. Trust and rapport must be established; before all else, do not violate that trust.
3. Gradualism—do things nonprecipitously and carefully.
4. Do not kill with kindness.
5. Work with assets.
6. Respect resistance.
7. Do not move people if it can be avoided and if it is against their will.

*One of us (RNB) was the consulting psychiatrist of the Washington project, excellently directed by George Roby, MSW. Dr. Jack Kleh and Mrs. Virginia Lehmann were the medical and legal consultants, respectively. See U. S. Department of Health, Education, and Welfare, Social and Rehabilitative Service, Community Services Administration: Report of the National Protective Services Project for Older Adults, HEW Publication No. (SRS) 72-23008, 1971.

In Blenkner's intriguing work, upsetting to some, she and her colleagues found that the protected group compared to the control group had higher rates of institutionalization and death. They attribute this to hopelessness (We would add helplessness engendered by *things being done for* people.) Members of the protected group were institutionalized earlier than they would otherwise have been and "contrary to intent . . . did not . . . prove protective of the older person although it did relieve collaterals and community agents." We believe it essential that studies be designed to confirm or refute the Benjamin Rose studies. In the meantime we favor continuing intervention but take seriously this injunction of Blenkner et al. "We should . . . question our present prescriptions and strategies of treatment. Is our dosage too strong, our intervention too overwhelming, our takeover too final?"

PRE-HOSPITAL ADMISSION SCREENING*

In 1965 the Langley-Porter Institute and the California State Department of Mental Hygiene established a pilot program to screen elderly persons on the brink of commitment to state mental hospitals. It was hoped that the project would provide *alternatives* to hospitalization and promote the proper care of the elderly outside the institution.

Innovations included the following:

1. Screening of persons over 65 years of age when involuntary commitment is under consideration
2. Screening in the patient's home by a team physician, psychiatrist, and social worker
3. Appropriate alternatives, including placement, to provide for total needs of the patient

One California study by Simon and Low-

*We are much indebted here to the review of the San Francisco Geriatric Screening Project contained in Mental health care and the elderly: shortcomings in public policy. Report of the U. S. Senate Special Committee on Aging, Washington, D. C., 1971, U. S. Government Printing Office.

enthal* showed that a common cause of commitment was acute brain syndrome. This disorder is a temporary but reversible mental disturbance, usually brought about by malnutrition, uncontrolled diabetes, decompensated heart disease, and other diseases. Since the reversible brain syndrome is closely related to physical illness, it could be treated in a general hospital, with continuing care at home or in a protective care facility (nursing home or convalescent home). It would then not be necessary for such persons to be committed for treatment in a mental hospital.

State institutions could effectively conduct screening in the hospitals themselves and then make proper alternative placement if necessary. Baltimore and some other cities have programs similar to that of San Francisco.

CONCLUSION

The Committee on Aging of the Group for the Advancement of Psychiatry (GAP) has taken the lead in pointing out the deficiencies in the report (*Action for Mental Health*) of the Joint Commission on Mental Illness and in American mental health care for the elderly. It has offered constructive proposals for community care and a series of publications on the subject.†

Although GAP has emphasized service in the community, it has called for a range of services and facilities including institutionalization to meet the realities of old age:

> Old people need a broad range of treatment settings. They must not be lumped into one category. In-depth evaluation must be done before the treatment process is started. Once an elderly patient is sent down one road it is difficult to divert him to another. . . . It is our position that the psychiatric hospital is an integral and necessary component of the therapeutic continuum for elderly psychiatric patients just as quality nursing home care is ideal for elderly medical patients. . . . We favor the development of comprehensive diagnostic and treatment centers, however, at each point along the sequence of neighborhood health centers, community mental health centers, and hospitals. Irreversibility must never be casually (and stereotypically) assumed.*

Mental health workers and the people they serve seek to maintain the older person at home so long as it is wise and appropriate. To effectively do so our communities must develop the necessary services. When reality dictates, however, both workers and older people must share in the decision to accept institutional care. The difficulty of that decision would be lightened by vast improvements in our nation's facilities.

---

*Lowenthal, Marjorie Fiske: Lives in distress, New York, 1964, Basic Books, Inc.

†Group for the Advancement of Psychiatry, Publications Office, 419 Park Avenue, South, New York, N. Y. 10016.

*Group for the Advancement of Psychiatry: Toward a public policy on health care of the elderly, Report No. 79, 1970, pp. 663-664.

REFERENCES

Bahn, Anita K.: Outpatient population of psychiatric clinics, Maryland, 1958–1959, Public Health Monograph No. 65, Washington, D. C., 1959, U. S. Department of Health, Education, and Welfare.

Blenkner, Margaret, Bloom, M., Wasser, Edna, and Nielson, Margaret: Protective services for old people: findings from the Benjamin Rose Institute study, Social Casework **52**:483-522, 1971.

Butler, R. N., and Sulliman, Lillian G.: Psychiatric contact with the community-resident, emotionally disturbed elderly, Journal of Nervous and Mental Diseases **137**:180-186, 1963.

Daniels, R. S., and Kahn, R. L.: Community mental health and programs for the aged, Geriatrics **23**:121-125, 1968.

Gaitz, C. M., and Baer, P. E.: Placement of elderly psychiatric patients, Journal of the American Geriatrics Society **19**:601-613, 1971.

Glasscote, P. M., Sussex, J. J., Cumming, E., and Smith, L. R.: The community mental health center: an interim appraisal, Washington, D. C., 1969, The Joint Information Service of the American Psychiatric Association and the National Association for Mental Health.

Gossett, Helen M.: Restoring identity to socially deprived and depersonalized older people, Bulletin of the Institute of Gerontology **15** (supp.):3-6, April, 1968.

Gossett, Helen M.: Augmenting and preserving the functioning capacities of aging persons in extended-care facilities, Bulletin of the Institute of Gerontology **15**(supp.):3-6, May, 1968.

Grigorian, H. M.: Geriatric psychiatry in a community mental health center. In Robertson, R.

H., editor: Proceedings of the thirteenth annual meeting, 1967, The Medical Society of St. Elizabeths Hospital.

Group for the Advancement of Psychiatry: Crisis in psychiatric hospitalization, Report No. 72, 1969.

Group for the Advancement of Psychiatry: The aged and community mental health: a guide to program development, Report No. 80, 1971.

Hollingshead, A. B., and Redlich, F. C.: Social class and mental illness, New York, 1958, John Wiley & Sons, Inc.

Joint Commission on Mental Illness and Health: Action for mental health, final report of the Commission, New York, 1961, Basic Books, Inc.

Kaplan, Jerome: A social program for older people, Minneapolis, 1953, University of Minnesota Press.

Kramer, M., Taube, C., and Starr, S.: Patterns of use of psychiatric facilities by the aged: current status, trends, and implications. In Simon, A., and Epstein, L. J., editors: Aging and modern society, Psychiatric Research Report No. 23, Washington, D. C., 1968, American Psychiatric Association.

Kubie, Lawrence S.: Need for a new subdiscipline in the medical profession, Archives of Neurology and Psychiatry **78**:283-293, 1957.

Kutner, B., Fanshel, D., Togo, Alice M., and Langner, T. S.: Five hundred over sixty: a community survey on aging, New York, 1957, Russell Sage Foundation.

Lehmann, V., and Mathiasen, Geneva: Guardianship and protective services for older people, New York, 1963, National Council on Aging Press.

Levenson, A. I.: Organizational patterns of community mental health centers. In Bellack, L., and Barten, H. H., editors: Progress in community mental health, vol. 1, New York, 1969, Grune & Stratton, Inc.

MacMillan, Duncan: Mental health services for the aged, a British approach, Canada's Mental Health, pp. 1-17, June, 1967.

Markson, Elizabeth, Kwoh, Ada, Cumming, J., and Cumming, Elaine: Alternatives to hospitalization for psychiatrically ill geriatric patients. In Special Section, Psychiatry and the elderly, The American Journal of Psychiatry **127**:1055-1062, 1971.

Moses, Dorothy V., and Lake, Carolyn S.: Geriatrics in the baccalaureate nursing curriculum, Nursing Outlook **16**:41-43, July, 1968.

Office of Research and Statistics, Social Security Administration: Financing mental health care under Medicare and Medicaid, Research Report No. 37, Washington, D. C., 1971, U. S. Government Printing Office.

Padula, Helen: Developing day care for older people: a technical assistance monograph prepared for the Office of Economic Opportunity, National Council on the Aging, Washington, D. C., Sept., 1972.

Reed, Louis, Myers, Evelyn, and Scheidemandel, Patricia: Health insurance and psychiatric care: utilization and cost, Washington, D. C., 1972, American Psychiatric Association.

Robertson, Wm. F., and Pitt, B.: The role of a day hospital in geriatric psychiatry, British Journal of Psychiatry **111**:635-640, 1965.

Rodstein, M.: Accidents among the aged: incidence, causes and prevention, Journal of Chronic Diseases **17**:515-526, 1964.

Special Committee on Aging, U. S. Senate: Alternatives to nursing home care: a proposal, prepared by staff specialists at the Levinson Gerontological Policy Institute, Brandeis University, Waltham, Mass. (Dr. Robert Morris, Director): Washington, D. C., 1971, U. S. Government Printing Office.

Special Committee on Aging, U. S. Senate: Home health services in the United States, Washington, D. C., 1972, U. S. Government Printing Office.

Special Committee on Aging, U. S. Senate, Report: Mental health care and the elderly: shortcomings in public policy, Washington, D. C., 1971, U. S. Government Printing Office.

Townsend, Peter: The family life of old people: an inquiry in east London, Glencoe, Ill., 1957, Free Press.

Townsend, Peter: The last refuge, London, 1962, Routledge & Kegan Paul.

Vickery, Florence B.: How to work with older people, Division of Recreation, Department of Natural Resources, State of California, Publication 59-3, 1960.

Wagner, Gertrude W.: Group meals for senior citizens in a community setting: a procedural manual, New York, 1972, The Hudson Guild Senior Association.

Whitehead, Anthony: In the service of old age, The welfare of psychogeriatric patients, Baltimore, 1970, Penguin Books.

Zimberg, S.: The psychiatrist and medical home care; geriatric psychiatry and the Harlem community, American Journal of Psychiatry **127**: 1062-1067, 1971.

11

PROPER INSTITUTIONAL CARE

Our definition of institutional care includes any care (medical, psychiatric, or social) given to older people *not* residing in their own homes or the homes of family and friends. Although efforts should be directed toward helping the mentally and/or physically ill older person remain independent and in his own home, there are many situations in which it simply not possible or advisable to do so. Active outpatient treatment may fail and short- or long-term institutional care is required.* Present means of financing care, the inadequacy of facilities and services, and deficiencies in number and training of manpower are among the obstacles to the provision of the spectrum of services and facilities needed to dovetail with the wide range of psychiatric/medical/social states of old people. Once again, as in other chapters, we will be describing what is presently available, balancing this against what would be ideal. Emergency shelter, acute and chronic hospitalization (both medical and psychiatric), nursing homes, homes for the aged, and foster care homes are the basic forms of institutional care utilized by the older population. We shall be examining what each of these has to offer, both in kind and in quality of service.

*The Group for the Advancement of Psychiatry took issue with the premise that "the only good psychiatry is treatment in the community." Their 1969 report entitled "Crisis in psychiatric hospitalization" was a "protest against a current bandwagon movement" that is exemplified by such slogans as "Keep patients out of psychiatric hospitals as much as you can" and "Use the psychiatric ward of a general hospital instead of a mental hospital." GAP stressed "the vital role of the psychiatric hospital in a continuum of comprehensive psychiatric treatment." They based their criticism of "the movement away from the psychiatric hospital" on both theoretical and clinical considerations. As a clinical result of uncritical acceptance, these slogans lead to diagnostic and treatment errors, they contended. Readmission rates increase. A large number of semifunctioning individuals are immobilized through misuse of medications.

DECISION TO INSTITUTIONALIZE AN OLDER PERSON

The unfavorable reputation of American institutions for the elderly combines with the natural reluctance of old people to leave their homes and communities; and the result is active or passive (and often justifiable) resistance to admission. An elderly woman recently came to our attention because she kept an arsenal of guns at home to use on herself or others if someone came to take her to a nursing home or mental hospital. Increased morbidity, disorientation, and mortality have been associated with the movement of people to institutions, since the aged are particularly vulnerable to the stress of sudden change. Thus the decision to institutionalize must be made conservatively and with care to fully prepare and cushion the individual against the inevitable shock.*

When is institutionalization indicated?

The need for medical care in an institution is fairly apparent and based on a physi-

*To provide an understanding of the impact of institutional care upon people, Erving Goffman's powerful essay, "On the characteristics of total institutions" (1957), should be required reading, along with Stanton and Schwartz's classic study, "The mental hospital" (1956).

cian's recommendation. However, it has not been possible to construct strict criteria for voluntary admission and involuntary commitment to state and private psychiatric hospitals; and the criteria for nursing homes and homes for the aged are even more nebulous and indefinite.

Lowenthal has identified five factors that influence the decision to place elderly, mentally ill persons in a hospital—some of which are relevant also for other chronic care facilities:

1. Disturbances in thinking and feeling, such as delusions or depressions
2. Physical illness
3. Potentially harmful behavior, such as confusion or unmanageability
4. Harmful behavior, such as refusing necessary medical care, or actual violence to others
5. Environmental factors, such as the unavailability or incapacity of a responsible other person to care for the patient*

It is immediately clear that adequate social supports such as home care services could prevent the institutionalization of a portion of the above described elderly. Medical hospitalization would be more appropriate for others, and a differentiation should be made between long-term and short-term needs for care. The outline below† illustrates an effort to build criteria for mental hospitalization of the aged.

I. Clearly appropriate for admission
   A. Those with functional psychoses and without significant physical illness or disability, for whom outpatient treatment is not feasible
      Examples
      1. Patients receiving psychiatric treatment in the community who require brief periods of protection from the consequences of their behavior during episodes of acute disturbance or depression (e.g., suicide, homicide, spending sprees, refusal to eat)
      2. Chronically mentally ill patients who need protection and management, as well as treatment, during prolonged periods of disruptive or disorganized behavior, and require regular and frequent attendance of a physician
   B. Alcoholics without significant physical illness or disability who, following detoxification, need a period of inpatient treatment for their alcoholism
   C. Those with severe organic brain disease whose usual behavior, intractable to medication, is too disturbing to be managed at home or in another facility
      Examples
      The physically aggressive patient, fire setter, eloper, or person otherwise dangerous to himself or others when physically able to carry out his potentially destructive behavior

II. Clearly inappropriate for admission
   A. Those with acute brain syndrome, symptomatic of a grave physical illness, requiring urgent admission to a general hospital
   B. Those who are moribund or comatose
   C. Those with major medical problems and minor mental symptoms
      Examples
      Patients who become mildly confused or disturbed as a result of or in conjunction with recent head injury, cardiovascular disease, diabetes, metabolic disturbance, terminal malignancy, etc. (Psychiatric consultation might be utilized, if required, rather than mental hospital admission.)
   D. Those with inconsequential lapses of memory and mild disorientation as a result of chronic brain syndrome, who are more effectively treated or managed in their own homes or, if necessary, in a foster home, home for the aged, etc. (A state mental hospital has little to offer and, in view of the large wards in most state mental hospitals, may aggravate the patient's confusion.)
   E. Those who need only adequate living accommodations, with economic or other social support services

As a footnote to the discussion above, it is important to remember that self-destructive or suicidal behavior in the elderly may be a slow process associated with prolonged and intense grief, loneliness, and progressive organic disease and manifesting itself in malnutrition, failure to take medicine, and other forms of deteriorating self-care.

---

*Lowenthal, Marjorie F.: Lives in distress, New York, 1964, Basic Books, Inc.

†This outline (somewhat paraphrased) illustrates the effort of one state (Maryland) to establish guidelines. (Helen Padula, Coordinator, Services to the Aged, Maryland.) Maryland was influenced by a preceding New York State effort. We emphasize that this is merely a guideline and should not be used in a rigid, immutable manner.

Advisability of voluntary admission

Wherever possible, the old person—like persons of any age—should participate fully in all decisions regarding himself, including those of institutionalization. The family, of course, should also be closely involved. Making the decision to admit a person to a nursing home, a home for the aged, or a hospital can be extremely difficult, since all these facilities are so disliked and feared by both the elderly and their families.

> Almost all older people view the move to a home for the aged or to a nursing home with fear and hostility. . . . All old people—without exception—believe that the move to an institution is the prelude to death. . . . [The old person] sees the move to an institution as a decisive change in living arrangements, the last change he will experience before he dies. . . . Finally, no matter what the extenuating circumstances, the older person who has children interprets the move to an institution as rejection by his children.*

Considerable change should be made regarding the concept of care, preparation of the older person and his family, and longevity of residents in such a facility. Many people could be admitted much later if they were given more support at home. In addition, there should always be an expectation and actual possibility of discharge and return home, with response to treatment and changes in the person's condition and circumstances.

Involuntary commitment (applies to state and private psychiatric facilities)

Admission to any institution should ideally be voluntary, but there are some circumstances that may require commitment against a person's wishes. Extreme civil libertarians urge that legal involuntary commitment to mental hospitals be done away with (but, strangely, have not commented on the de facto assignment of old people into nursing homes and related facilities—without any of the protections afforded in connection with admission to mental hospitals). Others insist that people who are a danger to themselves or to others need the protection of commitment procedure. Such procedures are not uniform from state to state, but in general the legal justification for action is (1) imminent physical danger to self, (2) imminent physical danger to others, or (3) a clear and present need of immediate care or treatment.

Doctors are the only practitioners who are allowed to perform commitment proceedings. Since a large percentage of the United States population has no access to a psychiatrist, the family physician is, by default, pressed into service in times of psychiatric emergency. Many doctors fear signing commitment papers, because of possible malpractice suits. The following are some of the safeguards to remember when commitment is under consideration—for the protection of both the older person and his doctor:

1. Know and observe laws regarding involuntary commitment. Get to know the local judge or clerk of court available for assistance and advice. Examine the patient within the legal time limit before signing papers.
2. Avoid shortcuts in examination (see discussion of the legal examination in Chapter 9). Watch for sedatives by giving the person time to recover. If the person is comatose, decide if this is medically or psychiatrically caused. If psychiatric, double check again at a later time.
3. Remember that taking the word of relatives is always risky.
4. Avoid personal conflict of interest.
5. Avoid use of force (e.g., injections, electroshock treatment).
6. Avoid illegal transportation. Most states rule that only a policeman can transport someone against his will.*

---

*From Shanas, Ethel: The health of older people: a social survey, Cambridge, Mass, 1962, Harvard University Press.

*In some jurisdictions (for example, the District of Columbia) where liability insurance is lacking or inadequate, the police themselves fear legal action.

7. Avoid institutions that are unfamiliar. Get to know all local facilities.
8. Avoid acting alone when consultation is available.

The informal, nonprotesting admission or emergency admission procedure is helpful when the person is too confused to comprehend what is happening.

DIFFERENT KINDS OF SHORT- AND LONG-TERM INSTITUTIONAL CARE

Emergency care

Many older people remain in their homes until an acute psychiatric and/or medical crisis occurs necessitating emergency care. Emergency rooms of hospitals have become the primary mode of providing initial care; this means, of course, that the patient must transport himself or be transported to the hospital independently, or must obtain the services of an ambulance. Fire departments, police, and rescue squads all may provide ambulance services, depending upon the particular community, with fire departments the most commonly involved. As we mentioned earlier, psychiatric emergencies are regulated differently from locale to locale, and in a number of communities only the police can legally transport such a patient.

Ambulance service staffs can range all the way from untrained volunteers to paramedics with modern, mobile intensive care units (MICU) that transmit physiological data from the field to the hospital through telemetry. In some countries, such as France, Ireland, Russia, and even in some parts of the United States, physicians have staffed mobile coronary care units. However, personnel training* and financing of emergency care are problems; for example, Medicare does not cover ambulance services.

Although emergency care in the United States has been generally poor, there are winds of change in communities like Miami where many older people reside. Improvements will reduce disabilities in all ages and there is no doubt, according to various studies, that many more lives could be saved. Unfortunately, even in emergency rooms age prejudice exists; Sudnow found both private and public hospitals responding less favorably to older than to younger persons.*

*The traditional American Red Cross training is not adequate. A pamphlet on the training of ambulance personnel may be obtained from the National Academy of Sciences, 2101 Constitution Avenue, N.W. Washington, D. C. 20418.

Emergency shelter

One of the saddest problems is that of passing the buck by shunting the old person from one place to another. "Decisions" are made by avoidance, by taking minimal responsibility, and by failing to consult with the patient, his family, and (often) the family doctor. Voluntary hospitals are renowned for their ethically dubious practice of dropping the "Medicare patient" on the doorsteps of the municipal hospital.

Emergency shelter admission is mandatory and should be available in any and all hospitals—to allow, at the very least, for a period of decision-making. This is as true for the so-called "social admissions" (the person may have no place to sleep, etc.) as it is for medical and psychiatric episodes. Not only is the brief admission useful to effect a proper diagnostic work-up, but also during that time therapy can begin and changes may be seen that may alter the original diagnostic impression and individual treatment program. The idea of hospitalization for several days in a unit attached to the emergency room of the hospital, for crisis intervention in all age groups, would be a step forward in evolving comprehensive social, medical, and psychiatric care in our general hospitals. Physicians, police, judges, and other community agents as well as families are frequently at a loss to know where to take an older person for comprehensive diagnostic attention. Complete diagnostic evaluations and a therapeutic trial should precede any admission to long-term mental hospitals or nursing home facilities.

*Sudnow, David: Passing on: the social organization of dying, Englewood Cliffs, N. J., 1967, Prentice-Hall, Inc.

Acute hospitalization

The term "acute hospitalization" usually applies to hospital stays lasting from a few days to three months, during which diagnosis and treatment take place simultaneously.* Transient confusional states (reversible brain syndromes) and functional disorders can respond to acute care, sometimes with dramatically positive results.

Psychiatric units in profit-making or in voluntary general hospitals usually provide short-term psychiatric care independent of age; in other words, when an older person is able to pay, he is more likely to receive the same degree of care as that given to other ages. If it is believed (either correctly or mistakenly) that the person is suffering from a chronic brain syndrome, he will at least receive decent care until transfer elsewhere is arranged. Private mental hospitals also do effective work in the acute hospitalization of older persons. In addition the inservice units of community mental health centers (usually public hospitals), as well as municipal, county, and state hospitals, provide this service with varying degrees of quality. Preadmission screening units, whether in the community or in general or state mental hospitals (see Chapter 10), should be alert to the disorders that can respond to acute hospitalization.

During acute hospitalization it is important to maintain orientation—through unrestricted visiting hours, personal belongings and the like, and family liaison. Home pressures, unattended pets and plants belonging to older persons, and mail (especially Social Security, pension, and public assistance checks) may need attention from hospital social aides or community agencies.

Chronic hospitalization

Organic brain damage is the major psychiatric reason for permanent hospitalization. Persons with chronic physical conditions (e.g., stroke victims) may be admitted to chronic disease and geriatric hospitals even though many such persons have accompanying or previously existing mental problems.

In 1968, 120,000 persons over 65 were residents of state and county mental hospitals, with an additional 15,000 in private mental hospitals and 3,000 in Veterans Administration hospitals. Approximately two thirds of these persons were first admitted at age 65 or older, and the remaining one third were hospitalized at a younger age. Females outnumber males two to one in private mental hospitals, whereas in state and county hospitals the sex ratio is about 100 females to 97 males. In contrast, the VA hospital population is almost exclusively male.

Private mental hospitals, both voluntary nonprofit and profit-making, offer care that is of adequate to high quality, at high prices, and thus they are beyond the resources of all but a few elderly. The Veterans Administration provides services to a predominately male population that includes Spanish-American and World War I and II veterans. There are 166 VA hospitals throughout the country as well as regional offices, domiciliary care, nursing homes (the Soldiers Home in Washington, D. C., being the first established), and outpatient clinics. The Veterans Administration states that it "has the most comprehensive program for continued treatment and follow-up of the aging patient to be found anywhere in the free world."* By law, the VA must provide medical care for 25 million veterans whose average age in 1972 was 45. In the same year, 1972, there where 2 million over 65, but by 1992 there will be 7 million as World War II veterans grow older.

State and county mental hospitals have been the center of long-standing controversy

*The work of Cosin in England, with patients moving in and out of the hospital, depending on their condition at given times, is illustrative of good care.

*Dr. Paul A. C. Haber, Deputy Assistant Chief, Medical Director for Professional Services. The VA has conducted a Normative Aging Study at the VA outpatient clinic in Boston since 1963, beginning with 2,135 men. See Aging and Human Development, special issue, 1972.

and we have come full circle in our attempts to provide proper mental health care. When the American social reformer Dorothea Lynde Dix (1802-1887) began her efforts, there were practically no hospitals for the mentally ill. The first American asylum for mental patients was established in Williamsburg, Virginia, in 1773, and it was the only such "state hospital" of its kind for fifty years. Toward the mid-nineteenth century, the belief grew that the mentally and emotionally ill could be helped and that the state owed them help. Miss Dix pressed the idea of hospital care. A state-by-state system of hospitals was established, which now has come increasingly under criticism because of the quality of care and the basic concepts of treatment that they represent. With cries of "bring the patient back to the community," we seem panicked into an unfortunate and precipitous course of dismantling the hospital system without establishing valid alternatives.

It can be argued that there is no reason for chronic hospitalization, since nursing homes and other facilities could provide the appropriate care. See the overview presented in Chapter 4. Many older people are in mental institutions not because they need to be but simply because there is on other facility for them. But paralleling the studies purporting to show that old people need not be in mental hospitals are reports that old people need not be in nursing homes. Old people seem never to belong anywhere! Yet there is a grain of truth in all these points of view. Old people frequently are misplaced; many could remain at home with supportive services. For those who do require permanent residential treatment for medical and/or psychiatric reasons, there is only a narrow range of choices available, which may not fit their particular situations. Neither present-day nursing homes nor mental hospitals can escape justly deserved criticism. The financing arrangements, often politically inspired, that support the growing nursing home industry have led to numbers of older persons with chronic brain syndromes being given custodial care in nursing homes rather than mental hospitals.* However such homes do not even offer the services of the admittedly inadequate hospitals. Many are unsafe in terms of fire protection and patient supervision. They may provide poor nursing and medical care, little or no psychiatric care, and minimal rehabilitation and recreation. Living in a nursing home is too often like being confined to a motel (in fact a number of homes seem designed for quick renovation into motels, should the present clientele prove unprofitable). State mental hospitals, on the other hand, generally have a mixed age range of people, more grounds than typical nursing home facilities, a larger number of staff, more activities and social programs, theaters, churches, gymnasiums, job opportunities (including sheltered workshops), gardening, and stores. There is an atmosphere of greater hustle and bustle, more like that of a community. Safety and fire security regulations are usually more strictly enforced. If the massive mental hospitals could be refurbished or be physically moved out of their usually geographical location (far from the community), if the "back wards" were abolished and all custodial care replaced with active treatment programs, and if admissions, periods of residence, and discharges became more fluid and flexible procedures aimed at integration with family and community life, then the concept of the mental hospital might become accepted by old people, their families, and professionals. As it is now, the mental hospital symbolizes being "old and crazy" whereas the nursing home means that one is "old, incapacitated, and about to die." Neither represents a positive approach to mental health care.

Foster care

"Foster care" originated as foster parent programs for children; efforts to encourage families to take in old people who are unrelated to them have never been very suc-

*Stotsky's studies concern the possible significant variables affecting the adjustment of state mental hospital patients in nursing homes and the kinds of patients who seem best able to use this kind of care.

cessful, presumably because old people are not so "attractive" as children. Foster care has become a euphemism for foster family care and really describes, in many areas, an underfinanced, unregulated, unprofessional series of "homes" operated for profit. Since some states have sought to reduce state mental hospital rolls, many old people—usually long-term and predominately schizophrenic patients—have been transferred, often indiscriminately, into foster care, intermediate care, and other so-called nursing homes.*

The passive, supine, nontroublemakers are most likely to be chosen for these dubious exchanges, since foster care and personal care homes will take only tractable persons who have minimal nursing needs. The average payment through welfare to such "homes" in 1970 was $125 per month; that is $4 daily—hardly enough to provide decent food and the basic amenities, let alone medical, psychiatric, and social care. Safety and fire inspections are notoriously negligent:

> The chief D. C. fire marshall yesterday ordered the immediate inspection of all foster care homes used by St. Elizabeths Hospital after two patients died early yesterday in a fire at one such home in Southeast Washington.
>
> THE WASHINGTON POST
> *December 15, 1971*

Nursing homes

Almost a million older people live in nursing homes in the United States, and these homes have received considerable adverse attention from legislators, the press, and the general public. We wish to emphasize that there are a number of fine commercial nursing homes* that give good care to the elderly, and we would hope to encourage and support their efforts. However, a significantly larger number of homes are correctly described as human dumping grounds and even as "halfway houses somewhere between society and the cemetery."† We shall be focusing here on the deficiencies of nursing home care—not in order to moralize but to present the reader with a picture of what remains to be acomplished in upgrading patient care.‡ We shall also provide a brief description of some of the reasons why nursing home care has evolved into its present form.

Categories of nursing homes and the financing of patient care

Commercial nursing homes are of course available to people who can afford to pay for their own care. However, because costs of care have risen so precipitously,§ a number of financing mechanisms have been created to assist the great majority of people who could not otherwise afford care. There continue to be many problems; for example,

---

*Butler, Goldfarb, Weinberg, and others have protested indiscriminate transfers to unacceptable settings. (Trends in long-term care. Hearings before the Subcommittee on Long-term Care of the Special Committee on Aging, U. S. Senate, Dec. 17, 1970.) The vulnerability of the aged to death or illness as a result of transfer ("transfer mortality") is a serious cause for concern. (Butler, R. N.: Immediate and long-range dangers to transfer of elderly patients from state hospitals to community facilities. Guest editorial in The Gerontologist **10:** winter, 1970. Also see Killian, E. C.: Effect of geriatric transfers on mortality rates, Social Work **15:** 19-26, 1970; there are numerous papers showing the same mortal and morbid effects.) Lieberman's studies have shown that a year or more of preparation may be necessary to increase survival during the first six months in an institution, even when the institution is adequate. (Lieberman, M. A.: Psychological effects of institutionalization, Journal of Gerontology **23:**343-353, 1968.)

Of course movement of patients is not necessarily an evil in itself. Some facilities are so terrible that transfer is humane. *Where* the person is being moved to is important. For instance, in Pennsylvania in 1967, a program was developed at the South Mountain Geriatric Center. Patients were moved out of the state mental hospitals and into this facility designed exclusively for the use of old people. Favorable results have been reported. (Cohen, E. S., and Kraft, A. C.: The restorative potential of elderly long-term residents of mental hospitals. Presented at twentieth annual meeting, Gerontological Society, St. Petersburg, Fla., Nov. 9, 1967.)

*Often called "proprietary" homes.

†Former Congressman David Pyror (D-Ark.).

‡A special debt is owed to Senator Frank Moss (D-Utah), ably assisted by staff director, Frank Frantz, of the U. S. Senate Subcommittee on Long-term Care, for its pioneer hearings on nursing homes in the pre-Medicare period.

§Some nursing home fees range up to and even beyond $1,000 a month.

middle-income people may have too much income to be eligible for assistance but not enough to pay for care by themselves.

The various categories of nursing homes, which are directly defined by their federal and state financing, do not always clarify the actual kind and amount of service offered. Therefore, one must check on the *actual* service rendered (e.g., how *much* nursing care) in a particular home, regardless of category.

Extended care facilities (Medicare)

An extended care facility (ECF) is more a function than a structure. (An ECF may be a separate institution such as a nursing home or be part of other institutions such as a hospital or home for the aged.) It does not offer long-term care but, rather, care extended beyond hospitalization for a specific period of illness. The patient is expected to return to independent living after convalescence and/or rehabilitation. Thus an ECF is an extension of hospital care with a probability of discharge. ECFs derive from Medicare legislation and are financed on a cost-reimbursement basis by the federal government. Retroactive denials of benefits have been common as the government has cut back on the terms of its original commitment. Patients are entitled by law to payments for up to 100 days of care and a lifetime reserve of 60 days, but regulations regarding eligibility have become increasingly restrictive.

Skilled nursing care facilities (Medicaid)

Skilled nursing home (SNH) is a Medicaid-derived term and refers to long-term, unlimited nursing home care without the requirement of previous hospitalization. Both long-term convalescent patients and those with terminal illnesses are eligible for admission. Financing is provided by a federal-state, cost-sharing program administered by the states. Again, as in ECFs, there have been retroactive denials of benefits, leaving some patients and their families with unexpected, enormous bills to pay. The term "skilled nursing home" often suggests more skill than is actually present; there may be no registered nurse on duty. Moreover the term implies that there are patients who may need or get along with "unskilled nursing," a dubious eventuality as far as older people are concerned.

Skilled nursing facilities

The 1972 Social Security Amendments created a single definition and set of standards for ECFs and SNHs. A new category, "skilled nursing facility," was introduced. However, one must be familiar with the older terminology described above.

Intermediate care facilities

An intermediate care facility (ICF) may approximate what the public has in mind when it refers to a "nursing home." The ICF is designed for people who theoretically need "less than a skilled nursing home . . . but more than a custodial or residential home." Personal care, simple medical care, and intermittent nursing care are the services under the jurisdiction of ICFs. This care for those who cannot afford to pay is federally funded through Medicaid, and the ICFs are subject to federal rather than state standards. Paradoxically, although policy makers were interested in the ICFs' cost-cutting potential, costs may be actually larger than in SNHs. (For example, the ICFs have in the past been paid the same amount as SNHs for providing less care.) Financially the rates of both SNHs and ICFs are negotiated rather than based on costs (as in the case of ECFs).

Financing of nursing homes

In discussing nursing home care it is important to clarify a few points about the commercial nursing home industry. The United States is one of the few countries in the world where the care of the sick elderly has become "big business," run primarily for commercial gain. The number of nursing homes has proliferated in the last ten years.

> The nursing home industry consists of 23,000 homes with more than a million beds. About 90% of the homes are profit-making, some owned by large chains with publicly sold stock. Others have nonprofit sponsors such as churches and commu-

nity organizations. A total of $2.5 billion was spent on nursing home care in fiscal 1969, of which the federal government paid $1.8 billion (through Medicare and Medicaid). It (the federal government) also supports the growth of the industry through FHA insurance and Hill-Burton grants-in-aid for construction and private loans from the Small Business Administration.

These 23,000 homes are more than twice the number than existed ten years ago. In the same period, the number of beds tripled. This growth began partly in response to the increasing demand for beds as the aging population increased, and was accelerated by the passage of Medicare and Medicaid. Guaranteed payments to nursing homes convinced investors that it was a no-lose proposition. By 1969, Wall Street considered nursing homes a glamour industry. Investments came from real estate developers, insurance men, and others outside the health field.* [Authors' note: Physicians, despite obvious conflict of interests, have invested in and own nursing homes.]

In 1970 and 1971 many nursing homes withdrew from the Medicare program that had so encouraged their growth. Some did so because they had not met standards (and a number of them could not afford to do so even if they had wished to) whereas others were frustrated and impatient with the bureaucratic confusion, laborious and contradictory rules and regulations from the federal government, retroactive denial of claims, and other administrative difficulties. It must also be noted that these institutions have had to adapt to rapidly changing federal law—the Kerr-Mills, Vendor Medical Programs, and Medicare. On the other hand, cases have been documented in which the nursing homes overbilled, billed for services never delivered, billed after a patient's death, and double-billed to different governmental programs for the same patient. The government has also charged that services were overutilized, thus costing more than originally anticipated.

Conditions in nursing homes

There are, as we have said, some excellent homes in which emphasis is on meeting patients' needs in every way possible within financial limits. But the remainder of homes run the gamut from filthy and unsafe to clean but cheerless and depressing. The worst of the homes are firetraps, with filthy living conditions and neglect of patient care. Other homes are stylized, motellike, antiseptically clean horrors—patients sit in numb silence with dejected faces or pace endlessly down hallways. There may be little commotion or communication except for the one-way mumble of television. Nutrition is often inadequate. Poor food-handling standards have resulted in food poisoning such as in the July, 1970 *Salmonella* epidemic in a nursing home in Baltimore, Maryland, where 107 patients became ill and 25 died. Personal abuse on the part of the staff toward patients can occur because the older people are ill, vulnerable, and unable to defend themselves and the staff may be untrained, unmotivated, and improperly supervised. The majority of nursing home administrators themselves have had no specific training directly related to their work. This is changing, happily. There is a shortage of physician services, skilled nursing care, dental care, social services, and psychiatric care.* Patients often are overmedicated and deprived of any responsibility or decision-making on their own behalf.

Nursing home standards

Individual nursing homes are subject to state and/or federal standards, depending on their financing, but the federal government gives enforcement functions to the states. Homes that do not meet standards are often allowed to remain "temporarily" open, and the explanation given is that patients would have no other place to go. Basic fire and safety standards may go unheeded and nursing home disasters are inevitable under the circumstances.

As the result of a 1972 directive by the President, the Health, Education, and Welfare Department has established a new office to oversee all HEW programs relating to

*National Council on Aging, William Fitch, Director: Older Americans: special handling required, June, 1971.

*Solon, J. A.: Nursing home and medical care. In DeGroot, L. J., editor: Medical care: social and organization aspects, Springfield, Ill., 1966, Charles C Thomas, Publisher.

nursing homes. The Office of Nursing Home Affairs (ONHA) is responsible for coordinating efforts by different agencies in the department to upgrade standards nationwide for the benefit of the almost 1 million Americans living in nursing homes. Establishment of ONHA and the appointment of Mrs. Marie Callender to head it means that for the first time a single official is responsible for pulling together different HEW nursing home efforts into a single coordinated program.

The list below gives the President's eight-point nursing home program,* announced in 1971.

1. Training state nursing home inspectors
2. Completion of federal support of state inspections under Medicaid
3. Consolidation of enforcement activities
4. Strengthening federal enforcement
5. Short-term training for professional and paraprofessional nursing home personnel
6. Assistance for state investigative units
7. Comprehensive review of long-term care
8. Cracking down on substandard nursing homes

Mental health specialists should know the character and deficiencies of nursing homes to which they refer people.†

Patient characteristics

The average age of nursing home residents is 78 years; two thirds are women and 96% are white. Some 85% to 90% of persons who enter nursing homes do not leave them alive. The average length of stay is 1.1 years, with one third dying within the first year and another third between the first and third years. The final third live three or more years.

As with all of the institutions for the elderly, "large numbers of the disabled are forced into nursing homes . . . at a very high charge to the public treasury simply because public programs could not give attention to alternative ways of meeting their needs outside of institutions."* A 1971 study by Brandeis University's Levinson Gerontological Policy Institute of nursing home inhabitants in Massachusetts showed that (of 100 persons) 37 needed full-time skilled nursing care, 26 needed minimally supervised "living," 23 could get along at home with periodic home visits by nurses, and 14 needed nothing. We have discussed, in Chapter 10, some of the alternatives to institutionalization.

The numbers of people in nursing homes who suffer from psychiatric disorders have been variously estimated; Goldfarb, for example, in 1962, found that 87% of patients showed significant evidence of chronic brain syndrome. As we have emphasized previously, persons with chronic physical disorders generally have psychiatric symptom manifestations. Added to these patients are the numbers of people now being transferred from mental institutions.† Nursing homes tend to select persons with the kinds of psychiatric symptoms that cause the least problems. Suicidal, boisterous, or hostile persons are likely to be rejected along with those who wander off, smoke in bed, or are addicted to drugs or alcohol. The tractable, de-

*From President Nixon's message on aging to Congress, March 23, 1972.

†The confidential character of nursing home inspection reports at the Department of Health, Education, and Welfare was challenged in April, 1972, when Malvin Schechter, the Washington editor of Hospital Practice magazine, brought a freedom-of-information suit against HEW Secretary Elliot L. Richardson. (States, also, do not provide inspection reports.) It now seems almost certain that information regarding nursing homes will be available to the public as a result of Mr. Schechter's efforts.

Schechter has also written the following excellent reports on nursing home deficiencies: (Of carpets, patient safety, and decision-making at HEW, Hospital Practice **6**:33, 1971) and (Nursing home fires: the anatomy of a tragedy, Hospital Practice **7**:139, 1972).

*Alternatives to nursing home care: a proposal, U. S. Senate Special Committee on Aging. Prepared by Levinson Gerontological Policy Institute (Robert Morris, Director), Brandeis University, Waltham, Mass., Oct., 1971, Washington, D. C., 1971, U. S. Government Printing Office.

†Kramer, M., Taube, C., and Starr, S.: Patterns of use of psychiatric facilities by the aged: current status, trends, and implications, Proceedings of the American Psychiatric Association Regional Research Conference on Aging, "Aging in Modern Society," 1967.

pressed, withdrawn persons are more acceptable, as well as those with incontinence and definite nursing needs.

Selecting a nursing home

Mental health personnel should be thoroughly familiar with any nursing homes to which they refer older people and their families. Visits to the nursing home in question are useful in order to talk to staff, observe the home and its operations, and view the patients firsthand. Families can contact local agencies (usually public health departments) and physicians who may be able to give an idea of the quality of individual homes. Local health and welfare councils, welfare departments and mental health associations may provide help in selection. Proper placement must, of course, be based on a comprehensive evaluation of the older person's condition and needs.

Homes for the aging

Homes for the aging are voluntary, nonprofit institutions, usually sectarian (religious) but sometimes under the auspices of benevolent and fraternal associations, trusts, or municipalities. See Table 11-1.

They are not at this time totally satisfactory community resources because many of them have not yet achieved full social responsibility. Religious, fraternal, and trust homes tend to be very selective in their admissions, and persons without some wealth and a sustaining family are more likely to be rejected. The homes ordinarily exclude the overtly mentally ill, the severely mentally impaired, and the acutely or notably physically ill. When illnesses develop after admission, transfer to municipal, county, and state facilities is probable because most homes for the aging have insufficient services and personnel to provide the necessary care. Members of minority groups are generally excluded through overt or covert means; less than 3% of residents are black. (Failure to comply with Title VI of the Civil Rights Act has left some homes out of Medicare.) Waiting periods for admission are long—several months to several years. Persons on waiting lists are not usually provided with outreach services although these services are developing in some areas.

Since homes for the aging do depend upon voluntary contributions, it is understandable how difficult it has been for them to offer a range of services on a multilevel basis in accordance with the changing medical and psychiatric statuses of older people. There is growing public support for diversion of public taxpayers' money from the commercial nursing home industry* to nonprofit homes. Table 11-2 describes the percentage of various kinds of institutional homes used by the elderly.

There are beginning to be major progressive changes as homes for the aging move

*Increasingly, homes for the aging have nursing home components.

Table 11-1. Kinds of nonprofit homes for the aging*

Type	Number of homes	Average number of beds	Total number of patients
Religious	1,500	84	117,180
Governmental (municipal)	670	105	63,000
Others (benevolent, fraternal, trust)	1,225	60	66,150
Summary	3,395		246,330

*Based on data from Frank Zelenka, American Association of Homes for the Aging; from Selected institutional characteristics of long-term care facilities, Department of Health Care Administration, George Washington University Long-term Care Monograph No. 4, Jan., 1970.

away from the limited historic connotations of "old age homes." A few have evolved into *campuses* where a wide spectrum of services and facilities is created to give progressive, graduated care. It has long been realized that older individuals do not fall neatly into institutional categories. Many can and should stay at home, if provided with supportive services. Living "independently" in apartments can be possible if medical services and ready access to hospital facilities are provided. And many can live in a home for the aging or a nursing home rather than a state hospital if such facilities offer therapeutic programs and can draw upon personnel usually found in a hospital. How can all of these services be offered? The Philadelphia Geriatric Center has included all the combinations suggested above in one city block; a hospital, the Home for the Jewish Aged (which was the parent institution), two residential apartment buildings, a research institute, and several small-unit, intermediate boarding facilities. A day care center for the elderly exists in another part of the city.

Other homes for the aging have moved beyond their physical structure into the community. Social services, Meals-on-Wheels, and day care centers are developing in some areas. "Drop-in" centers with recreational service, arts, and crafts may occasionally be found along with sheltered workshops. Unfortunately it is all too rare that religious organizations have formed coalitions with each other or with nonsectarian organizations to pool their resources and services and thus offer more than each could do alone. One would also hope that religious institutions would become greater sources of advocacy and moral force on behalf of the elderly.

Table 11-2. Percentages and kinds of institutional homes

Homes	Percent
Commercial nursing homes	79
Voluntary nonprofit homes for aging: nursing homes and "campus" complexes (religious, benevolent, fraternal, and trust)	14
Governmental homes (federal, state, county, and municipal)	7

Some homes do accept the so-called senile patient. The Menorah Home and Hospital for the Aged in Brooklyn, New York, a 526-bed institution with 300 senile residents and 500 outpatients, has pioneered in the provision of psychiatric and mental health services for the aged. In 1957 Menorah founded a Geriatric Guidance Clinic and also established the first day center in a home for the aged (with a membership of 250 older people living in the community).

Other exemplary institutions, some of which approximate the campus-type of environment are the Carmelite Homes (the Mary Manning Walsh Home* of New York City and St. Josephs of Trumbull, Connecticut), the Isabella Home Geriatric Center in New York City, and the Avery Convalescent Center in Hartford, Connecticut.

FINANCING INSTITUTIONAL CARE

Personal and economic costs of mental diseases are staggering.† One estimate for 1968 ran over $20 billion, or 2.4% of the Gross National Product per year.‡ A tragic way of cutting costs would be to place older mental patients outside the mainstream of psychiatric care. Therefore a truly appropriate national health plan must cover long-term and terminal care for the psychiatrically and physically impaired patient. Two thirds of our nation's health bill is for chronic illness (two thirds of $70 billion in 1970). Yet most health insurance plans have tried to sidestep

*Bernadette de Lourdes, Mother: Where somebody cares: the Mary Manning Walsh Home and its program for complete care of the aging, a descriptive account of modern concepts in action. New York, 1959, G. P. Putman's Sons.

†For example, a private nursing home can cost $1,200 a month and some families pay another $1,000 a month to obtain a 24-hour private duty nurse in the nursing home. Private mental hospitals may cost $2,000 monthly.

‡Conley, Ronald W., Conwell, Margaret, and Willner, Shirley G.: The cost of mental illness: 1968. Statistical Note No. 30, National Institute of Mental Health, Washington, D. C., Oct., 1970.

the issue or leave it to the states. Individuals and their families can rarely meet the high costs.

Historically the care and treatment of the mentally ill has been left to the individual states. The first federal assistance was offered to the states in the National Mental Health Act of 1946. Part of the Medicaid legislation with significance for mental health was sponsored by Senator Russell Long in 1965. It permits federal financial assistance for persons in the group age 65 and over who are patients in institutions for mental diseases. It is a companion piece to the Title XVIII (Medicare) legislation, which provides specifically for those older persons with acute brain disorders and other mental illnesses who can be expected to respond to relatively brief but intensive treatment in mental hospitals.* The Long Amendment also makes provisions for the very many aged who are suffering from chronic disorders, either organic or functional, and who need long-term continued care in state mental health facilities. In expressing the intent of the Amendment, the Senate Committee on Finance stated that it:

> . . . wishes to insure that the additional Federal funds to be made available to the States under the provisions of the bill will assist the over-all improvement of mental health services in the State. State and local funds now being used for institutional care of the aged will be released as a result of the bill, but there is great need for increased professional services in hospitals and for development of alternate methods of care outside the hospitals. To accomplish this, States may have to reallocate their expenditures for mental health to promote new methods of treatment and care. The committee bill provides that the States will receive additional Federal funds only to the extent that a showing is made to the satisfaction of the Secretary that total expenditures of the States or its political subdivisions from their own funds for mental health services are increased.†

However, millions of dollars in Medicaid payments have not resulted in better programs or higher medical standards. In most states, monies designated by law for the improvement of the care of elderly mental patients in state hospitals go into the state general revenue fund and are seldom seen by the hospitals.

The loophole in the legislation that allows this misuse of funds is the "maintenance of state effort" clause which, for example, required a state to maintain a budget for mental health programs in 1969 that would "exceed" what was spent in any quarter in the fiscal year ending June 30, 1965. Two major problems exist in respect to the clause (Section 1903b). First: It is a matter of legal interpretation as to whether the "extent that" the state must excede the previous budget *includes* the federal payments. Second: For all practical purposes, even if the stricter interpretation is accepted, the various commissioners for mental health would ask for budgetary increases anyway, merely to combat rising costs. Thus there is no guarantee that programs involving patient care will be improved, but rather that the federal government is simply paying the increased overhead. The money, in other words, is not earmarked in any significant way, and the intention of Congress that matching funds be spent in developing and implementing a comprehensive mental health program cannot be enforced under the current statute. A tightening up of the ambiguous language is necessary. Federal funds should be paid only when the state shows evidence of expenditures in personnel, equipment, and program development that improve mental health services.

FAMILY REACTION TO INSTITUTIONALIZATION

Families often need help in dealing with their feelings about an older family member's going to an institution. Social service departments in institutions are especially important in maintaining liaison with relatives. Many family members are extremely ambivalent, both because of the negative reputation of institutional care and because of their own

---

*Theoretically, the Medicaid legislation is supposed to cover the medically indigent of all ages, not all of whom are on welfare.

†From U. S. Senate Committee on Finance. Social Security Amendments of 1965: Report to accompany H.R. 6675, June 30, 1965, Washington, D. C., 1965, U. S. Government Printing Office, p. 149.

feelings of failing or abandoning the person. Some experience a sense of relief about which they later feel guilty. Families who care (as opposed to those who reject the older person—a less common category) often experience a grief reaction upon admission as though the person had already died. This "death" may be more traumatic than the actual death of the older person later on. In some cases family members may actually stop visiting the person because of inability to tolerate their own grief and ambivalence. We feel that there should be a built-in expectation and real possibility of discharge and return home so that families are not subtly encouraged to cut themselves off emotionally. Families need to be advised that some of the very supportive things they can do for an older person are to visit frequently, take the person on outings and weekends at home if possible, become involved with the institution by getting to know the staff and administrative personnel, and provide the extra amenities and attention that only a family can give.

The actual day of admission of an older person is often handled insensitively, the person simply being "deposited" without any transition or preparation. This shock approach can result in increased illness and even death; certainly it is questionable psychologically. We advise flexibility and individualization; some persons indeed respond best to a firm, quick (but humane) admission, while many others need to take their time, to absorb things slowly with a good deal of support. The inauguration of day programs, preliminary admissions for weekends or during times when families want to go away on vacation, and provisions for family or friends to sleep in the institution (nearby or even in the same room) when the older person is anxious and frightened could soften the suddenness and harshness of admission. Family and friends could be allowed and encouraged to serve as volunteers in institutional activities, from socializing to performing simple services for residents including their relative. Children and grandchildren should be given access to the person; a little life and noise in most institutions would be a vast improvement. In general there should be much more fluidity between the institution and the community.

Group and individual therapy with families can be useful in helping to resolve long-term family conflicts and short-term reactions to institutionalization. See Chapter 12 for further discussion of therapy.

OTHER FACTORS IN INSTITUTIONAL CARE

Right to treatment*

A second legal concept beyond the question of involuntary admission discussed earlier is the "right to treatment." It is difficult to balance the right to freedom with the right to treatment. A Federal District Court for Alabama has ruled that patients committed involuntarily to a mental hospital through noncriminal procedures have a constitutional right to "adequate and effective treatment." The court further found that the state was failing to provide adequate treatment to the several thousand patients who had been civilly committed to Bryce Hospital in Tuscaloosa. The ruling was made as a result of a class action suit initiated by guardians of patients at Bryce and by certain hospital employees. It was stated that the Constitution requires adequate and effective treatment, because without it the hospital is transformed into a penitentiary where one could be held indefinitely without conviction for any offense. The court ordered a report from the hospital within 90 days which must include: a precise definition of the mission and functions of the hospital and a specific plan to deliver adequate treatment to patients.†

---

*We are indebted here to the work of Charles Halpern and his brief in the Wyatt vs. Stickney case in Alabama concerning the right to treatment (Amici's proposed standards for adequate treatment, Jan. 21, 1972).

†Ricky Wyatt et al. v. Dr. Stonewall B. Stickney et al., U. S. Court for Middle Dist. of Ala., Northern Div., Action No. 3195-N. (It is unfortunate that the American Psychiatric Association has not supported the enforcement of the right to treatment for persons suffering from mental and emotional disorders. See 1967 Position Statement of the American Psychiatric Association.)

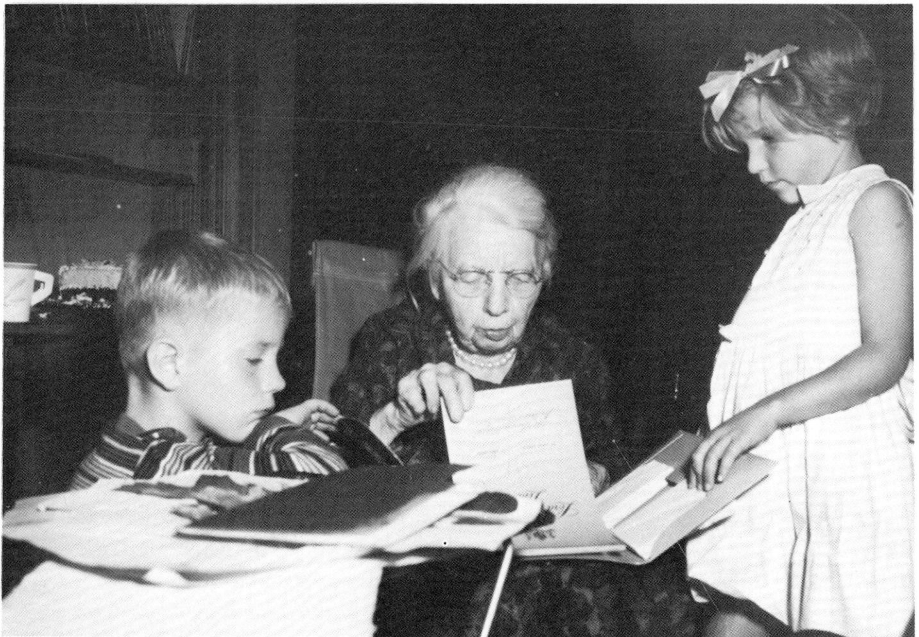

Young visitors: an older person's privilege and right.

Photo by Russell Lewis.

Individual treatment plans

The right to treatment must involve an individual treatment plan for each patient:

> The need for an individualized treatment plan cannot be over-emphasized. Without such a plan, there can be no evidence that the hospital has singled out the patient for treatment as an individual with his own unique problems.*

Preliminary diagnostic formulation and individualized treatment plans should be accomplished within twelve hours of admission to any kind of hospital or institution. Reception units or special psycho-geriatric units should be available for brief hospitalizations, perhaps three to five days up to three to six weeks, to facilitate proper diagnosis and in the cases of reversible brain syndrome and functional disorders, definitive treatment. The staff should avoid a mental "set" regarding treatability or length of hospitalization. Experience has emphasized that trials at treatment constitute a major part of evaluation; for example, considerable time should be given to make certain that a seemingly fixed and permanent organic brain disorder is not a refractory depression.

Periodic and comprehensive reevaluation is important. Patients who arrive with one condition may develop others during their stay. Changes in psychiatric symptoms are often due to physical changes that the patient himself may be unable to report.

Other patient rights and privileges

The many and pervasive aspects of authoritarianism seen in our hospitals and institutions are facets of infantilization and serve the needs of the providers rather than those served. The goal should be the least restrictive conditions necessary to achieve the purposes of institutionalization. Patients' rights must be preserved in very specific ways. Commitment or voluntary admission to a mental hospital or "assignment" to a nursing home should not per se abrogate the right to manage affairs, to sign contracts, to hold professional, occupational, or vehicle

---

*From Bazelon, Judge David: Implementing the right to treatment, University of Chicago Law Review, pp. 742 and 746, 1969.

operator's licenses, to marry or obtain a divorce, to register and vote, and to make a will. Patients should not be placed incommunicado. Visitation (including small children) and telephone communications should be permitted at all times (a 24-hour basis) except when there are clear indications that such communications and visitations promote disturbances in the patient, which are untherapeutic and harmful at a *particular* time. Any limit upon such contact must be periodically reviewed, and renewal or continuation must not be automatic.

Patients must have the unrestricted right to receive sealed mail except when responsible staff personnel can clearly defend restriction on the basis of an individualized patient plan. Again, periodic review must occur.

Privacy* and space to move are other rights. Privacy is obviously qualitative as well as quantitative, and the availability of at least four hours a day alone should be made. No multipatient room should exceed four persons. There must be a minimum of 80 square feet of floor space per patient, with soundproofing, screens or curtains, and at least one toilet, lavatory, shower or tub for each six persons. A comfortable, attractive day room area (40 square feet per patient) with reading lamps, tables, chairs, and recreational facilities is considered necessary, and a dining room area should include 10 square feet per patient.

Food, abundantly and attractively served, is another patient right, unless medically restricted. The diet must, at minimum, provide the Recommended Daily Dietary Allowance developed by the National Academy of Science. Opportunities for snack times and raiding an icebox, as well as moderate use of alcohol within medical limits, are psychologically beneficial.

The money available to the older person (from public assistance funds and Social Security checks to private funds) must be safeguarded as there is presently no assurance of this after institutionalization, particularly if a family is not involved.*

*Lawton, M. P., and Bader, Jeanne: Wish for privacy by young and old, Journal of Gerontology **25**:48-54, 1970.

Persons should not be stripped of their clothing and made into "patients" with shoddy institutional apparel. Patients have the right to wear their own clothes and have their own possessions with them unless this is legitimately considered dangerous. Personal possessions and clothing help to maintain orientation, self-respect, and identity. Personnel are advised also to avoid calling persons by their first or "pet" names, as this too implies loss of dignity and infantilization. Further, patients should not be on "display" for the amusement of others.

On an institutional visit we were introduced by the chief nurse to an 87-year-old woman. The nurse who, of course, insisted upon being referred to as Mrs. L. by the patients, said "Jane, sing your song for the visitors." "Jane," who had formerly been a teacher of some repute, obediently belted out a popular song. Such callous disregard for patient dignity is perhaps not common but it does occur all too frequently.

All persons should have access to clergymen and religious services of their choice.

Physical environment

The environment of hospitals, nursing homes, and other institutions is ripe for change. Clever minds could be put to work to design aesthetic and prosthetic environments that would help to compensate for mental and physical losses. Wandering patients who are now often restrained could be encouraged through the use of color coding, the buddy system, and adequate staff to orient themselves. Maximum security atmospheres could be reduced by such devices as attractive wooden fences, gates, and even shrubbery rather than iron bars. (Few geriatric patients break out of institutions! They merely need something to restrain them.)

Protection from accidents and fires needs to be improved, and all institutions should be subject to the Life Safety Code of the Na-

*Needed are public guardianships in all our states to provide some measure of legal protection for the low-income elderly.

tional Fire Protection Association. Air conditioning in summer and control of temperature and humidity in winter are crucial, since older people cannot withstand extreme atmospheric conditions. Excessive numbers of older people die during heat waves.

With the advent of plastic and electronic devices that may be under either direct or remote control, much can be done to make up for deficiencies in ambulation, audition, vision, and general stimulation.* Safety devices such as grab bars, call buttons, and nonslip floors are essential. Calendars, clocks (set to the *correct* time!), and mirrors are useful orientation devices. The general environment should be reasonably calm but alive with stimuli, lest reactivity become extinguished. Good illumination and colorful decorations are helpful. Beauty parlors, barber shops, and canteens add variety; music should be available but not, because of the Goldstein catastrophic reaction (Chapter 9), constantly blaring, Muzak-fashion. Outdoor activities such as gardening and perhaps even caring for pets in mini-zoos on institutional grounds can be extremely therapeutic.

Physicians' care

All institutions should have physicians with central responsibility and commensurate authority to override private doctors of individual patients if necessary. These physicians should plan the general medical program (routine tests, dental care, immunizations), conduct regular rounds, prescribe medications, respond to emergencies, and be available for consultations with families. Each physican must beware that he or she does not function for the convenience of the institution rather than providing service to patients (for example, prescribing excessive medication may relieve the staff but make "zombies" out of patients). The physician himself should be under review by all staff members, regarding his judgments.

*Butler, R. N.: Research and clinical observations on the psychological reactions to physical changes with age, Mayo Clinic Proceedings 42:596-619, 1967.

Nursing care

Nursing of the older patient requires flexibility, good humor without ridicule, and respect without distancing.* Wolanin has described nursing staff reactions to incontinence, difficult self-feeding, obscene language, and other unpleasant behaviors.† Basic individualized knowledge of the patient is crucial‡ and in keeping with our stress upon comprehensive evaluation. The list below notes problems frequently presented by nursing staffs to medical and psychiatric consultants on the rare occasions when they are called in to nursing homes and homes for the aged.

1. Depression
2. Confusion or other symptoms of acute or chronic brain syndrome
3. Paranoid delusions
4. Noisiness
5. Restlessness or wandering
6. Combativeness
7. Inappropriate dependency on staff
8. Persistent talk of a wish to die
9. Incontinence
10. Families who are unjustifiably critical or demanding of the institution

Bed rest can be dangerous, replicating all the untoward effects of chronic, debilitating illnesses: cardiovascular, respiratory, metabolic, and neuromuscular changes. To illustrate, with decreased respiration can come hypostatic pneumonia, and with immobility a decrease in strength of muscles and weakening of bones (osteoporosis) may occur. People should be ambulated quickly, even after operations.

Bedsores (also called decubiti, trophic ulcers, or pressure sores) can develop quickly, especially in the bedridden, debilitated el-

*Jaeger, Dorothea, and Simmons, L. W.: Humor in nurse-patient relationships. In The aged ill: coping with problems in geriatric care, New York, 1970, Appleton-Century-Crofts.

†Wolanin, M. O.: They called the patient repulsive, American Journal of Nursing 64:173-175, 1964.

‡Gubersky, B.: Geriatric nursing. In Cowdry, E. V., editor: The care of the geriatric patient, St. Louis, 1958, The C. V. Mosby Co.

derly. Such sores occur at pressure points—the bony areas of elbows, hips, and heels, and the buttocks—and are the result of reduced blood supply caused by the body's weight. Persons who are not turned in bed, who are malnourished or anemic (vitamin C deficiency and low protein intake are most dangerous), or who have been allowed to lie in urine until the skin macerates may develop infections in the sores. These infections are indolent, causing little or no pain. Care should include ambulation, rotation of the patient, cleanliness and dryness, avoidance of oversedation, and checking of pressure points for early signs of redness. Physiotherapy through overhead trapeze and activity as well as active and passive exercises, including massage, are indicated. Paraplegic patients may need to be placed in frames that turn (Stryker frames). Indwelling catheters may be necessary to control urinary incontinence. Foam rubber, air mattresses and water beds, pillows, and sheepskin sheets are useful. When an ulcer has developed, it should be cleaned (debridement). Trypsin, an enzymatic digestive agent, along with topical antibiotics (e.g., neomycin) is appropriate.

Incontinence refers to the inability to control bladder and/or bowel. The condition may be permanent as a result of severe injury, central nervous system disease, chronic infections, etc. At other times it is temporary and reversible, related to anxiety, pain, hostility, and inadequate attention. Even persons with organic brain damage may be able to improve control.* A careful evaluation and correct assessment as to cause must be made, and a plan for treatment built and kept. Emotional aspects should be dealt with through psychotherapy and staff involvement. The incontinent patient with no permanent physical damage can often be retrained. In urinary incontinence one begins by giving the patient the bedpan or urinal regularly on schedule to develop a habit (e.g., every two hours or on rising, after eating, and before bedtime). In bowel retraining, proper timing is also of the essence. Good dieting helps. Passive exercises for the bedridden (bending the knees and pressing the thighs against the abdomen) can sometimes stimulate the urge to defecate. Walking and other efforts to improve muscle tone help. Adult gauze diapers and underpads should be used and frequently changed until control improves.

Staff morale and dedication is another crucial consideration. Decent care for all patients, rich or poor, depends upon the goodwill and skill of all levels of staff; yet much of the time the poor working conditions, low pay, low status, and lack of inservice and outside training for nursing personnel have been ignored. Like many other groups providing human services (police, firemen, teachers, government workers), nursing personnel were not allowed to strike, for obvious reasons—namely, the welfare of patients. Yet this moral pressure has amounted to a kind of moral blackmail. Walkouts have occurred in some localities. One would have to suppose that the anger and feelings of exploitation on the part of staff get communicated to patients in active or passive forms.

Much of the actual care of patients in mental hospitals and nursing homes falls upon nursing assistants and aides. Adequate pay, continuing education, and opportunities for promotion should be mandatory if good staff morale is to be maintained.* All staff should be included in the planning and carrying out of treatment with patients.†

Patient restraint

Physical and chemical (by drugs) restraint and seclusions must be avoided ex-

*Wilson, T. S.: Incontinence of the urine in the aged, Lancet 2:374-377, 1948.

*See Jackson, Hobart: Bridging continuing education and mental health in long-term skilled institutional care for the elderly, presented at a 1972 conference of the same name.

†Shore writes of practical experiences with various kinds of staff meetings in old age homes. See Shore, Herbert: You can have more effective staff meetings, Professional Nursing Homes, Nov., 1962.

cept under true emergency conditions. Restraints (called "poseys") are not a substitute for personal contact to alleviate the anxiety that often causes the physical agitation. Restraint or seclusion should never exceed two hours without review and rewriting of the order by a physician. Medications must be under constant monitoring and not be used as chemical straightjackets.

Medical and psychiatric experimentation

The Ten Commandments of Medical Research Involving Human Subjects, as employed by the National Institute of Health, should be in effect. No experimental research on elderly patients is permissible without express and informed consent, given after consultation with legal counsel. The volunteer should be made fully aware of the risks and benefits of the experiment and his right to terminate the experiment at any time. Similarly, any unusual, hazardous, and/or experimental treatment procedures such as new drugs or lobotomy must be introduced only after express and informed consent and consultation with counsel.

Institutional neurosis

Institutional neurosis can occur in hospitals, nursing homes, prisons, or anywhere that persons are removed from society and live in a rigid, isolated community. It can also develop in the person's own home if he is isolated. The symptoms are erosion of personality, overdependence, expressionless facies, automatic behavior, and loss of interest in the outside world. Immediate and long-term effects of military or concentration camp imprisonment have been described, much of which applies also to isolated institutions for the old.*

*Segal, H. A.: Initial psychiatric findings of recently repatriated prisoners of war, The American Journal of Psychiatry **111**:358, 1954. See also Kral, V. A.: Psychiatric observations under severe chronic stress, The American Journal of Psychiatry **108**:3, 1951.

Age and sex segregation

Sexual segregation is a very questionable practice. It is cruel to automatically rule out heterosexual (or homosexual) activities with spouses or other consenting adults, including other patients, as long as no clear physical or psychological danger is present. One of us (RNB) participated in studies at Chestnut Lodge in 1958-1959, which did not segregate patients by sex and allowed freedom and privacy for sexual activities. Old people should not be scolded for masturbation. Masturbation is a normal sexual outlet, and staff members in institutions may need help in overcoming their own anxieties about patients' use of this outlet. Conjugal visits with spouses should be encouraged.

There is question about the wisdom of age-segregation treatment facilities. It is argued that when the elderly are placed in age-integrated wards of hospitals they receive less staff attention and may be injured by young, aggressive patients. On the other hand, restriction to an age-segregated unit can end up with monotony and difficulties in recruiting and keeping well-trained, dedicated staff. Some studies have indicated that older persons show greater improvement in age-integrated facilities.

Reality-orientation, remotivation, and rehabilitation programs

Reality-orientation*

James C. Folsom first organized a "reality-orientation program" in Winter Veterans Administration Hospital in Topeka, Kansas, in 1958. The bulk of the work is done by the nursing assistants who spend the most time with the patients. Folsom feels patients are not ready for remotivation until they have gone through the reality-orientation classes. The program is ideally suited for patients

*Taulbee, Lucille, and Folsom, James: Reality orientation for geriatric patients, Hospital and Community Psychiatry **17**:133-135, 1966. See also Reality orientation: a technique to rehabilitate elderly and brain damaged patients, Hospital and Community Psychiatry Service of the American Psychiatric Association, 1969.

who have been institutionalized for long periods of time or have moderate to severe organic brain impairment.*

During the classes which have four patients each the instructor presents basic personal and current information over and over to each patient, beginning with the patient's name, where he is, and the date. Only when he has relearned these basic facts is the patient presented with other facts such as his age, home town and former occupation.

Remotivation

Remotivation has been defined as a "means of reaching the large number of long-term, chronic patients residing in large mental hospitals, who do not seem to want to move toward improvement or discharge."† Remotivation must be followed by activities leading toward rehabilitation, such as occupational and recreational therapy, the industrial programs, and finally vocational and social rehabilitation. It has also been applied to nursing homes. Any effort to stimulate and encourage social participation is undoubtedly therapeutic. Arts and crafts and group activities such as movies or games or singing are important because they offer human contact. Remotivation or any program must be carefully evaluated to avoid infantilization.

The remotivation technique‡ consists essentially of the following five steps, which the psychiatric aide uses with small groups of ten to fifteen patients:

1. *The climate of acceptance*—establishing a warm friendly relationship in the group
2. *A bridge to reality*—reading of objective poetry, current events, etc.
3. *Sharing the world*—development of the topic, introduced above, through planned objective questions, use of props, etc.
4. *An appreciation of the work of the world*—designed to stimulate the patients to think about work in relation to themselves
5. *The climate of appreciation*—expression of enjoyment at getting together, etc.

As Robert S. Garber, Chairman, APA Remotivation Project Advisory Committee wrote:

Each patient has sick roles and healthy roles. The sick ones have come to dominate his life, but the healthy roles are not entirely dead. I as a psychiatrist deal mainly with the sick roles. You as remotivators are in touch with the health roles.*

Rehabilitation

Mental hospital and nursing home programs could benefit immeasurably from the availability of rehabilitation as a medical specialty (physiatry), one of the significant developments of twentieth century health care. An important model is the Institute of Rehabilitation Medicine in New York (part of New York University's Medical Center), founded and directed by Dr. Howard Rusk since 1948. The blind, the deaf, the retarded, the hemiplegic, the paraplegic, those suffering from Parkinson's disease can benefit from rehabilitative programs. We have reviewed physical, occupational, and speech therapies in Chapter 10.

Work therapy and sheltered workshops

"Work therapy" is appropriate only as a truly therapeutic activity and not as compulsory and uncompensated housekeeping and maintenance chores that save the institution money. Patients may volunteer to do work for the institution but should be compensated in accordance with the minimum wage laws of the Fair Labor Standards Act, 29 U.S.C. No. 206 as amended, 1966. Patients who are physically able should, however, make their own beds, dress themselves, and perform other acts ordinarily encompassed under the rubric of self-care.

---

*Sensory training programs, in which the institutionalized geriatric patient is stimulated to use the five senses, exist in a few places. See Downey, G. W.: Sensory training reawakens patients to life, Modern Nursing Home 27:62, 1971.

†Bechenstein, N. I.: Enhancing the gains; remotivation, a first step to restoration, Hospital and Community Psychiatry 7:115-116, April, 1966.

‡Remotivation kits for nursing homes and for mental hospitals, 1968, are available through the American Psychiatric Association, Washington, D. C.

*From Garber, R. S.: A psychiatrist's view of remotivation, Mental Hospitals 16:219-221, Aug., 1965.

The handicapped, including the aged, for instance in homes for the aged, may participate in "sheltered workshops."*

Sheltered workshop—a work-oriented rehabilitation facility with controlled working environment and individualized vocational goals, which utilizes work experiences and related services for assisting the handicapped person to progress toward normal living and a productive vocational status.†

This kind of shop gives an opportunity to make some modest money, as well as providing activity and promoting pride. Because industries pay on a piece basis it is economically feasible for them. Packaging, stuffing, stapling, tag stringing, and various types of simple repetitive assembling are examples of activities.

At the Philadelphia Geriatric Center "the workshop is one of our most successful therapeutic enterprises of all activities in the home; it is the one with the greatest competition for places, and there is always a waiting list and people who wish to put in more than usual possible time per person."‡ The Riverdale Home in New York conducts a large program.

Patient government

There are many legitimate complaints—about food, lack of entertainment, nursing care—legitimate not only because in too many instances the complaints are valid but also because of the deep frustration and grief associated with institutionalization and the understandable need to ventilate feelings. Patient government, joint patient-staff conferences, and the presence of older people on the boards of trustees of hospitals and homes for the aging should be standard and not just window-dressing. Old people would do well to be their own ombudsmen and check up on the conditions and treatment in institutions.

*See "Sheltered workshops and homebound programs," a handbook, first edition, 1972, The National Committee on Sheltered Workshops and Homebound Programs (15 W. 16th St., New York), p. 3. See also Shore, Herbert: The sheltered workshop, Professional Nursing Home, Feb., 1966. And see Rehabilitation Services Administration, Social and Rehabilitative Service, U. S. Department of Health, Education, and Welfare: Standard for rehabilitation facilities and sheltered workshops, 1969.

†Official definition adopted by the National Association of Sheltered Workshops and Homebound Programs, Oct., 1959. (This organization has been renamed the International Association of Rehabilitative Facilities, 5530 Wisconsin Ave., Washington, D. C. 20015.)

‡Personal communication, Dr. M. Powell Lawton, Philadelphia Geriatric Center, Philadelphia, Pa.

Volunteers

Volunteers are often said to be more problems than they are worth. On the other hand, with careful selection one can assemble a loyal, conscientious group of people who are a valuable adjunct to the quality of an institution.* The Red Cross Gray Ladies are an example of a well-trained volunteer group. Most institutions are wary of volunteers—some with good reason, since they do not want their weaknesses exposed to the public.

Research

It is imperative that research be built into institutions. Research in this field should be of two kinds: studies concerned with enhancing the understanding of old age and chronic illness, and studies dealing with improvement in services. Rarely is research done in nonprofit or commercial homes.† The Philadelphia Geriatric Center is an example of a voluntary institution that has developed a fine research program.

*Shore, H.: How to get better results with volunteers, Professional Nursing Home, March, 1963.

†The Kramer Foundation (Palatine, Illinois) is a not-for-profit corporation organized to carry out research and educational projects with emphasis on the medical and psychological aspects of nursing home care.

REFERENCES

American Psychiatric Association: Position statement on the question of adequacy of treatment, American Journal of Psychiatry 123:1458-1460, 1967.

Bennett, Ruth G., and Nahemow, L.: Institutional totality and criteria of social adjustment in residential settings for the aged, Journal of Social Issues 21:44-78, 1965.

Blau, D., Kettell, Marjorie, Arth, M., Smith, Jacqueline W., and Oppenheim, D.: Psychiatric hospitalization of the aged, Geriatrics **21**:204-210, 1966.

Brody, Elaine M.: Follow-up study of applicants and non-applicants in voluntary homes, The Gerontologist **9**:187-196, 1969.

Brody, Elaine M., and Spark, G. M.: Institutionalization of the aged: a family crisis, Family Process **5**:76-90, 1966.

Brudno, J. J.: Group programs with adult offspring of newly admitted residents in a geriatric setting, Journal of the American Geriatrics Society **12**:385-394, 1964.

Butler, R. N.: Immediate and long-range dangers to transfer of elderly patients from state hospitals to community facilities (guest editorial), The Gerontologist **10**:259-260, 1970.

Charitable Research Foundation: Effective standards for institutional care of the infirm aged, Wilmington, Del., 1959, The Charitable Research Foundation.

Coons, Dorothy H., Gottesman, L. E., and Donahue, Wilma: A therapeutic milieu for geriatric patients, Ann Arbor, 1969, Institute of Gerontology, University of Michigan.

Cosin, L. Z., Mort, Margaret, Post, F., Westropp, Celia, and Williams, Moyra: Experimental treatment of persistent senile confusion, The International Journal of Social Psychiatry **4**:24-42, 1958.

Donahue, Wilma: Action programs to prevent, reduce or improve institutionalization. Mental health care and the elderly: shortcomings in public policy. Report by the Special Committee, U. S. Senate, Washington, D. C., 1971, U. S. Government Printing Office.

Droubay, E. H.: Blue is for bathrooms. . . colors guide geriatric patients, Mental Hospitals **15**: 386-390, 1964.

Evans, Frances M.: Psychosocial nursing, New York, 1971, The Macmillan Co.

Freeman, J. T., editor: Clinical features of the older patient, Springfield, Ill., 1965, Charles C Thomas, Publisher.

Freeman, J. T.: Physicians and long-term care facilities, Journal of the American Geriatrics Society **19**:847-859, 1971.

Friedman, J. H., and Lehrman, N. S.: New geriatric admision policy in a state mental hospital, Journal of the American Geriatrics Society **17**:1086-1091, 1969.

Galpern, Marie, Turner, Helen, and Goldfarb, Alvin: The psychiatric evaluation of applicants for a home for aged, Social Casework **33**:152-160, 1952.

Geschickter, C. F.: Some fundamental aspects of the aging process. In VA research in aging prospectus, Washington, D. C., 1959, U. S. Veterans Administration.

Goffman, Erving: Asylums, New York, 1961, Anchor Paperback.

Goldfarb, A. I.: Institutional care of the aged. In Busse, E. W., and Pfeiffer, E., editors: Behavior and adaption in late life, Boston, 1969, Little, Brown & Co.

Goldfarb, A. I.: The orientation of staff in a home for the aged, Mental Hygiene **37**:76-83, Jan., 1953.

Gottesman, L. E.: Resocialization of the geriatric mental patient, American Journal of Public Health **55**:1964-1970, 1965.

Halpern, C.: A practicing lawyer views the right to treatment, The Georgetown Law Journal **57**: 782-817, 1969.

Hammerman, Jerome, and Shore, Herbert: Value, rationale, use and implications of a classification system for residents in a home for the aged, The Gerontologist **4**:141-148, 1964.

Jaeger, Dorothea, and Simmons, Leo W.: The aged ill: coping with problems in geriatric care, New York, 1970, Appleton-Century-Crofts.

Kahana, Eva, and Kahana, B.: Therapeutic potential of age integration: effects of age-integrated hospital environments on elderly psychiatric patients, Archives of General Psychiatry **23**:20-29, 1970.

Kobrynski, B., and Miller, A. D.: The role of the state hospital in the care of the elderly, Journal of the American Geriatrics Society **18**:210-219, 1970.

Kramer, C. H.: Total therapeutic situation for aged, Geriatric Focus **5**:1, 1966.

Lawton, M. P., and Brody, Elaine M.: Assessment of older people: self-maintaining and instrumental activities of daily living, The Gerontologist **9**:179-186, 1969.

Lehrman, N. S., and Friedman, J. H.: A treatment-focused geriatric program in a state mental hospital, Journal of the American Geriatrics Society **17**:1092-1096, 1969.

Lindsley, O. R.: Geriatric behavioral prosthetics. In Kastenbaum, R., editor: New thoughts on old age, New York, 1964, Springer Publishing Co., Inc.

Lowenthal, Marjorie F.: Lives in distress, New York, 1964, Basic Books, Inc.

Moses, Dorothy V., and Lake, Carolyn S.: Geriatrics in the bacculaureate nursing curriculum, Nursing Outlook **16**:41-43, 1968.

Nader, R.: Old age: the last segregation, New York, 1971, Grossman Publishers, Inc.

National Committee on Aging: Standards of care for older people in institutions (3 volumes); vol. 1. Suggested standards for homes for the aged and nursing homes; vol. 2. Methods of establishing and maintaining standards in homes; vol. 3. Bridging the gap between existing practices and desirable goals, 1953 and 1954, National Council on the Aging.

Nicholson, Edna E.: Planning new institutional facilities for long term care, New York, 1956, G. P. Putnam's Sons.

Office of Research and Statistics, Social Security Administration: Financing mental health care under medicare and medicaid, Research Report No. 37, U. S. Department of Health, Education and Welfare, 1971.

Querido, A.: Experiment in public health, Bulletin of the World Federation of Mental Health **6**: 203-216, 1954.

Randall, Ollie A.: A 20th century philosophy for homes for the aged, New York, 1949, National Social Welfare Assembly.

Reingold, J., Wolk, R., and Schwartz, Shirley: A gerontological sheltered workshop: the aged person's attitudes toward money, Journal of the Geriatrics Society **19**:315-331, 1971.

Rudd, T. N.: The nursing of the elderly sick, Philadelphia, 1964, J. B. Lippincott Co.

Rypins, R. F., and Clark, Mary Lou: A screening project for the geriatric mentally ill. Appraisals to determine suitable care facilities, California Medicine **109**:273-278, 1968.

Shore, Herbert, and Leeds, Morton: Geriatric institutional management, New York, 1964, G. P. Putnam's Sons.

Solon, J. A., Roberts, D. W., Krueger, D. E., and Baney, Anna M.: Nursing homes, their patients and their care, Public Health Monograph No. 46, Washington, D. C., 1957, U. S. Government Printing Office.

Stanton, A. H., and Schwartz, M. S.: The mental hospital, New York, 1954, Basic Books, Inc.

Stevens, M. K.: Geriatric nursing for the practical nurse, Philadelphia, 1965, W. B. Saunders Co.

Stotsky, B. A.: A controlled study of factors in the successful adjustment of mental patients to nursing homes, American Journal of Psychiatry **123**:1243-1251, 1967.

Stotsky, B. A.: Nursing home or mental hospital—which is better for the geriatric mental patient, Journal of Geriatric Psychology **111**:113-117, 1967.

Stotsky, B. A.: The elderly patient, New York, 1968, Grune & Stratton, Inc.

Thompson, P. W.: Principles, rules of thumb, or ways of looking at jobs with long-term patients, Journal of the American Geriatrics Society **17**: 1074-1080, 1969.

Waisman, A. D., and Hackett, T.: Psychosis after surgery, New England Journal of Medicine **259**: 1284-1289, 1958.

Wilner, D. M., and Hefferin, Elizabeth: Older patients in United States public mental hospitals: a national survey of administrative opinions, Journal of the American Geriatrics Society **17**: 822-843, 1969.

Worcester, Alfred: Care of the aged, the dying and the dead, ed. 2, Springfield, 1961, Charles C Thomas, Publisher.

Zelditch, Morris: The home for the aged, 1957. Available at Council of Jewish Federations and Welfare Funds, 729 Seventh Avenue, New York.

12
PSYCHOTHERAPY AND ENVIRONMENTAL THERAPY

In this chapter we will review the common modalities of *psychotherapy*—individual, group, family—and shall also consider *environmental therapy,* under which we include the location and mobilization of resources, advocacy, consultative services, and encouragement of political activity on the part of older people.

We have already considered the roles of the mental health specialists and the team concept in Chapter 8 on therapeutic principles. All forms of environmental and psychotherapy can be provided by the mental health team as a functioning unit (in varied combinations of therapists, older people, family members or groups) or by individual therapists from all of the disciplines.

INDIVIDUAL PSYCHOTHERAPY

Individual psychotherapy is *least* available to old people and yet should be part of any therapeutic relationship. The older person needs the opportunity to talk and to have a listener. He needs the therapist's support in his or her effort to "seize the day" and build a "life" during the remaining time available.*

A survey in the Washington metropolitan area revealed minimal contact in private practice between therapists and older persons.† Public clinics‡ also reported low rates of contact of any kind, but especially little in the way of psychotherapeutic work. Although the studies cited were done some time ago, the findings still remain true today. Psychiatrists, social workers, psychologists, mental health teams, and other therapists do not see many old people; when they do, the purposes are usually diagnostic and the effort is "disposition."

Old age is the period in life with the greatest number of profound crises, often occurring in multiples and with high frequency. The critical psychological events in this age group are the familiar human emotional reactions to death and grief, diseases and disabilities. Depression and anxiety escalate, defensive behavior is seen, earlier personality components may reappear in exaggerated forms, and newly formed functional states are frequently noted. These conditions require psychotherapeutic efforts, indepth as well as supportive.

The terms "good" and "poor" candidates for psychotherapy should be questioned, especially the implication that a number of people should not be offered treatment because they cannot "use" it. We wonder how this judgment can be made before treatment has begun. Some older people who meet all the criteria for "good" candidates fail to find therapy helpful, whereas "poor" candidates may show unexpected response and results. The test of objectivity is the willingness to give adequate trials to *all* persons without allowing our theories, prejudices, and fears to interfere. Theories in any case can

*See "The shameless old lady" (Appendix on motion pictures), based on a play by Bertolt Brecht in which an elderly widow makes the most of the last eighteen months of her life.

†Butler, R. N., and Sulliman, Lillian G.: Psychiatric contact with the community-resident, emotionally disturbed elderly, Journal of Nervous and Mental Disease **137**:180-186, 1963.

‡Bahn, Anita K.: Outpatient population of psychiatric clinics, Maryland, 1958-59, Public Health Monograph, No. 65, 1959, U. S. Department of Health, Education, and Welfare.

be masterful camouflages. For example, Freud was preoccupied with death and pessimistic about old age. His work reflects his avoidance of the issues of late life and his decision to explain the human personality only in terms of the early years. Ironically we would barely know of him had he died before the age of forty, since his finest work was done in the postmeridian period of his life.

We submit, on the grounds of clinical experience, that the elderly, if not brain-damaged, are greatly receptive to psychotherapy and can in no way be considered "poor candidates." They often exhibit a strong drive to resolve problems, to put their lives in order, and to find satisfactions and a "second chance." Their capacity to change has been demonstrated in many instances; the fact that older people spontaneously begin reviewing their lives in a way similar to psychotherapy is indicative of the manner in which this process is part of the natural course of late life. Even the brain-damaged elderly can gain from psychotherapy as Goldfarb, among others, has demonstrated.

Any evidence pointing toward older people as untreatable is usually to be found in the minds of therapists rather than in empirical studies. Powerful forces of countertransference and cultural prejudice are at work, including personal fear and despair over death. Therapeutic pessimism and nihilism are inappropriate, invalid, and inhumane. The old, like the young, can gain from insight and understanding, from objectivity and empathy. Biology is not destiny in old age any more than in youth. Personal history and culture are of profound importance.

Theoretical considerations

Freud and the vast majority of his followers ruled out psychoanalysis for the aged without ever testing its usefulness. Abraham raised some objections to this general negativism, reporting upon five persons he called "old" who were in their fifties. He and Jelliffe stated the "age of the neurosis" is more important than the age of the patient. Grotjahn reported upon analytic work with a 71-year old case of "senile brain disease." Wayne, Meerloo, Gitelson, Alexander, Atkin, Kaufman were among those who first described some limited psychotherapeutic efforts with old people.

Goldfarb, Greenleigh, Linden, Weinberg, Butler, and others have devoted substantial amounts of their public and private clinical work to older people. Goldfarb's "brief therapy"* and Linden's work with group therapy became the best known of these efforts in therapy.

Because of the tendency of old people to review their lives, to seek meaning, to deal with death, there is an obvious existential component to any therapeutic work with them. Yet existential therapists have not demonstrated great interest. We have found ideas of Buber† (the importance of relationship with others) and Frankl‡ (the possibilities within the confines of the "death camp") to be particularly useful for older people. All forms of psychotherapy—"uncovering" to "supportive" and Freudian to Jungian to Rogerian—can contribute to both a better understanding of the psychology and psychotherapy of old age (for therapy is a major source of knowledge) as well as to the direct help for people. Psychoanalytic concepts, Skinner's ideas regarding conditioning and the extinction of dysfunctional patterns of behavior, and Jung's stages of development§

*Goldfarb emphasizes the dependent relationships of elderly patients (comparing them with early parent-child relationships). The physician assumes the role of parent figure pressed upon him by the patient. Thus sometimes the therapist will be seen as a scapegoat and sometimes as the omnipotent helper.

†Buber, Martin: The William Alanson White Memorial Lectures, Fourth Series, Psychiatry **20**:95-129, 1957.

‡Frankl, Victor: From death camp to existentialism (1959). In Man's search for meaning, New York, 1963, Washington Square Press, Inc.

§It is interesting that two thirds of Jung's practice was made up of middle-aged and older persons, whereas Freud's private practice was composed of younger patients. These differences may help to account for variations in theoretical emphases with Freud's therapy concentrating on youth and sex while Jung emphasized individuation and creativity.

all apply to the elderly condition. What is obviously needed is an integrated and eclectic utilization of all contemporary personality theories and practices, including the life cycle perspective of human life. The complexities of late life require complex therapy.

Common themes in psychotherapy with older persons

New starts and second chances

Old people often express a wish to undo some of the patterns of their life, to unritualize behavior and give some newness to their experiences. These people speak of the monotony or dryness of their experiences, a kind of "salt losing its savor" feeling. This should be met not just with feeble efforts to regain what has been lost but to build new interests and new possibilities.

Death in disguise

Some older people have resolved their personal feelings about death. Others manage to deny death without serious emotional consequences. But a number of older people need help, first in recognizing the source of their anxieties and fears (namely death) and then in reaching some degree of accommodation with the inevitable. Therapists must be able to recognize disguised fears of death. For example, one man spoke of "running toward that man and then I saw him and I slowed down to a walk." He was referring to death. In his attempts to revitalize his life, the spectre of death presented him with an omnious impediment which he had to face before therapy could continue in the direction he wanted to go.

Keen awareness of time

There is an obvious concern with time when it is clear that the remaining days are running short. Younger therapists often have great difficulty understanding what it means *not* to think in terms of a future. We must take our cues from older people who have faced this issue squarely; the development of a sense of immediacy, of the here-and-now, of presentness—all aid in the evolution of a sense of simple enjoyment and tranquility, which we have called elementality.

Grief and restitution

Psychotherapy in old age must deal with grief, with losses of loved ones, and with dysfunctioning of one's own body and its parts. Efforts at restitution are crucial. One of the most important goals in therapy is helping the older person find a secure confidant either in his family or in his circle of friends and acquaintances.

Guilt and atonement

> We have left undone those things which we ought to have done; and we have done those things which we ought not to have done.

The 51st Psalm opens with "Miserere, mei Deus" (Have mercy upon me, O God). The cry for mercy, indeed for clemency, in the face of death must be heard. But the therapist does not have it within his power to "grant" mercy or bring full alleviation of the distress. One can listen, really listen, bear witness, be able, as it were, to attest to the realities of the life described, and thus help give meaning and validity to that life. Reconciliation may be possible with spouses, siblings, children, friends.

Reality must be central. If this globe were the center of the universe and not, as Copernicus insisted, only part of the solar system, it would be easier in some ways to deal with. If there were simple alignments between our drives, our moral strictures, and the workings of the world, if Freud were dead wrong, we could move merrily along. If aging and disability did not exist, if lives were not filled up with malevolence, acts of violence, and real wrongs done to others and oneself, then we could simply reassure the old people who are sick with guilt. But psychotherapy in old age is a therapy of atonement as well as of restitution. One cannot deny cruel and thoughtless acts, falsely reassuring that all is irrational Freudian guilt. Facing genuine guilt as well as the attrition of the person's physical and emotional world is what makes psychotherapy with the aging an intellectually and emotionally powerful experience. The therapist cannot win out against death, but he can win out *for* life, for a sense of the real, for the kind of growth that truly matters, dealing as it does with the evaluation of ways to love—and hate—with the meanings of human conduct, with an appreciation of human nature and the succession of the generations.

Autonomy versus identity

Identity, while an important concept, has been found to be difficult to study in various age groups. In our clinical experience autonomy should be separated out from identity as a concept. The so-called "identity crisis" of the adolescent is as much a problem of establishing freedom and achieving responsibility and self-sufficiency (autonomy) as it is one of identity ("self-sameness"), if not more so. Erikson deals with only one side of this issue:

> The term identity expresses. . . mutual relation in that it connotes both a persistent sameness within oneself (selfsameness) and a persistent sharing of some kind of essential character with others.*

In old age (data, for instance, from interviews before the mirror; see Chapter 9) most healthy people find themselves essentially the same as they have always been. With emerging medical (changes in body schema) and psychiatric problems (depression) the sense of self goes through reevaluation, but again more crucial is the problem of autonomy. For example, there is the question "Can I survive independently without being a burden?" It is true, of course, that if one's identity is closely bound to autonomy, the two merge, as it were, together. The person, for instance, whose identity has been that of a dependent person may find it easier to accept illness and institutionalization than the so-called independent autonomous person whose identity has been structured accordingly. The latter may suffer the more in dependent situations despite a "sound" identity by usual standards. Thus it is autonomy that may be more decisive as a determinant of human behavior than identity at various ages, depending upon circumstances.

*From Erikson, E. H.: The problem of ego identity. In Identity and the life cycle, Psychological Issues 1:101-164, 1959.

With respect to the life review,* identity and autonomy are equally important. But here again we find our experiences at variance with Erikson but for a different reason. We find that the old often wish to escape their identities and that the fatalistic acceptance proposed by Erikson in his bipolar view of ego identity versus despair is not universal.

Therapeutic issues

Am I a "patient"?

Insight into one's condition—that is, agreement that one has a psychiatric condition—is held by many to be a crucial prognostic indicator. On the other hand, humiliative labeling as a patient and all too willing acceptance of the "sick role" are questionable too. We believe it is important that appraisal be flexible and individualized. For some a useful agreement can be made to share in an effort to deal with an "illness," or "emotional problem," while for others it seems more functionally useful to see that the person receives important mental health services without their being identified in that way. With older people, as with all ages, it is as critical to identify and encourage areas of health as it is to clarify problems. Many beautifully "diagnosed" persons never reach their full potential in treatment because the therapist failed to recognize and utilize their strengths and assets in the therapeutic process.

Significance of certain illusions

The therapist must not in any way be destructive of the processes of illusion and

*The University of Chicago Committee on Human Development has pursued studies of reminiscence. See Gorney, J. E.: Experiencing and age; patterns of reminiscence among the elderly (unpublished Ph.D. dissertation, 1968) and Falk, J. M.: The organization of remembered life experience in old age: its relation to subsequent adaptive capacity and to age (unpublished Ph.D. dissertation, 1969). See also Havighurst, R. J., and Glasser, R.: An exploratory study of reminiscence, Journal of Gerontology **27**:245-253, 1972.

denial needed by older people. One must discuss the fact of death, the facts of loss, and the problems of grief, but always in the context of possibilities, restitution, and resolution. The same principle applies in work with persons of all ages; one must work compassionately and carefully to understand and encourage a realistic lowering of defenses rather than attacking them overtly.

Question of "cures"

Jung wrote, "The serious problems in life are never fully solved. If ever they should appear to be so, it is a sure sign that something has been lost. The meaning and purpose of a problem seems to lie not in its solution but in our working at it incessantly." The struggle, the need for change, and the opportunity for change—the really profound problems, the deeper intricacies of human existence—are genuine problems and subject to alteration up to the point of death.

Value of listening

It is imperative to listen attentively, to bear witness, to heed the telltale echoes of the past, to pick up the flatness of speech where distant feelings have died, to observe outbursts of unresolved issues in lives, and to empathize with the irreconcilable. When the older patient is garrulous, continually reminiscing, importunate, and querulous, the fact is that talk is necessary and listening by another mandatory. (One must also listen to silences.)

Worth of one therapeutic session

In the best of therapy each session must involve active work, thinking through, building hypotheses, persistently searching out ways to assist the person. This is especially true for the older person for whom there may be only one session available (because of impending death, physical weaknesses, or lack of access, financially or transportation-wise, to the therapist). When this is the case much can be done in a short time.

One Jungian analyst, Mrs. Florida Scott-Maxwell, wrote:

> A farmer's wife came and told a tragic story where nothing could be done, but her compassion and strength made it possible to continue. As usual with these cases, I asked if she would care to come again; she looked a little surprised, and said, "There is no need, I've told you everything." She had only wanted to confide in someone she respected, in case there was more she could do, and not to be so alone in her hard life. . . One visit was enough for her.*

The brief amount of time must be measured in terms of the quality of the experience rather than the quantity.

Telephone psychotherapy

Because of the financial and physical limitations of old people the therapist should be very flexible about the use of the telephone in conducting psychotherapy.†

> One 75-year-old man, with a history of heart attacks and continuing angina, would talk by phone when he could not travel. Even then he might have to interrupt his sessions to place a nitroglycerin tablet under his tongue. He never took obvious "advantage" of the situation and attended some 90% of his sessions in person.

Telephone outreach therapy is preferable to denial of the therapy for the homebound old person. (Fees for phone calls have been controversial in private psychotherapy but may be justified *when prearranged* because therapists are ordinarily paid on a time basis rather than a fee-for-service basis.)

Self-confrontation and the use of memory aids

Self-confrontation has been used in research and in clinical practice for various age groups and diagnostic categories.‡ Still and motion pictures as well as audio and video tapes recordings have been employed.

---

*From The measure of my days, New York, 1968, A. A. Knopf. [Note: Mrs. Scott-Maxwell was in her eighties and still working as a therapist at the time she wrote the above book.]

†Unfortunately, some 6 million old people—three out of every ten—do not have telephones, reminding us again of the penury of old age.

‡Paul, N. L.: Effects of playback on family members of their own previously recorded conjoint therapy material, Psychiatric Research Report 20, 1966, American Psychiatric Association.

Such techniques could be especially valuable, we believe, in work with older people individually and in family therapy. We have used photo albums, the mirror, and tape recorder; but we (and others) have not yet taken full advantage of the technological possibilities.

The need for self-definition in the life review and the problem of memory argue for the value to the patient of being able to take tape recordings home, for instance, for further listening and reflection. This would also encourage an active participation in the therapeutic process, not a passive, dependent position. As Norman Paul has said, "Confrontation with the discrepancy between the inner self-image and the observable self permits one to become an active agent in evaluating one's own strengths and weaknesses in interpersonal relations, the discovery of which represents both an extension of the educational process and a challenge for all."

Providing direct instructions, for instance, written or taped, for medication schedules and the statement of general principles and specifics may be useful for the older patient so long as not done with an aura of patronization.

Psychotherapy and public policy

We do not wish to further belabor the lack of Medicare coverage of mental and emotional problems, but we must, for the obvious reason that these facts militate against the provision of the specific treatments we are outlining. In addition, insurance supplementary to Medicare often excludes mental, psychoneurotic, and personality disorders.

Intensive outpatient psychotherapy (e.g., psychoanalysis) is considered a luxury on Capitol Hill and elsewhere. It is usually employed with the upper-income groups, not the poor. The cost of ambulatory psychiatric care in the high option Blue Cross–Blue Shield program in Washington was $2.15 in 1969, for insured persons. Some consider this high. Most national health insurance (NHI) plans under consideration provide limited coverage for mental illness. The more generous provide approximately 30 to 90 days for inpatient care and up to 20 outpatient visits to private physicians per year. These provisions tend to be discriminatory with regard to coverage for mental illness as compared to other illnesses.

An American Psychiatric Association study entitled "Health Insurance and Psychiatric Care: Utilization and Cost"* indicates that coverage for mental illness is widespread in existing private insurance plans, that utilization of these benefits is relatively low in comparison with those for all other conditions, and that costs of coverage of mental conditions would undoubtedly be supportable under NHI. For example, charges for hospital inpatient care for mental conditions range from 3% to 6% of charges for inpatient hospital care for all other conditions. Under a specific plan like the high option Blue Cross–Blue Shield plan for federal employees, total costs of care for mental conditions, both inpatient and outpatient, equaled 6.4% of benefits paid for all other conditions. In 1969, benefit payments for ambulatory care for mental illness under the federal employees' high option Blue Cross–Blue Shield plan were $2.15 per person, as stated, and total benefits for psychiatric care were $7.07 per person.

Evidence shows that greater availability of psychotherapy on an outpatient basis would reduce chronicity and disability in psychiatric states and reduce the need for general medical care. There are rare studies (one involving Group Health of Washington, a prepaid group practice) that show a decrease in the use of medical facilities when outpatient psychotherapeutic services are introduced.†

GROUP THERAPY

Group experience for older people

Group therapy is a very valuable procedure that should be widely used in all insti-

*Reed, L. S., Myers, Evelyn S., and Scheidemandel, P. D.: Health insurance and psychiatric care: utilization and cost, Washington, D. C., 1972, American Psychiatric Association.

†Goldberg, I. D., Krautz, Goldie, and Lock, B. Z.: Effect of a short-term outpatient psychiatric therapy benefit on the utilization of medical services in a prepaid group practice medical program, Medical Care 7:419-428, 1970.

tutions (nursing homes, hospitals, etc.) and outpatient services. It utilizes psychotherapeutic principles and techniques from individual psychotherapy as well as techniques directly derived from group process.*

Group therapy has been more widely used in work with the elderly in and out of institutions than is generally realized or reflected in professional and scientific literature. This is partly a function of necessity, an outgrowth of the disinterest of many therapists in individual therapy with old people. It is also selected as economical. Volunteers have been "trained" to conduct group therapy as well as administrators, aides, nurses, social workers, psychologists and psychiatrists. Usually sociability and emotional catharsis are the main objectives, but in the institutional setting the "management" of behavior is a major consideration. The need of providers of services to control the disturbed and upset feelings and actions of their patients needs to be questioned. Where group therapy endeavors to understand and not simply "control," it is certainly preferable to chemical restraint through tranquilizer-straightjacketing. Group therapy can also be evolved for the staff of institutions and agencies to help them work through their negative (often unconscious) attitudes about the elderly. Social agencies, community and day centers, and "golden age" or "senior citizens" groups offer group psychotherapy to community-resident elderly. The utilization rate of "golden age" or "senior citizens" centers and clubs is relatively low, and they probably attract the more gregarious older people. The goal of these groups is usually the growth and satisfaction of participating members through positive social experiences. Group workers also develop recreational, cultural, social, and educational graup activities in the larger community.

Group therapy has been used with preretirement and retirement problems but, in general, governmental and private preretirement programs fail to deal adequately with psychological and interpersonal aspects of retirement. They tend to stress financial planning and the like.

As with group therapy in general, the role of the leader in a group of older persons may be active or passive and involve various activities, from the passive one of listening to the active ones of questioning, explaining, teaching, protecting, reassuring, confronting. Some prefer to use the term "therapist" rather than "leader," for the latter sets certain expectations. Some consider the central role to be serving as catalyst of emotional interchange while protecting individuals and the group from excessively destructive anger and disruptive anxiety.

Not all groups need leaders:

> In the city of Washington one of us (RNB) founded a group for older professionals and executives, with several intents: to provide an activist, advocacy group on behalf of the elderly and to provide a setting for mutual mental and emotional interchange. In effect, it became a "leaderless" group. It has never had a professional paid leader and, having begun in 1965, it was still in existence and lively when this volume went to press.

Groups have to have momentum and vitality to maintain continuity and reduce absences and dropouts. Selection of members is critical. We argue for heterogeneity in every way possible. Age-integrated groups minimize the sense of isolation of the older person. Indeed, such group members may "forget" the factor of age. Topics in groups composed largely of old people tend to be illness, death, loneliness, family conflict; age-integrated groups are more likely to deal with the whole range of the life cycle, enabling older members to review and renew their own experiences and values.

Group therapy should be used with the

*Ten curative factors in group therapy as listed by Yalom in his excellent text on group psychotherapy are the following.

1. Imparting of information
2. Instillation of hope
3. Universality
4. Altruism
5. The corrective recapitulation of the primary family group
6. Development of socializing techniques
7. Imitative behavior
8. Interpersonal behavior
9. Group cohesiveness
10. Catharsis

families of old people. When an old person is admitted to an institution, for example, family members often experience profound conflicts. In one sense, they are already experiencing the death of their older relative and the first grief reaction (the later actual death and later grief reactions may actually have less impact). Work with relatives helps ameliorate guilt and grief and build liaison for visitation, home stays, and discharge when possible.

Group therapy should not be viewed as second-rate to individual psychotherapy. Group therapy has its own applicability and is a powerful instrument of itself. Both individual and group therapy may be usefully combined in work with the same person. The person may need the opportunity for reviewing his life on an individual basis and preparing for the impending encounter with death while at the same time gaining much from the continuing human interchange and the range of emotions—love to hate—that a well-functioning group can provide.

Some persons benefit from participating in more than one group. One such man, in his late years, found his "rap sessions" eye-opening because of the differences in the way he was seen by two groups.

Silver introduced group therapy with senile patients in 1950.* He found a party atmosphere important—with milk, cookies, and music. Problems with memory and attention were severe in his group. But it was Linden who first described an organized program of group therapy, in 1953. Goldfarb stressed working with new residents of homes to assist with orientation.

"Age-integrated, life crisis" group therapy†

Since 1970 we have conducted and studied four age-integrated life crisis groups (eight to ten members each) with one contrasting middle-age group. We have experimented with age integration (age range from 15 years to 80 and above), believing that age segregation as practiced in our society leaves very little opportunity for the rich exchange of feeling, experience, and support possible between generations. "Life crisis" refers to the near-normal to pathological reactions to adolescence, education, married or single life, divorce, parenthood, work and retirement, widowhood, illness, and impending death. Thus such groups are concerned not only with the intrinsic psychiatric disorders but also with preventive and remedial treatment of people as they pass through the usual vicissitudes of the life cycle. Criteria for membership include absence of active psychosis and presence of a life crisis (acute, subacute, or chronic). Reactions to life crises follow traditional diagnostic categories, of course, including depression, anxiety states, hysterical reactions, obsessive compulsive and passive-aggressive reactions, hypochondriasis, alcoholism, and mild drug use. Groups of six, eight, ten members each are formed—balanced for age, sex, and personality dynamics. They meet once a week for an hour and a half. We have found it useful to have male and female cotherapists from different disciplines to provide both a psychodynamic and a sociological orientation for each group as well as opportunities for transference. Individual membership in a group averages about two years and new group members are asked to commit themselves to a minimum of three months' participation.

The life cycle crises approach to group therapy needs to be neither strictly encounter nor strictly psychoanalytic. Rather it is equally concerned with the interaction among and between group members, as determined by reality and the past histories of each member, and with the individual problems of each member. The goal is the amelioration of suffering, the overcoming of disability, and the opportunity for new experiences of intimacy and self-fulfillment. Emphasis is on the verbalization of emotions, but natural

---

*Silver, A.: Group psychotherapy with senile psychiatric patients, Geriatrics 5:147-150, 1950.

†Butler, R. N., and Lewis, Myrna I.: The role of the elderly in a new treatment form: age-integrated life crisis group therapy. Abstract published by the 9th International Congress of Gerontology, Kiev, U. S. S. R., July, 1972.

physical expression of course occurs. Expression of both anger and positive feelings is encouraged—not for a mere defusing of feeling but as a step toward constructive resolution of problems and a positive life experience.

Patients often continue in individual psychotherapy with the referring doctor. When this is not feasible, individual therapy may still be encouraged along with group therapy, either with one of the co-therapists or with someone else. However, absence of such therapy does not preclude participation in groups.

Regarding the elderly, some of the phenomena we have observed have included (1) pseudo "senility," (2) a "Peter Pan" syndrome (refusal to grow up), and (3) leadership being preempted by the middle-aged, with neglect or "mascoting" of elderly and young (necessitating therapeutic intervention). Unique contributions of the elderly include models for growing older, solutions for loss and grief, creative use of reminiscence, historic empathy, and a sense of the entire life cycle. Possibilities for psychological growth continue to the end of life.

Case notes on 70-year-old woman:

> Repeated hospital admission for psychiatric depression. Living in retirement village. No genuine financial worries but not rich. Episodes characterized by increasing depression, hopelessness, remorse, insomnia, and anorexia (no appetite). Attributes her illness to worry over daughter, who is subject to manic-depressive disease and hospitalizations.
>
> Gives impression of quiet elderly lady who moves and talks little, nearly mute. Face looks grief-stricken and full of worry. Hand-wringing. No signs of organic failure. Slow but appropriate answers. Denies suicidal thought but wishes she were dead.
>
> In life crises group it comes out that she believes in hereditary and physiological basis of emotional illnesses—and hence blames self for daughter's troubles. Also describes for first time an affair with a married man, conducted at 67 after death of her own husband. She feels unfaithful, disloyal. Over the year she has become increasingly bright-eyed and alert, listening with interest to the sexual experiences of younger group members and eliciting their views of her own life.

FAMILY THERAPY

The family, if there is one, should of course be involved in any work with an older person unless circumstances dictate otherwise. There should also always be clarification as to who constitutes the "patient." Sometimes the older person is "brought in" by a son or daughter and it is quickly apparent that it is the adult child who needs help. Issues in family therapy include the need for decisions about the older person, feelings of guilt and abandonment, old family conflicts, and the need to provide continuing care and involvement with the older member. The therapist may decide to see the entire family together—not only those living in the household but also those living separately.

Older marital couples may also need counseling concerning marital problems, confrontations with serious illness and approaching death, and concerns about children and grandchildren.

BEHAVIORAL MODIFICATION AND THERAPY*

Only Lindsley, in 1964, has developed a theoretical prospectus for the application of operant conditioning (pioneered by B. F. Skinner) to the elderly institutionalized person.† But the various elderly populations, inpatient or outpatient, have not been studied and treated according to either "behavioral modification" or "behavioral therapy." The former is the practical application of operant conditioning and includes, for example, the use of token economy (reinforcing behavior by reward). Behavioral therapy, pioneered by Wolpe, includes aversion techniques (the use of noxious stimuli).

ENVIRONMENTAL THERAPY

We are using the term "environmental therapy" to encompass the development of

*We are indebted to Dr. Harold Weiner of St. Elizabeths Hospital, Washington, D. C., for his comments on these approaches.

†Lindsley, O. R.: Geriatric behavior prosthetics. In Kastenbaum, R., editor: New thoughts on old age, New York, 1964, Springer Publishing, Inc.

age awareness, social participation,* mobilization of community resources, and even registration drives, job placement, direct advocacy, consultative services, and political organization. The courage of so many old people in the community is striking, since they must struggle against a system marked by fragmentation and indifference. Self-respect and dignity in old age obviously does not follow from felt and actual powerlessness. Consequently we regard self-assertion in all the above forms, including political activism, as supportive of good mental health.

Age awareness and acceptance

We do not mean to be facetious in saying that "old age is beautiful" (it could be but often is not); however, it is important to encourage age awareness and acceptance. Gray hair need not be dyed. Old people should not have to "think" or "act young."

Prejudice against age has led men and women in business, the professions, politics, and everyday life to seek plastic surgery to eliminate the stigma of age. Face-lifting operations are frequently undertaken at great expense for dubious reasons.

People should neither be compelled nor feel compelled to misrepresent their age for employment or social purposes. A significant number of the elderly refuse to even identify with people their own age or with the problems that come with age. The well-to-do are especially prone to this, preferring to think of themselves as "different" from the poverty-striken elderly all around them. Yet unless they are extremely wealthy, they too can be devastated financially by just one major illness or period of adversity.

In order to begin to confront the realistic difficulties of late life old people must first recognize their age, accept it, and even take pride in it. Secondly, they must recognize themselves in others of their age, empathize with common experiences, and realize "we are all in this thing together" in spite of economic differences, cultural or social backgrounds, or social status. When one is old, there is really no effective way to escape the effects of a culture that denigrates age. The most effective defense is a united challenge that combines practical, direct action with psychological support—both from others and to and from each other.

Mobilization of community resources

In previous chapters we have stressed the role of the mental health worker in effectively "hustling the system" on behalf of their patients/clients. These persons should also be helped to utilize the system (for example, see discussion of registration drives). Social and family agencies could play leading roles in putting pressure on other voluntary agencies as well as institutions of government. For instance, a family agency should insist that community mental health centers (CMHCs) provide outreach care for elderly patients.

In the District of Columbia in 1971 the Jewish Social Service Agency was told that one CMHC did not accept patients over 60. A complaint was lodged through the city's Advisory Committee on Aging, and the exclusion ended.

Community workers can help fabricate networks of care within the community. Friends, the neighborhood storekeeper, druggist, and others have all been involved by mental health staff in looking out for the older person. This must be done, of course, with two perspectives in mind—that the privacy of the person not be compromised and that the network be used for strengthening the status of the person rather than undermining it through infantilization.

Organized sources of information and referral, especially true clearinghouses, should be "forced" into creation via district Social Security offices, voluntary agencies, state commissions on aging, and the like.

In the remainder of this chapter we shall be focusing on specific ways to mobilize the

*Cavan's study, now often overlooked, with its sizable sample of 2,988 subjects demonstrated the vast importance of social factors to adjustment. See Cavan, Ruth S.: Personal adjustment in old age. In Lansing, A. H., editor: Cowdry's problems of aging, ed. 3, Baltimore, 1952, The Williams & Wilkins Co.

community through efforts made by the mental health worker or made directly by the older person himself.

Registration drives

Registration drives are among important efforts that mental health workers can initiate or support. Cloward and Piven* helped generate the idea of registering all eligible recipients for various income and service programs so they could in fact benefit from whatever the programs were offering. George Wiley has expanded on this thought with the National Welfare Rights Organization, which has now become a nationwide movement of welfare recipients. In effect this is working "within" the system, yet it is something the system never quite anticipated. The operations Medicare Alert and FIND (Friendless, Isolated, Needy, Disabled) were outreach programs for the elderly. The first registered older people for Medicare B (for doctors' coverage); the second resulted in the study "The Golden Years: A Tarnished Myth" done by the National Council on the Aging, demonstrating the enormous needs and poverty of the elderly. Workers in specific cities have set up outreach programs designed to get the low-income elderly in touch with the material benefits to which they are entitled under existing state and federal legislation. The work of Benefit Alert† in Philadelphia is illustrative. It is important to stress, however, that (to quote Brody et al.) "Prosthetic devices such as Benefit Alert are no substitute for structural changes in program"; these simply make it less easy to ignore the elderly, since they are demonstrating their need and eligibility for services and benefits.

*Cloward and Piven argued in 1966 (Cloward, Richard A., and Piven, Frances F.: The weight of the poor. . . a strategy to end poverty, The Nation **202**:510-517, 1966) that "adding all eligible persons to the welfare rolls would generate a financial crisis of such magnitude that the federal government would be pressured to respond with a plan for a guaranteed annual income." An Advisory Council on Public Welfare the same year suggested, as had others, a "national floor under assistance payments" and federal, rather than state, responsibility for public welfare program studies and financing (Advisory Council on Public Welfare: Having the power we have the duty. Report to the Secretary of Health, Education, and Welfare, Washington, D. C., 1966, U. S. Government Printing Office).

†Brody, S. J., Finkle, H., and Hirsch, C.: Benefit Alert: outreach program for aged, Social Work **17**:14-23, 1972.

Employment

If old people are so delighted with retirement, how come older-age employment services are overloaded with applicants?

For example: The Arlington (Virginia) Senior Adult Counseling and Employment Service placed 30 to 40 applicants a month in 1971 but always had a backlog of 100 people waiting.

Some old people need the money because the Social Security or pension checks just will not stretch far enough.* Some want to get out of the house to occupy their time. Many want the "meaningfulness" of work.† So long as work and money have such profound financial, social, personal, and ethical significance, it is illusory to deny their importance to health, both physical and mental. Some old people are told to do volunteer work—advice that is indeed helpful to some but naive in instances where economic survival is at issue. Arbitrary retirement is often cruel and of questionable constitutionality. It is anticipated that there will be increasing numbers of legal suits testing the right of any person, regardless of age, to employment.

Unemployment hangs over the head of many people who are over 50 years of age. An instance of this was seen in 1963 when the Studebaker Corporation announced the

*Of the $60 billion in aggregate income that old people received in 1970, about 30% was earned by them. Self-employment is often of necessity "bootleg" work: typing, babysitting, housecleaning, handyman services (electrical and carpentry skills), etc., which is *not* reported as income so as to avoid imperiling Social Security pensions.

†Friedmann, E. A., and Havighurst, R. J.: The meaning of work and retirement, Chicago, 1954, University of Chicago Press.

end of automotive production in its South Bend, Indiana facilities. The company plant shutdown affected nearly 10% of the area's total work force of 90,000 people. More than half of those laid off were over 50 years of age. The entire community rallied together with state and federal agencies. The successful Project ABLE (Ability Based on Long Experience) was an experimental action and demonstration program supported through the Department of Labor's Office of Manpower, Automation and Training. It showed that large numbers of unemployed older workers can be returned to productive employment through mobilization of the community, individual counseling, and job development and opportunities. South Bend itself recovered.*

Several laws were enacted in 1971 to relieve the unemployment difficulties of older workers. Public Law 91-593 authorized recognition of the first week in May as National Employ the Older Worker Week. The 1970 Employment Security Amendments (Public Law 91-373) established "extended benefits" during periods of high unemployment for those whose regular unemployment compensation entitlement has been exhausted. Provisions for a "midcareer service" were included in the Employment and Manpower Act of 1970, which was vetoed by the President. These provisions would have provided training, retraining, counseling, and other needed services for middle-aged and older workers.

The Senior Opportunities Services (SOS) program of the Office of Economic Opportunity is intended to identify and meet the needs of persons over 60, with projects that serve and/or employ older persons predominately. The various projects include community action programs to provide employment opportunities, home health services, assistance in the Food Stamp plan, and outreach and referral services. As much as possible these activities are staffed by older citizens, paid or volunteer. OEO's Senior Aides and Senior Community Service Aides are engaged in such activities as homemaker and health assistance, nutrition, institutional care, home repair, child care, and social service administration.

Operation Mainstream, an employment program for chronically unemployed, operates two programs especially for older people: Green Thumb, which involves beautification by planting—for men; and Green Light, which employs aides in libraries, schools, and day care centers—for women.

Age discrimination in employment is directly related to unemployment. The Age Discrimination in Employment Act is administered by the Department of Labor, Wage and Hour Administration, in 350 offices throughout the nation (see listings in the telephone directory). This Act has not been enforced adequately and applies only to persons under 65. People over 65 are totally unprotected by law although some through individual and class legal efforts are attempting to challenge this. Typical ways in which employers avoid hiring the older person are to declare that the person is "overqualified," "unskilled," less needful of a job as compared to the young, and less reliable and flexible. Most of this is false and the rest could easily be remedied through, for example, training programs that accept the person over 50 years of age.

Job placement requires vocational evaluation and counseling as critical first steps. The U. S. Employment Service (USES) has been very disappointing in its feeble efforts to place older workers, but pressure should nonetheless be placed upon USES and its various offices. There are Federal Job Information Centers (in various cities), which give advice and information on federal job opportunities. The Women's Bureau in the Department of Labor has taken some interest in the job plight of older women and can offer advice. Various communities offer privately sponsored, nonprofit, over-60 em-

*United Community Service of St. Joseph County, Inc. Project ABLE (Ability Based on Long Experience). Final Report Contract No. MDS37-64, Older Worker Employment, South Bend, Ind., Dec., 1965.

ployment and counseling services and agencies. In some there are forty-plus clubs for finding employment after age 40. For the handicapped and elderly, sheltered workshops may be available (See Chapter 11.) In Appendix C we have outlined various governmental programs to which older people can apply (some being specifically designed for the low-income elderly).

Advocacy

Advocacy includes use of all means at our disposal, from direct action to moral persuasion, to effectively represent the needs and grievances of older people. The contributions of Saul Alinsky and Ralph Nader should be known to the mental health worker. Class-action cases are essential, for instance, to mandamus (to compel) better treatment in state mental hospitals* and other governmental facilities. Legal and protective services,† private conservatorships, and public guardianships are essential—not only to protect older people but also to advance their causes, for better housing, in administrative and judicial reviews regarding Social Security and Medicare claims, et cetera. Contemporary grievance mechanisms are being overhauled and improved following court cases.

Nursing home deficiencies must not be covered up by local, state, or federal governments. The Freedom of Information Act should compel the Social Security Administration to reveal the names of specific institutions with their specific deficiencies.

Individual older people have a variety of rights to be protected such an contractual and testamentary rights. Tenant rights have become increasingly important.

The Group for the Advancement of Psychiatry has argued that every community mental health center should have an advocate for the aged, a spokesman "in negotiations with other agencies or governmental counseling."

There already exist various advocates for old people. Some churches have lay commissions and special ministries to the aging. Cities and states have advisory committees and commissions. (By 1965 most states had small units with responsibility for planning, coordinating, and evaluation programs and for making recommendations.) In 1971, 20 state commissions on aging were independently responsible to governors; 19 were placed within multipurpose departments (e.g., Human Resources), in social welfare departments, 6 others had varied special status, etc. Massachusetts created a cabinet-level Department of Elder Affairs in 1971 to oversee all programs for the elderly. The new Department has authority over such functions as Old Age Assistance, Disability Assistance, and the provision of a program for income maintenance (formerly functions of the Welfare Department); over licensing and inspection of nursing homes, rest homes, and similar facilities for the elderly (formerly the responsibility of the Department of Public Health); and over construction and administration of housing and transportation services for the elderly (which previously had been vested in the Department of Community Affairs).

For advocacy to mean anything there must be *accountability*. Challenging of authority must be balanced by "reactions" from the challenged; otherwise the "system" is not working. There has been a crescendo of complaints about the unresponsiveness of the system under which we live. We do not wish to perpetuate any romantic illusions about "working within" the system. We have not been impressed with great progress on behalf of old people in the last decades—nor on behalf of minority or other groups. There has been only a 1% change in the distribution of wealth between 1950 and 1970, to take one major indicator. To work at all on the problems of the elderly, as with all groups that have suffered or are suffering injustices, one must be willing to be angry and outraged, depressed and despairing; but

*Wyatt versus Stickney, Alabama, 1971-1972.

†Neighborhood legal services, Legal Aid societies, public defenders, public-interest law firms, and protective services are available for the legal needs of the old.

always ready and spoiling for a struggle. In short, affirmation, anger, and despair in due proportion are appropriate emotions.*

The Swedish concept of ombudsman has been proposed for application in the United States. (An ombudsman in Scandinavia is a mediator who protects the rights of individual citizens and works with governmental agencies to assure fair representation.) Ralph Nader started a Retired Professional Action Corps, which endeavors to put public-interest law at the disposal of old people. We believe old people themselves should take leadership. They should make unannounced visits to nursing homes. When they do not wish to retire, they should be willing to refuse to leave their jobs. There are countless ways in which they could challenge the myths and prejudices against old age.

Consumer fraud and quackery are a serious problem because old people are especially vulnerable.† Many have chronic ailments that seem never to get better. Hard-earned savings may be lost to exploitative medical fakers, land salesmen, hearing aid salesmen, and so forth. In 1966 the U. S. Senate Special Committee on Aging published a report on "frauds and misinterpretations affecting the elderly."

The human desire for magic cures and salvation runs deep. In late life additional factors, ranging from brain damage to grief, add to the vulnerability. Public consumer education is not sufficient. Direct advice and discussion by the various service professions and vocations—mental health workers to physicians—carry considerable weight. But legislation, more than we presently have, is necessary and its strict enforcement is mandatory. Illustrative legislation is the Interstate Land Sales Full Disclosure Act.

Consultative services

Consultative services should be standard to agencies, homes, religious organizations, and so forth. The list below describes the major users of consultation regarding the problems of elderly people.

1. Nursing homes
2. Homes for the aged
3. Nonpsychiatrist physicians
4. General hospital inpatient and outpatient sections
5. Boarding homes, public housing for the aged, and similar residential concentrations
6. Public assistance departments, including their sections for protective service for the elderly
7. Clergymen
8. Senior citizen centers
9. Industry and government
10. Homemaker and home health aide agencies
11. Visiting nurses and public health nurses
12. Planning bodies, such as model cities boards, senior citizen councils, commissions on aging, housing authorities

Generally speaking, consultative relationships to such institutions and agencies provide evaluation and recommendations concerning the institution itself, its staff, or those it serves. The following list further delineates this general observation and offers some models of consultation.

1. *Administrative consultation.* The center consultant meets with the home administrator, usually to discuss staff problems but sometimes family or financial problems. The focus is on organization and decision-making.
2. *Staff (milieu) consultation.* The center consultant meets with staff groups to discuss and interpret the psychological importance of events in the home which affect staff and patient group behavior.
3. *Client-centered case consultation.* The center consultant discusses a specific case with a staff group or individual. Focus is on the patient.

---

*Joan Colebrook wrote movingly about urban renewal in the South End of Boston (Colebrook, Joan: A reporter at large: the renewal, New Yorker, Jan. 1, 1966). She observed: "Social workers were trying to provide some moral support for impoverished and isolated older people who found themselves in the way of the bulldozer." She was writing about old people trying to survive in their run-down neighborhoods with abandoned and substandard housing, garbage-strewn empty lots, dimly lighted streets. They were subjected to mugging and purse-snatching. When urban renewal began, it happened that the possessions of a lifetime were at times thrown into the streets if an older person was in a hospital or for some other reason not able to be home. She also observed some relocation deaths.

†See Butler, R. N.: Why are older consumers so susceptible? Geriatrics 23:83-88, 1968.

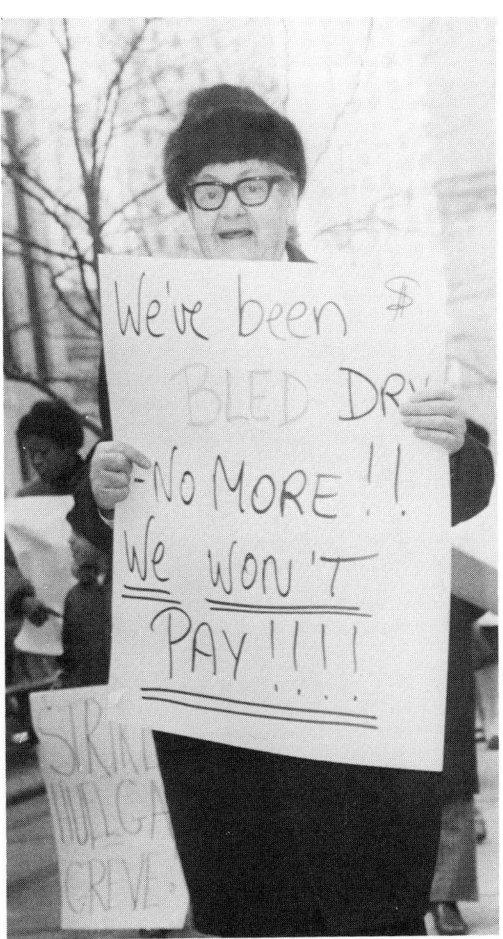

Self-respect follows self-assertion.

Photo by M. DeChiara.

4. *Consultee-centered consultation.* The focus of discussion is the patient, but the center consultant keeps the staff members' countertransference in mind during the discussion.
5. *Didactic meetings.* These allow for an organized presentation of basic psychological principles. Many staff have a keen interest in such learning.*

Political organizations

Having some sense of power and political participation is therapeutic; the active seeking of objectives may not always be successful but the process itself can be a source of satisfaction and increased self-esteem. The elderly are beginning to be more active politically and may soon vote more consistently as a power block (they constitute 17% of the vote). The National Council of Senior Citizens and the American Association of Retired Persons (the two largest organizations for older people) have lobbied for more favorable Social Security benefits, medicare, housing, and other areas of concern. A much smaller but more militant group calls itself the Gray Panthers.

*From Group for the Advancement of Psychiatry: The aged and community mental health: a guide to program development. Formulated by the Committee on Aging, vol. 8, No. 81, Nov., 1971.

REFERENCES

Abraham, K.: The applicability of psycho-analytic treatment to patients at an advanced age. In Selected Papers of Psychoanalysis, London, 1949, Hogarth Press.

Beattie, W. M., Jr.: New perspectives in social welfare research in gerontology (editorial), The Gerontologist **2**:66, 1962.

Blank, Marie Latz: Recent research findings on practice with the aging, Social Casework, pp. 382-389, 1971.

Blau, D.: Role of community physicians in the psychiatric hospitalization of aged patients, Journal of Gerontology **16**:399-400, 1962.

Brody, Elaine M., and Spark, Geraldine M.: Institutionalization of the aged: a family crisis, Family Process **5**:76-90, 1966.

Butler, Robert N.: Intensive psychotherapy for the hospitalized aged, Geriatrics **15**:644-653, 1960.

Community Services Society of New York: The Senior Advisory Service for Public Housing Tenants: final report, New York, 1969.

Gellhorn, W.: Ombudsmen and elderly citizens' protection in nine countries, Cambridge, Mass., 1966, Harvard University Press.

Ginzberg, Raphael: Geriatric ward psychiatry. Techniques in the psychological management of elderly psychotics, American Journal of Psychiatry **110**:296-300, 1953.

Goldfarb, Alvin I.: Psychotherapy of aged persons. IV. One aspect of the therapeutic situation with aged patients, Psychoanalytic Review **42**:100-187, 1955.

Goldfarb, Alvin I.: Group therapy with the old and aged. In Kaplan, H. I., and Saddock, B. J., editors: Comprehensive group psychotherapy, Baltimore, 1971, The Williams & Wilkins Co.

Grotjahn, M.: Psychoanalytic investigation of a 71 year old man with senile dementia, Psychoanalytic Quarterly **9**:80-97, 1940.

Jelliffe, S. E.: The old age factor in psychoanalytical therapy, Medical Journal and Record **121**: 7-12, 1925.

Kaufman, M. Ralph: The psychoanalytic point of view: old age and aging, The American Journal of Orthopsychiatry **10**:73-79, 1940.

Klein, Wilma H., LeShan, Eda J., and Furman, S. S.: Promoting mental health of older people through group methods. a practical guide, New York, 1965, Mental Health Materials Center, Inc.

Kubie, Susan H., and Landau, Gertrude: Group work with the aged, New York, 1953, International Universities Press.

Legal research and services for the elderly: A handbook of model state statutes, Washington, D. C., 1971, National Council of Senior Citizens.

Lehmann, Virginia: You, the law and retirement, 1966, U. S. Department of Health Education, and Welfare.

Linden, Maurice E.: Group psychotherapy with institutionalized senile women: study in gerontology in human relations, International Journal of Group Psychotherapy **3**:150-151, 1953.

Martin, Lillien J.: A handbook for old age counselors, San Francisco, 1944, Geertz Printing Co.

Meerloo, J. A. M.: Transference and resistance in geriatric psychotherapy, Psychoanalytic Review **42**:72-82, 1955.

Miller, M. B.: The chronically ill aged, family conflict, and family medicine, Journal of the American Geriatrics Society **17**:950-961, 1969.

National Council on the Aging: Resources for the aging: an action handbook, New York, 1969.

Payne, J.: Ombudsman roles for social workers, Social Work **17**:94-100, 1972.

Rechtschaffen, A.: Psychotherapy with geriatric patients: a review of the literature, Journal of Gerontology **14**:73-84, 1959.

Ryder, Margaret B.: Case work with the aged paent and his adult children, The Family **26**: 243-250, 1945.

Stern, K.: Problems encountered in an old age counseling center. In Shock, N. W., editor: Problems of aging, New York, 1948-1949, Josiah Macy, Jr., Foundation.

Wolff, K.: Group psychotherapy with geriatric patients in a mental hospital, Journal of the American Geriatrics Society **5**:13, 1957.

Yalom, Irvin D.: The therapy and practice of group psychotherapy, New York, 1970, Basic Books, Inc.

13
DRUG AND ELECTROSHOCK THERAPY

Drugs, judiciously employed, can be of supportive value in the treatment of anxiety, severe agitation, and depression in old age. They should not, however, represent the sole form of treatment given to any elderly person. When possible, other approaches to the amelioration of symptoms should be tried first: various forms of psychotherapy, social activities, physical exercise. If drugs are nonetheless deemed necessary, they should be administered only as one component of an organized treatment plan.

There is considerable evidence to support the view that we have an "overmedicated society." Much concern, of course, is voiced about use of drugs in the youth culture and about barbiturate, tranquilizer, and alcohol consumption among the middle-aged. But old age has its own drug problems resulting from high usages of tranquilizers, sedatives, and hypnotics. To some degree these medications reflect the greater anxiety, depression, and insomnia found in older people. But they also point to the anxiety of doctors and other health personnel, their impatience with old people (to whom they would rather give a pill than to listen), and their own need for instant gratification (treatment results). Unfortunately drugs reinforce some of the slowing observed in old people, aggravate a sense of aging and depression, and can contribute to or directly cause acute and chronic brain syndromes. We will emphasize some of the untoward side effects and complications of drug therapy while acknowledging the legitimate use of medications in a carefully thought out and monitored treatment plan. But in general we submit that the medical profession's penchant for chemotherapy with the elderly should be restrained.

DRUG TREATMENT

Antidepressants

These include the tricyclic compounds and the monoamine oxidase inhibitors (MAOIs). We recommend against the use of the monoamine oxidase* inhibitors. These mood elevators have profound side effects, including orthostatic hypotension, inhibition of ejaculation, weakness, and hypertensive crisis associated with the concurrent intake of certain food substances such as cheese.

The MAOIs include isocarboxazide (Marplan), nialamide (Niamid), phenelzine sulfate (Nardil) and tranylcypromine (Parnate).†

The other group, the dibenzazepine derivatives (tricyclic compounds), mix badly with the MAOIs. Their antidepressant effects are not remarkable but are regarded as established. The most popular are amitriptyline (Elavil) and imipramine (Tofranil). Ten days of Elavil at 150 mg. daily in divided doses is probably an adequate course. With Elavil the patient may feel worse for the first two to five days, rather than better.

Strokes and myocardial infarctions ("coronaries") have been reported with this class of medication, the tricyclic compounds. They should not be given within two weeks after

*An important central nervous system enzyme.

†We will first give the generic name for purposes of prescription. Because advertising has been so successful in introducing people to drugs, we will also give the most common trade name(s) in parentheses.

discontinuing an MAOI, since hyperpyretic (high-fever) crises and deaths have occurred. They must be used cautiously in patients with a history of urinary retention or with narrow-angle glaucoma or increased intraocular pressure. Physical and mental performance, as in automobile driving or operating machinery, may be affected.

It is also important to understand the patient's life history and defenses before prescribing antidepressant drugs. Suppression of a symptom—be it depression or anxiety—may be undesirable. For instance, in a depression viewed as a maladaptative expression of grief, the release of suppressed grief will have a more enduring value than drug-suppressed depression. No drug can substitute for a lost loved one, as therapeutic counseling and the forging of new relationships can.

Included among the tricyclic compounds is desipramine (Norpramin). The mechanisms of its established effects against depression are not known. Desipramine is supposed to be a metabolite of imipramine and was therefore presumed to act more quickly. This has not proved out. A therapeutic trial may demonstrate that an apparent case of senile brain disease is an endogenous depression. One must observe carefully for orthostatic hypotension.

Amitriptyline has a tranquilizing component and so is especially indicated in anxious depression. The antidepressant effect of this agent may be apparent in four days, or perhaps not before three or four weeks. For mild depressions in the elderly the dosage is 25 mg. t.i.d. to 25 mg. b.i.d. and 50 mg. at bedtime. Begin at 10 mg. t.i.d. and 20 mg. at bedtime. For severe depressions, rapidly build up to 150 to 200 mg. daily. As much as 250 mg. can be given to a heavily built person.

With *imipramine* the dosage is 30 to 100 mg. daily, in divided doses, and should start at 10 mg. t.i.d. and be increased gradually. Four to eight weeks is a reasonable trial; most patients who are going to respond do so in the first two weeks.

Methylphenidate (Ritalin) is a mild central nervous stimulant that counteracts physical and mental fatigue while having only slight effect on blood pressure and respiration. Its potency is intermediate between amphetamines and caffeine. It is useful only in mild depression and then only in a limited number of cases. We have found it useful in some instances of mild early chronic brain syndromes. It is sometimes helpful in counteracting drug-induced lethargy resulting from barbiturates, tranquilizers, antihistamines, and anticonvulsants. There is reported effectiveness against "apathetic or withdrawn senile behavior." One must be wary of using this drug, however, since it may aggravate anxiety and tension. Glaucoma is a contraindication. Begin with 10 to 15 mg. daily in divided doses, preferably taken 30 to 45 minutes before meals; 20 to 30 mg. is the maximum for the elderly.

Lithium carbonate has been an effective agent in the treatment of patients of all ages with manic-depressive illness. Dosages range from 300 mg. once daily up to 600 mg. q.i.d. Among the elderly, one encounters hypomanic states that often respond to lithium with much smaller amounts than would ordinarily be anticipated. Effective doses may be as low as 300 mg. once daily to 600 mg. twice daily. Hypomanic states and bipolar depressions are most susceptible to lithium therapy.* Evidence for the treatment of depressive states is less impressive. One must be certain there is adequate kidney excretion because of the small margin between the therapeutic and toxic doses.† In older people on low-sodium diets and on diuretics the need for caution is increased. However, after one has followed the patient for some time one may reduce the monitoring of lithium blood levels. Begin on a once-per-week basis; then once every one to six months. Blood samples should be taken in the early morning (8 to 9 A.M.) prior to the first dose of lithium. Brain damage is a contraindication. Clinical signs of toxicity include diarrhea, vomiting, tremor, mild ataxia,

---

*According to Dr. Zigmond Lebensohn, who has an extensive clinical experience with lithium.

†Van Der Velde, C. D.: Toxicity of lithium carbonate in elderly patients, American Journal of Psychiatry **127**:1075-1077, 1971.

drowsiness, muscular weakness, slurred speech, and confusion.

Tranquilizers

Theoretically, tranquilizers are regarded as an improvement over sedatives by virtue of alleviating anxiety with less mental impairment. Physical addiction is not a serious problem but emotional dependence upon tranquilizers is not uncommon.

There is an overprescribing of tranquilizers. Moreover, higher and higher dosages may be given because of developing tolerances and frustration over results.* Such practices are dangerous—for the patient may suffer unnecesary complications and untoward side effects. The drugs are also expensive for the older person. Additionally one should follow the dosage of psychotropic drugs indicated by the Food and Drug Administration (FDA) as a protection against malpractice.

Tranquilizers often serve the provider of service rather than those served. Zombies are created by the phenothiazines in particular, such as chlorpromazine (Thorazine) and thioridazine (Mellaril). These drugs slow people so markedly that physical activity is greatly reduced, with resultant muscle atrophy. Chlordiazepoxide (Librium) and thioridazine (Mellaril), respectively, can adversely affect the libido (sexual desire and capacity).

We should also point out that not infrequently an elderly person is given a number of drugs simultaneously; for example, tranquilizers *and* antidepressants. This can be a dangerous practice.

Major tranquilizers

For the elderly the agent of choice among the major tranquilizers is *thioridazine* (Mellaril). It appears to be as effective as chlorpromazine, but it produces less extrapyramidal effect and only moderate sedative and hypotensive effects. It is useful against the anxiety associated with depression but one must beware of its possible depressive effects. Ejaculatory impotence is another possible side effect. Thioridazine is active against so-called senile (usually nocturnal) agitation and valuable against intractable pain. The dosage is 10 mg. b.i.d. to 100 mg. t.i.d.; usual dosage is 30 to 150 mg. daily.

All phenothiazines may potentiate central nervous system depressants (e.g., anesthetics, opiates, alcohol). Another danger of phenothiazines is that leukopenia can occur, so routine blood follow-up is indicated. Female patients seem to have a greater susceptibility to orthostatic hypotension (fall in blood pressure when standing erect). There are many side effects, of varying possible severity—dryness of the mouth, blurred vision, drowsiness, altered libido. The phenothiazines often produce extrapyramidal symptoms.

Haloperidol (Haldol) is the first of a new series of major tranquilizers, the butyrophenones. The patient must be warned of decreased thirst. Fatal cases of bronchopneumonia have been reported following use of all major tranquilizers including haloperidol. The mechanism is thought to be decreased thirst due to central nervous system inhibition followed by dehydration, hemoconcentration, and reduced pulmonary ventilation. The patient must be told not to drink alcohol and not to operate machinery or drive a car. Do not prescribe with anticoagulants. Parkinsonian symptoms can occur.

Be sure to explain the potential dosages and side effects of drugs to patients. Spell out the possible depressive and retarding effects of the phenothiazines and the likely occurrence of annoying symptoms such as dryness of the mouth. Forewarn the patient regarding hypotension and extrapyramidal symptoms. Indicate that antiparkinsonian agents are available.

Special caution must be exercised in using drugs with potentially suicidal patients, who may take large quantities and mixtures of tranquilizers and sedatives. Certain drugs should not be prescribed for a suicidal pa-

*The U. S. Senate Special Committee on Aging found in the states of Illinois, Ohio, and New Jersey in 1971 that 35% to 40% of all prescriptions for elderly consumers under Medicaid (the federal-state health program for the needy) were tranquilizers and sedatives.

tient. Glutethimide has a very low therapeutic-lethal ratio.

Minor tranquilizers

There are three widely used agents of the benzodiazepine series. chlordiazepoxide, diazepam, and oxazepam.

Chlordiazepoxide hydrochloride, N.F. (Librium) is of some value in the relief of anxiety and tension and is one of the most widely prescribed drugs in America. It can be useful for preoperative apprehension. In elderly and especially debilitated patients, begin with minimal dosage, to preclude ataxia or oversedation. Begin with 5 mg. up to twice daily (10 mg.) and do not exceed 5 mg. four times daily (20 mg. total dosage). Beware of potentiation by the phenothiazines and MAOIs. Both increased and decreased libido have been reported.

Diazepam (Valium) is somewhat useful in tension and anxiety states, particularly where muscular tension is notable. Because of its ability to relieve skeletal muscle spasm related to local inflammation of joints and muscles, it is advantageous to some elderly persons with arthritis. Lower doses in the range of 2 to 5 mg. for the elderly and debilitated are indicated. Begin with 2 to 2.5 mg. once or twice daily. Increase gradually only as needed. One should be cautious of potentiation by the phenothiazines, narcotics, barbiturates, MAOIs, and other antidepressants as well as alcohol. Patients should be warned about driving and hazardous occupations (e.g., putting shingles on the roof). Because of withdrawal symptoms, an abrupt discontinuation should not be undertaken.

Beware also of such side effects as excessive drowsiness, fatigue, ataxia, confusion, depression, hypotension, urinary retention, and changes in libido. The drug is contraindicated in the presence of acute narrow-angle (congestive) glaucoma.

With *oxazepam* (Serax), the initial dosage is 10 mg. three times daily. Any increases should be given with caution and not exceed 15 mg. three to four times daily.

The benzodiazepine derivatives are not of demonstrable superiority over the barbiturate series of sedatives. Phenobarbital, however, may provoke paradoxical excitatory reactions in some older patients and thus has to be tried carefully.

Meprobamate (Equanil; Miltown) is given for tension and anxiety but is probably no more effective than old-fashioned phenobarbital. Physical dependence can occur with either. Begin in the older age group with 200 to 400 mg. t.i.d., up to four times daily.

Other drugs

Cerebral vasodilators, cerebral stimulants, hormones, and anticoagulants are among other classes of drugs that have been recommended and sold for depressed, "senile," or deteriorated old people. They are of little clinical use and may be dangerous in some instances.

The antihistamines have not been of demonstrated value. Pentylenetetrazol and monosodium glutamate seem relatively safe but of uncertain efficiency. Nylidrin and papaverine (like alcohol) may increase cerebral blood flow, but that is no guarantee of clinical effectiveness.

Vitamins are useful when there are deficiencies. Hypovitaminosis must be carefully evaluated. Victims of pellagra (nicotinic acid deficiency) should receive by mouth 500 mg. up to three times daily as necessary. For old people a basic vitamin-mineral combination should be given to offset effects of the processing of foods, poor dietary habits, and low appetite related to loneliness and grief.

Hormones can be beneficial for the emotional well-being of postmenopausal women. In addition, the steroids contribute to basic bodily health and are valuable in supporting sexual capacities. (See Chapter 6 for recommended dosage.)

There is a continuing search for drugs to assist memory. The efficiency of ribonucleic acid in aiding memory has not been established. There are no specific drugs against the brain damage of organic disorders.

Alcohol as therapy

Wine has been widely recommended in geriatric medicine and in convalescent care.

It is the world's oldest tranquilizer. It gives pleasure, helps one sleep (valuable for use against insomnia), and reduces pain. Galen, the great Roman physician, called wine "the nurse of old age." Among the dessert wines, two to three ounces of port is useful for sleep.

One must beware, however, of the unfortunate potentiating or synergistic action of alcohol on other sedatives, tranquilizers, or narcotics. Sherry appears to stimulate the appetite and digestive processes, and its virtue in increasing sociability has been emphasized by Kastenbaum in his study at Cushing Hospital, Framington, Massachusetts.* Alcohol may also be useful for patients suffering from cerebral arteriosclerosis. However, it must be remembered that tolerance for alcohol decreases with old age; mental confusion and poor coordination can combine with alcohol to increase the risk of falling; and alcohol adversely influences sexual potency.

TREATMENT OF INSOMNIA

Insomnia may be seen in many emotional reactions—grief, anxiety, anger, severe depressions, and even as a consequence of sexual deprivation—and should be treated first by simple measures. See Chapter 14. Drugs for sleep (hypnotics) include barbiturates, which should generally be avoided in this age group because of the occasions of paradoxical stimulation. Phenobarbital, pentobarbital, and secobarbital are three popular barbiturates. Chloral hydrate is valuable. Nonbarbiturates include glutethimide (Doriden), methyprylon (Noludar), methaqualone (Quaalude), and ethchlorvynol (Placidyl); but tolerance, habituation, addiction, and, indeed, suicide can be the end results of excessive use of these nonbarbiturates as well.

Dosage:

Chloral hydrate	250 to 500 mg. (available in syrup as well as capsules)
Ethchlorvynol	500 mg.
Flurazepam	15 mg.
Glutethimide	250 to 500 mg.
Methaqualone	150 mg. (preferred dosage; 300 mg. may be necessary)
Methyprylon	300 mg.

*Kastenbaum, R.: Wine and fellowship in aging: an exploratory ACTION program, Journal of Human Relations 13:266-271, 1965.

Glutethimide has a small safety margin between hypnosis and acute overdosage. It is the least preferred of the nonbarbiturate hypnotics in old age.

Such side effects as dizziness, drowsiness, and light-headedness from some hypnotics are seen in the elderly or debilitated. Therefore, the initial dosage of flurazepam hydrochloride (Dalmane) to cite one example, should be 15 mg., rather than the usual adult dosage of 30 mg.

DANGERS AND SAFEGUARDS IN DRUG USE WITH THE ELDERLY

The *sedating effects* of twelve of the twenty most commonly used medications in persons over 65 (e.g., Librium, Doriden, phenobarbital) can cause serious problems, as we have stated. Older people who are experiencing a physical slowing of speed and coordination find these features exacerbated by a number of drugs. Some persons react with fear and depression, thinking they are failing fast or even dying. In fact various psychoactive agents have caused deaths in old people.

Drug metabolism is another factor, since the liver may have reduced blood flow in old people and thus the rate of drug detoxification may be slowed. Moreover, older people have a lower general bodily metabolism rate, prolonging drug action or creating exaggerated drug reactions. Kidney impairment can also affect excretion of the drug. The old have a relatively greater accumulation of drugs in body fat compared to younger people; therefore, drug effects may be prolonged because of this accumulation.

Iatrogenic brain syndromes are not uncommon. Doctors unwittingly produce reversible and, often unrecognized, irreversible brain syndromes. Tranquilizers and hypnotics are the most likely causes of such conditions, but steroids used in arthritis can cause organic brain disorders as well as hypomania and/or depression.

Finally, *tardive dyskinesia* is an affliction often associated with drug treatment. This condition appears more likely to occur in the aged although it is found at all ages. It is a serious malady, which appears to be an irreversible end result of phenothiazine therapy* and may develop only after the reduction or withdrawal of the offending drug. It is characterized by slow, rhythmic, and involuntary movements of the face and extremities. One may see chewing or gyrating of the jaws, grinning, lip-pursing, eye-blinking, "fly catcher" tongue, difficulty in swallowing, and/or spastic neck-stiffening. Winkleman and others feel it is more commonly seen in the brain-damaged; thus it is a reason for limiting use of the phenothiazines in old people with a brain syndrome.† Some persons also seem more sensitive to drugs than others.

We do not believe tranquilizers should be used in high dosages and we recommend that they be prescribed only for brief periods, related to specific symptoms such as anxiety. They should *not* be continued over extended periods. They should *not* be employed for the benefit of the therapist or the quiet serenity of the institution. In general it is wise to administer all drugs with caution in old age, beginning with low dosages and increasing gradually in a stepwise, progressive fashion when a higher dosage is definitely indicated. The patient must be under continuous clinical and laboratory surveillance. The basic work-up will have afforded baseline data. Complete blood counts should be repeated at least monthly. With use of the phenothiazines, liver tests, such as alkaline phosphatase and bilirubin, should also be followed.

The potential dangers, complications, and side effects should be carefully and fully explained to patients—both the annoying symptoms like dryness of the mouth, for instance, and the dangerous symptoms such as hypotension (low blood pressure and possible fainting) and extrapyramidal symptoms (parkinsonism).* Antiparkinsonian agents are available, with benztropine mesylate (Cogentin) and procyclidine (Kemadrin) most commonly used.† Special caution should be exercised in prescribing for possibly suicidal patients.

One of the important reasons for informing older people about the drugs they are taking is to help them distinguish side effects from other bodily changes. As we mentioned previously, we have found that old people may misinterpret the retarding effects of the tranquilizers as signs of aging. Doctors remain all too secretive about preparing patients for drug effects, partly because they fear the development of symptoms in suggestible persons. Many also simply do not wish to take the time. It is archaic to assume that "what the patient doesn't know won't hurt him," because often it does. One must help patients overcome fears of medications while simultaneously encouraging them to respect effects and dangers.

MENTAL HEALTH THERAPIST'S INVOLVEMENT IN DRUG THERAPY

The mental health therapist's own attitudes toward the use of drugs may influence their effects on older people. If the therapist is philosophically against drugs (feeling that people should resolve issues for themselves) or is anxious about their side effects and potential complications, he or she is likely to convey these concerns to the older person,

*Degenerative brain changes have also been held responsible.

†Dr. George Crane of the Spring Grove State Hospital of Maryland has emphasized the dangers of the phenothiazines—especially the danger of tardive dyskinesia. See Crane, G. E.: Tardive dyskinesia in patients treated with major neuroleptics, American Journal of Psychiatry **124** (supp.):40-48, 1968; Crane, G. E.: Persistence of neurological symptoms due to neuroleptic drugs, American Journal of Psychiatry **127**:1407-1410, 1971; Crane, G. E., and Gardner, R., Jr.: Psychotrophic drugs and dysfunctions of the basal ganglia: a multidisciplinary workshop, National Institute of Mental Health, Public Health Service Publication No. 1938, 1969.

*An estimated 1 million Americans (probably an underestimate) of all ages suffer untoward drug reactions yearly and 30,000 die.

†These agents do not appear to ameliorate tardive dyskinesia.

even when not stating them explicitly. Hopefully, the therapist can be open enough to appreciate the value of drugs that are judiciously employed. There are people who need the *immediate* support of the magical/real expectations of medicine and the "medicine man" (the power of the physician as well as the actual, chemically active drug effects). One rational way of reconciling the therapist's possibly negative feeling about drugs with occasions when people need them is to note that therapy is a *process,* an experience over time. At various points, drugs might maintain working men or women on their jobs or help parents with their parenthood. But in the overall therapeutic effort, drugs may become only a minor part.

However, even if the therapist is totally opposed to drugs, he should not deny his client/patient their usefulness but should collaborate with a physician who will administer the drug. Having separate "talking" and "drug" therapists may provoke some divided reactions in the person being treated, with manipulations in some instances, but such behavior can become a part of the treatment process.

At the Chestnut Lodge Sanitarium (Rockville, Maryland) patients were regularly assigned two doctors: the administrative physician, who made decisions about home visits, drugs, etc., and the therapeutic physician.*

Nonphysician mental health personnel should know what drugs an older person is taking, whether for physical or mental conditions. The *Physicians' Desk Reference,* although not ideal, is a source of information about the side effects and complications of all drugs. The *Merck Manual* also may be useful.

All mental health personnel should be familiar with a prescription and know how to interpret it. They may be called on to prepare prescriptions for the signature of the physician in some circumstances. Included here is a sample prescription form.

*See Stanton, A. H., and Schwartz, M. S.: The mental hospital, New York, 1954, Basic Books, Inc.

JAMES R. DOE, M.D.
1000 Henry Street, N.W.
Waco, Texas
Phone: 211-2111
BND No: AB3208036*

℞ (treatment)

Medicine (generic proposed) — Amount (per tablet, capsule, etc.)

Number

Sig. (directions):

Label in full as to contents

Rep: 0-1-2-3-4-5-PRN — M.D.

(signature)

*Note the BND (Bureau of Narcotics and Dangerous Drugs) number. Some medications, including narcotics, hypnotics, and some tranquilizers, are under such controls.

Prescription terms

1. Weights (amounts are usually expressed in milligrams, grams, or grains):

Milligram means one thousandth of a gram, roughly equivalent to 1/65th grain. It is usually abbreviated mg.

Gram is a unit of weight in the metric system. It is usually abbreviated g., gm., or Gm. It is equivalent to about 15.43 grains.

Grain is a unit of weight in the avoirdupois system. It is usually abbreviated gr. It is equivalent to 1/480 ounce and to 0.065 gram.

Ounce is 1/12 of a pound avoirdupois and is equivalent to 31.1 grams. The abbreviation for ounce is oz.

The metric system is preferred and the old English system is slowly being phased out.

2. Latin abbreviations:

℞ "Recipe."
Sig. to write. It means the directions for taking the drugs.
b.i.d. Bis in die, two times a day.
t.i.d. Ter in die, three times a day.
q.i.d. Quater in die, four times a day.
a.c. Antecibum, before meals
p.c. Post cibum, after meals.
h.s. Hora somni, before sleep.
prn Pro re nata, according to circumstances, rather than routine schedule.
sos Si opus sit, if necessary, if occasion requires
Rep. repeat.
q.h. Quaque hora, every hour.
q2h Quaque secunda hora, every second hour, etc.

Telephone prescriptions should always be checked later and countersigned. One must also be careful about pronunciation. The names of a number of drugs sound alike (e.g., the trade names Haldol and Halodrin, Elavil and Aldoril, Mebaral and Mellaren, Ritalin and Ismelin), among others:

To *label in full* is a sound practice in most cases. In the Americas, except for the United States, and in most of Europe, the law requires manufacturers to label all medicines with brand name, ingredients, and dosage as well as what the medicine is for, its side effects, full dosage range, and expiration date (if there is one). Until we have such laws in this country, the doctor should label in full and instruct the druggist on his prescription to do so. This is valuable for all ages, and especially so for old people with confusion and defects in memory.

There is another safety factor in adequate labeling. When the doctor cannot be reached or the pharmacist's records are in error, good labeling makes it possible to check on medications if allergic or other untoward reactions occur. The older person or another family member, often a child, may unwittingly take an overdose of a drug or take the wrong drug.

COST OF DRUGS

One should always think of cost in prescribing drugs for older persons. Medicare does not cover out-of-hospital prescription drugs, the largest single personal expenditure that the elderly must now meet almost entirely from their own resources.

Generic prescriptions help the pocketbooks of all patients, especially the elderly. For example, in 1971 reserpine,* which is the generic name of an antihypertensive drug, sold for $10 per 1,000 tablets, whereas Serpasil (reserpine by one brand name) sold for $49. Of some use is the *Handbook of Prescription Drugs* by Richard Burack (Pantheon Books' original publication in 1967, reprinted in 1970), which lists the generic drugs and explains how to obtain them.

*Beware of reserpine, for it is depressogenic. When you see a depressed person, check to see whether he or she is receiving reserpine for high blood pressure.

Discount drugs can be obtained by way of the National Council of Senior Citizens, the American Association of Retired Persons,* and some other organizations.

Drug packaging is another issue for older people. It would be useful if drug companies would use some special device in packaging drugs for old people, as they do with the "Pill," which aids the younger woman in remembering to take her contraceptives, through clever calendar dispensers. Such an aid would be invaluable in coping with the memory problems of late life.

OTHER FORMS OF PHYSICAL TREATMENT

Electroshock therapy (EST)

Ugo Cerletti, an Italian psychiatrist, in 1938 developed the use of electroshock to induce convulsion and loss of consciousness by placement of electrodes on the temporal areas of the skull.

If antidepressants in the context of a comprehensive psychotherapeutic plan have received an adequate trial without results, electroshock therapy is indicated in a severe, refractory depression.† Cases of clearly exogenous reactive depressions should not ordinarily be treated by EST. Psychometric tests (of intellectual function and memory) should be considered before the administering of EST, especially when organic brain damage is suspected.

After careful evaluation and under careful conditions, including the use of preshock sedation and muscle relaxants (such as Intocostrin) to avoid fractures, electroshock therapy can be quite effective against the depressions of old age. Effects on memory must be continually assessed, and the number of treatments should be minimal. Respiratory and cardiovascular complications may occur; neurological complications are

*William Hutton, Executive Director, National Council of Senior Citizens, and Bernard Nash, Executive Director, American Association of Retired Persons.

†Of course, drugs can be given concurrently.

rare. Care is strongly advised in instances of coronary occlusion, since fatalities have been reported.

In the presence of serious suicidal risk, it is not advisable to wait out drug trials. EST can often bring about prompt relief with a limited series of four to eight treatments. In severe and suicidal situations even a history of cerebrovascular accidents and/or myocardial infarctions (coronaries) is not a contraindication *per se.*

Unfortunately patients who have received electroshock treatment hesitate and resist returning to the doctor even years later if once again they develop serious depression. Fear and distaste of electroshock therapy are commonplace.

Hyperbaric oxygenation

Claims of improvement in chronic brain syndrome by hyperbaric oxygenation (oxygen administered under high pressure) are disputed.* Goldfarb, experienced in the assessment of older people, found no "improvement . . . in intellectual or social performance," and an "increase in physical activity, restlessness and aggressivity."†

*Jacobs, E. A., Winter, P. M., Alvis, H. A., and Small, S. M.: Hyperoxygenation effect on cognitive functioning in the aged, New England Journal of Medicine 281:753-757, 1969.

†Goldfarb, A. I., Hochstadt, N. J., Jacobson, J. H., II, and Weinstein, E. A.: Hyperbaric oxygen treatment of organic brain syndrome in aged persons, Journal of Gerontology 27:212-217, 1972.

REFERENCES

Burack, R.: Handbook of prescription drugs, New York, 1970, Pantheon Books, Inc.

Cole, J. O.: Methods for evaluating drug efficacy in geriatric-psychiatric disorders. In Levine, J., Schiels, B. C., and Bouthilet, L., editors: Principles and problems in establishing the efficacy of psychotropic agents, Public Health Service Pub. No. 2138, Washington, D. C., 1971, U. S. Government Printing Office.

Gallinek, A.: Electric convulsive therapy in geriatrics, New Jersey State Journal of Medicine 47:1233-1241, 1947.

Lifshitz, K., and Klein, N. S.: Psychopharmacological geriatrics. In Clark, W. G., and Del Guidice, J., editors: Principles of psychopharmacology, New York, 1970, Academic Press, Inc.

The Merck manual of diagnosis and therapy, ed. 12, Rahway, N. J., 1972, Merck, Sharp & Dohme Research Laboratories.

Physicians' desk reference to pharmaceutical specialties and biologicals, annual ed., Oradell, N. J., 1970, Medical Economics, Inc.

Prout, C. T., and Hamilton, D. M.: Results of electro-shock therapy in patients over 60 years of age, Bulletin of the New York Academy of Medicine 28:454-461, 1952.

Ray, O. S.: Tranquilizers and mood modifiers. In Ray, O. S., editor: Drugs, society and human behavior, St. Louis, 1972, The C. V. Mosby Co.

Tsuang, M. M., Lu, L. M., Stotsky, B. A., and Cole, J. O.: Haloperidol versus thioridazine for hospitalized psychogeriatric patients: double-blind study, Journal of the American Geriatrics Society 19:593-600, 1971.

14
TREATMENT OF SPECIFIC CONDITIONS

Some of the mental and emotional conditions that have been previously described are so crucial to mental health care in old age that we will focus specifically on their treatment in this chapter. Of special concern are the all-too-frequent organic brain syndromes, grief and depression, and paranoid states. Once again we emphasize the absolute necessity of diagnosing those conditions which are subject to improvement, especially the reversible brain syndromes and functional states. We shall also touch briefly on the treatment aspects of insomnia, parkinsonism, stroke, deafness, blindness, and emotional effects of retirement.

ORGANIC BRAIN SYNDROMES
Reversible (acute) brain syndromes

Many workers such as Cosin in Britain* have demonstrated the treatability of acute confusional states in the elderly. The work of Simon and his colleagues in the United States is a highly significant affirmation of the possibilities for the psychiatric care of old people. The 1959 Langley Porter studies provided information "quite different from that gathered in institutions for the chronically ill, and our results are more pertinent for the family physician or psychiatrist who deals first with the mentally disturbed aged patient."†

*Cosin, L. Z., Mort, Margaret, Post, F., Westropp, Celia, and Williams, Moyra: Experimental treatment of persistent senile confusion, The International Journal of Social Psychiatry 4:24-42, 1958.
†Simon, A., and Cahan, R. B.: The acute brain syndrome in geriatric patients. In Mandell, W. M., and Epstein, L. J., editors: Acute psychotic reaction. Psychiatric Research Reports of the American Psychiatric Association, Washington, D. C., 1966, American Psychiatric Association, p. 9.

Sound diagnosis is of the essence.* Persons with reversible brain syndromes must have early active treatment to enhance their likelihood of recovery. Whether the syndrome stands alone or is superimposed on a chronic brain syndrome, it is imperative that there be immediate treatment of the underlying acute pathophysiological disturbance. (One may have to send someone to look in the person's medicine chest to determine whether any drugs are responsible—for example, antihistamines, sold without prescription, can be a culprit. Nitrogen retention following upon urinary tract infection may be causative. See Chapter 5 for other possible contributory factors.) Thorough diagnosis requires a comprehensive evaluation and treatment center. At present the elderly are not likely to receive such care in the United States. As disreputable as state hospitals can be, it is still more likely that an older person will get an appropriate workup there than at a general hospital or community mental health center. An evaluation may not be done at all in a nursing home situation.

Treatment of the reversible brain syndrome includes maintenance of adequate fluid and caloric intake. Intravenous fluids (sodium chloride or dextrose) and tube feedings may be required. Oxygen inhala-

*One study (Ellenbogen, B. K.: Subarachnoid hemorrhage in the elderly, Gerontologica Clinica **12**:115-120, 1970) reported that of 72 patients with spontaneous subarachnoid hemorrhage, 37 were age 60 or over. Neck stiffness and disturbed consciousness were important signs. Uniformly, bloodstained cerebrospinal fluid was found on lumbar puncture.

tion may be necessary. Tranquilization, judiciously prescribed, can be most valuable; but this should not be continued beyond the immediate need. Preferred hypnotics are nonbarbiturates and chloral hydrate. Constipation to the point of impaction can cause reversible brain disorders. When laxatives are needed, we recommend senna concentrate.* In general, with conservative, supportive treatment, some 50% of patients with RBS's survive and can return home.

Advances in internal medicine and surgery aid in the prevention and treatment of reversible brain syndromes. To take just one example, the "black patch syndrome" (cataract deliria) after eye surgery has been reduced through careful preoperative preparation and efforts toward continuing orientation, with the presence of familiar persons and the use of familiar objects throughout the postoperative recovery period.

Chronic brain syndromes

There is no definitive treatment for the two major organic disorders of old age, cerebral arteriosclerosis and senile brain disease. Reversal or arrest is impossible with our present knowledge.† But much can be done for the patient by suitably adjusting the environment. Structuring of a medically and socially prosthetic milieu whether at home or in an institution is important. Simplification, order, the balancing of care versus self-care, the moderation of stimuli (avoiding the Goldstein catastrophic reaction), the provision of recreation and occupational therapy, and the utilization of objects, personnel, and techniques to preserve orientation are among general procedures of value. Home care services oriented toward the chronic brain syndrome patients can be excellent when available. Supportive individual and/or group psychotherapy for the patient and his family is often advisable. When agitation is present, one should first try the minor tranquilizers; then thioridazine (Mellaril) is the agent of choice (Chapter 13). We have already presented principles of home care (Chapter 10) and institutional care (Chapter 11).

GRIEF AND DEPRESSION

Depressive reactions

It is dismaying at times how refractory the depressions of later life can be. Nonetheless, depending on the type, degree, and duration, considerable relief is possible. With milder depressions associated with a sense of personal insignificance ("over the hill," "out to pasture"), the therapist should help the older person find a role, a place, an activity of authentic interest.

With the more serious depressions (death of loved one, serious illness, other loss), psychotherapy, drugs, and/or electroconvulsive therapy may be employed. The psychotherapeutic approach may not always be oriented toward insight, because insight might be unbearable. On the other hand, one must not conclude that supportive psychotherapy is the method of choice with older people. The person is likely to be preoccupied by his painful thoughts and feelings, so the help of another, a professional therapist or a friend, through open discussion may be very liberating. Particularly valuable is the release of anger, grief, and guilt. As with the milder depressive states, attention must also be given to the personal and social context. The possibility of suicide must be carefully weighed, particularly in the old man.

The masking of depression by traits subsumed under the wastebasket term "senility" has long been recognized. Psychotherapeutic intervention and electroshock therapy have demonstrated the "organic" simulation of

*Simple matters like fevers, some cathartics, and impactions can cause intellectual confusion. Drastic cathartics such as cascara, saline cathartics, and milk of magnesia can cause severe electrolyte imbalances. Standardized senna granules may be the best and safest laxative.

†Some investigators (Albrecht, Ruth: Social roles in the prevention of senility, Journal of Gerontology 6:380-386, 1951) feel that more appropriate social roles and activities would retard or even eliminate some forms of "senility." While this requires further study, it is a provocative point.

depression.* Anxiety is also masked by seemingly organic symptoms such as "rigidity," as Atkin pointed out.†

Anger, considered a crucial element in most depressions, is not a diagnostic entity yet perhaps should be.‡ There are many manifestations of anger—violence, cold hostility, sarcasm, defiance, tantalizing and teasing, sneering, passive obstructiveness (either dependent or aggressive), gossip, withdrawal, and, of course, self-destructive behavior to the point of suicide. We stress anger for several reasons in our therapeutic work. Anger must be confronted and expressed. However, the expression of anger is not enough, and, contrary to popular cant, is not a magical cure-all. Anger can be a cover for deeper problems that may be centered, for instance, around the need for intimacy and a profound sense of deprivation. These underlying problems must be brought out. Direct confrontation may be necessary.

It is also necessary to deal directly with feelings of helplessness. The woman who has nursed her dying husband is one illustration of the "giving up–given up" complex that Engel, Schmale, and Greene of the University of Rochester School of Medicine have described.§ (See Chapter 4.)

Helping the dying person

Psychotherapy and physical care

Dr. Melvin J. Krant, professor at Tufts University Medical School in Boston and director of a cancer unit, has written an article, "The organized care of the dying patient,"‖ which contains many ideas that could be adopted by other hospitals. He observed, "Helping someone die well should be conceived as a positive part of health care . . ."

His organization moves beyond the walls of the hospital, including home visits. Fundamentally, Krant and his co-workers and others who have contributed to the field concentrate on the elimination of camouflage from the care of the dying.

> A modern hospice was planned, built, and staffed under the guidance of Dr. Cicely Saunders to enable patients who are in the last states of their illness to have a peaceful and above all, a tranquil closure to life and to be supportive to the patients' relatives and friends in their bereavement. "Contrary to common belief, patients in the proper atmosphere, and helped by modern medicine and nursing, can be maintained in an alert and peaceful frame of mind to the last . . ."¶

In her work Elisabeth Kübler-Ross has not only delineated five stages in the psychology of dying but developed a therapeutic approach (Chapter 3). Analgesics are obviously important, but intractable pain and anxiety must be aided also through personal help. Some have advocated mind-expanding drugs such as LSD and also heroin, but these are not available for use in the United States and their desirability is questionable.

To work effectively with death and dying, the therapist and other staff should be part

---

*Clow, H. E.: Psychiatric factors in the rehabilitation of the aging, Mental Hygiene **34**:592-599, 1950.

Clow, H. E., and Allen, E. B.: A study of depressive states in the aging, Geriatrics **4**:11-17, 1949.

Kaufman, M. R.: Old age and aging: the psychoanalytic point of view, American Journal of Orthopsychiatry **10**:73-79, 1940.

Ehrenberg, R., and Gullingsrud, M. J.: Electroconvulsive therapy in elderly patients, American Journal of Psychiatry **11**:743-747, 1955.

†Atkin, S.: Discussion of the paper by M. R. Kaufman on old age and aging: the psychoanalytic point of view, American Journal of Orthopsychiatry **10**:79-83, 1940.

‡It may be a reflection of Western civilization that anxiety and depression are considered diagnostic entities but anger is not.

§Schmale, Jr., A. H.: Relationships of separation and depression to disease. I. A report on the hospitalized medical population, Psychosomatic Medicine **20**:259-277, 1958.

Greene, W. A.: Disease response to life stress, Journal of the American Medical Women's Association **20**:133-146, 1965.

Engel, G. L., and Schmale, Jr., A. H.: Psychoanalytic theory of somatic disorder: conversion, specificity, and the disease onset situation, Journal of the American Psychoanalytic Association **15**:344-365, 1967.

‖Krant, Melvin J.: The organized care of the dying patient, Hospital Practice **7**:101-108, 1972.

¶From editorial, St. Christopher's Hospice, Lawrie Park Road, London Nursing Times, July 28, 1967.

of ongoing seminars, workshops, staff conferences.

We do not agree with claims that "the time is short, too short for the attempt to start another life and to try out alternate roads to integrity." We find that the fundamental issues in life and consequently in psychotherapy—love, guilt and atonement, separation and integration—can be dealt with to the very end of life itself. It is imperative to encourage the life review and thus aid in the resolution of old as well as recent conflicts. Each person should have the opportunity to live as fully as possible up to the moment of his death. It is unthinking and cruel to write off as untreatable those people who have no dependable "future" as long as they have a "present" existence.

Allowing death

There are medicolegal considerations that go beyond psychotherapeutic efforts with the dying. Technical knowledge has made it possible to preserve life in persons who would have died in the past—and in the absence of apparent sentience—by artificial support of circulation, respiration, and nutrition.

Who is to make the decision to allow someone to die? Mental health personnel may be called upon to help make such a decision. The doctor may have moral concerns or be fearful about future litigation. Malpractice suits have skyrocketed. His training is appropriately directed toward the prolongation of life and it may be wise indeed for society to sustain that commitment in the medical profession.

The mental health specialist can help by individual or collective discussions with all pertinent participants: the person himself, if feasible, the family, the doctor, the clergyman, the lawyer, even business colleagues. One must check to see if the individual's house is in order and if appropriate arrangements have been made in the interest of the person, his family, and the "natural objects of his affection." He may *need* or desire to live only to complete certain personal and tax arrangements. Some persons and their families may want to sustain life until after a granddaughter is born, for example, or a favored grandchild has married.

Mental health workers' contributions should be in the nature of fact-finding—as to both the practical and the emotional aspects of the situation. The family should not be put into the difficult position of finally deciding, for the doctor has the ultimate responsibility. He must decide not to force-feed by tube or needle. But his decision and his conscience must derive from hard data, in the context of moral and legal situations.

The "right to die"

Why sustain a "vegetable life" at the suffering of the person and great expense to the family? Among many others, Walter C. Alvarez* has outlined the case for "passive euthanasia," letting people die who are suffering and beyond help. Pope Pius XII stated that when a person is in coma and is beyond recovery, there is no need to employ "extraordinary means" to keep him alive. An Episcopal priest has said, "The Christian obligation of everyone involved is primarily to administer to the person, not to the disease. I personally would like to see euthanasia available to those who want it. If the doctor is too dedicated to fighting the disease, he may forget the person." A Miami physician, Dr. Walter Sackett, who is also a member of Florida's legislature, introduced a "death with dignity bill." Many others however, feel it is impossible to predict death, that persons have recovered from comas, that tampering with death is sacrilegious, or that death itself is such an insult and tragedy that any compliance with it is inhumane. Thus we hear debate over the "right to die with dignity."

Ideally, there should be a panel to make the decision about death—made up of the patient, his family, his advisors, his doctor, an independent lawyer, theologian or clergyman, social worker. It is not simply a matter of taking a vote, but making a thoughtful decision. There is something

*The old man who wanted to die (editorial), Geriatrics **26**:57, 1971.

called a "Living Will,"* a document that a person can sign requesting that if he or she is unable to make decisions, doctors will honor his request by not prolonging his life. "Laws have to be very carefully written, otherwise you'll end up with human guinea pigs like they had in Nazi Germany," said Dr. Angelo D'Agostino, who is both a psychiatrist and a Jesuit priest.

Funeral arrangements

Unlike the Victorians, we do not see the "good funeral" and its obsequies as life's ultimate reward. It is generally accepted that the American funeral system is outrageously expensive and offers little in the way of meaningful psychological support to mourners (Mitford, 1963). Families are vulnerable to entrenched customs, the dubious approaches of some funeral directors, and the sense that they must "do right by" the deceased. The shock and grief of death is rapidly surcharged with guilt. In 1970 the average American funeral cost $1,000, including cemetery costs. This amount of money may bring comfort to funeral directors but does little to comfort those who may have already outstripped their resources on care of the person while he was alive.

Nonprofit memorial societies offer simple, dignified, and economical funeral arrangements, somewhere between $100 and $500.† They tend to make life easier for survivors and give the deceased some control over his own demise. These societies are organized as non-profit organizations, democratically controlled by their members.‡ They are usually initiated by a church or a ministerial association and occasionally by labor, civic, or educational groups. Most have lifetime membership fees of $10 to $15, plus a $5 records charge at the time of death.

One can write the Continental Association of Funeral and Memorial Societies at 59 East Van Buren Street, Chicago, Illinois 60605; or the Memorial Society Association of Canada at P. O. Box 4367, Vancouver, British Columbia. There are memorial societies in more than a hundred cities in the United States and Canada. (These societies do not sell funerals or cemetery lots in advance.)

Memorial services can offer valid "psychotherapy" for survivors. "In a funeral the center of attention is the dead body; the emphasis is on death. In a memorial service the center of concern is the personality of the individual who has died . . ." An honest appraisal of the deceased—with both liabilities and assets—can help the survivors work through their own complicated feelings, sometimes cast in an excessive idealization that may actually prolong grief.

In addition to earth burial and cremation, bequeathal to a medical school performs a valuable service* and saves expense. Only the Orthodox Jewish faith objects to bequeathal of one's body or of organs for transplant. With changing religious attitudes and the desire to spare survivors soaring funeral costs, there are now more bodies donated than needed by medical schools in some parts of the country. Some people—status-conscious to the end—want to leave their bodies to prestige schools like Harvard.

---

*One can write to the Euthanasia Educational Fund, 250 West 57th St., New York City, for free copies of what is called "A Living Will."

†Social Security provides a lump sum death benefit. This is a variable amount, which may be as much as three times the monthly benefit the deceased worker would have received if he had lived to retirement age, up to a maximum of $255.

‡A manual of simple burial, by Ernest Morgan, describes memorial societies in detail. (Obtainable from the Continental Association of Funeral and Memorial Societies.)

*Eye and temporal bone banks as well as the Kidney Foundation also give the person a sense of valued legacy. Usually only the corneas of old people are acceptable, however. There is now a Uniform Anatomical Gift Act or its equivalent in every state and most Canadian provinces. A Uniform Donor's Card filled out and signed by the donor and two witnesses (three in Florida) constitutes a legal document. The person now has final say over the disposition of his body. However, if a family strongly objects, most institutions will not go against its wishes.

Mourning*

Geoffrey Gorer observed that the majority of the people today are "without adequate guidance as to how to treat death and bereavement and without social help in coming to terms with grief and mourning."† He describes three distinct stages: the first, a short period of shock lasting for a few days; the second, a time of intense grief during which the mourner suffers psychological changes such as listlessness, disturbed sleep, failure of appetite, and loss of weight; and, third, a gradual reawakening to an interest in life. Gorer emphasizes that during the second phase, lasting six to twelve weeks, "the mourner is in more need of social support and assistance than at any time since infancy and early childhood."

It might be said: where depression is, let grief be. If grief is denied outlet, a depression is one of the possibilities. Insulation or denial of grief is not the sole cause of depression, of course, since ambivalence toward the deceased (that is, anger and conflict) complicates the usual course of grief. It is the task of therapy to help open up the grief process. For example, the widows or widowers should be encouraged to discuss whether they felt they did all that could be done. It is the goal of prevention to see that grief is never stopped up to begin with.

The impact of bereavement cannot be minimized. Rees and Lutkins have shown a greater mortality of survivors within six months of a loss than among controls of similar age.‡ Data on 4,486 widowers, 55 years of age and older, have been collected for a nine-year period following the death of their wives in 1957.§ Of these, 213 died during the first six months of bereavement, 40% above the expected rate for married men of the same age. Thereafter, the mortality rate fell gradually to that of married men and remained at about the same level. The greatest increase in mortality during the first six months was found in the widowers dying from coronary thrombosis and other arteriosclerotic and degenerative heart disease. There was also evidence of a true increase in mortality from other diseases, although the numbers of individual categories were too small for statistical analysis. In the first six months 22.5% of the deaths were from the same diagnostic group as the wife's death.

Perhaps even more painful to the older person than the death of a spouse is the loss of a grown child. This experience is more likely to occur the longer the older person lives. Many people consider such deaths to be against the laws of nature, and feelings can be extremely difficult to resolve.

Plight of the surviving spouse

There are the practical as well as the emotional problems associated with widowhood—relationships with in-laws, children, financial matters, governmental benefits, unwanted callers who read the death announcement in the papers. Some decisions, such as selling one's home, moving to a completely new location, etc., are best delayed until part of the mourning period is past and the person has greater perspective and energy at hand.

Widowhood, as a process, is often a year's emotional journey as one moves in fresh and painful memory through all the anniversaries and holidays that may have meant so much, even in conflict as well as in warmth. At least one year of anniversaries—birthdays, Thanksgiving, the Christmas season, Fourth of July, etc.—must often be experienced nostalgically and sadly before one is ready to again take up life wholeheartedly. The oldest and the youngest spouses may take even longer. Consolation is difficult and indeed may not be accepted at all. In therapy the task is to open up grief, uncover any

---

*See also Chapter 4.

†He feels that only the Orthodox Jew through formal ritual patterns of religious observance receives the comfort and discipline required to resolve grief.

‡Rees, W. D., and Lutkins, S. G.: Mortality of bereavement, British Medical Journal 4:13-16, 1967.

§Parkes, C. M., Benjamin, B., and Fitzgerald, R. G.: Broken heart: a statistical study of increased mortality among widowers, British Medical Journal 1:740-743, 1969.

complicating anger, help the person face his or her envy of married friends, develop new relationships, and find activities and meaning. A comfortable standard of living (so often absent) helps in the struggle against apathy and isolation. Because of social and cultural attitudes that have negated previous experience with finances, some widowed women often need considerable help, not only in obtaining but also in managing finances. (See Chapter 6.)

The widower may also have special problems. If he has been the typical husband, he may be totally unprepared to cook for himself, sew on buttons, etc. and will need concrete assistance in learning how to do things for himself.

Socially the surviving spouses may have a difficult time of it, especially women. They are often left out by old and good friends, for they are now "fifth wheels." If attractive, others' wives may shun them; if dreary and mournful, everyone will stay away. Self-pity and outrage at one's fate are futile, and action of a constructive sort must be encouraged to get the person back into contact with understanding but not patronizing people.

The Widow-to-Widow program was established in the Boston area as an experimental mental health program of preventive intervention directed at new widows and staffed by other widows. It is based on the premise that the best helper of a widow at the time of grief is another widow. Silverman wrote, "Since statistics indicate a higher risk of emotional and psychiatric disturbances among younger widowed women than is to be expected from the population at large, this program was established to find ways of reaching those women (all recently widowed and under the age of 60) to determine what services would ease their distress and grief and, thereby, lessen the possibility of their developing a psychiatric disorder."* With the program's emphasis on younger women we see again the prejudice, undoubtedly unwitting, that old people suffer less. It also has not been extended to widowers.

*From Silverman, Phyllis R.: The Widow-to-Widow program, Archives of the Foundation of Thanatology 2:133-135, 1970.

However, the idea is a promising one and could very well be set up in various communities, applying the concept to men as well as women, and at all ages. It is believed that the helping widows—and widowers—should receive a series of orienting lectures and participate in a continuing seminar in order to review available knowledge and to help work through the many painful feelings and countertransference reactions that occur.

Alcoholics Anonymous (for survivors who develop or who have had drinking problems) and Parents Without Partners are also self-help organizations that have been very useful. It is important to have professional skills on hand without at the same time downplaying or interfering with the "natural" talents of the nonprofessionals. Voluntarism, however valuable, must not be misused as a substitute for necessary professional services.

Silverman makes a good point, valued by us as a significant rationale for life crisis group psychotherapy. "Most mental health agencies serve those suffering from a defined psychiatric disorder, such as depression, rather than those in need of preventive services as they pass through a life crisis. This may be because most people suffering from the 'hazard of living' that occurs with the death of a spouse do not consult with such agencies unless a prior contact has been established."*

Post-Cana is the Catholic lay association for widows and widowers set up to "assist and promote the solution of those spiritual, parental, psychological, financial, social, and other problems arising directly or indirectly from the untimely death of a husband or wife."

Widowhood illustrates well the significance of employment counseling and placement to mental health. For both practical

*From Silverman, Phyllis R.: Ibid.

reasons (income reduction through widowhood) and the appropriate need for activity, work may be needed. There exist in some communities "Over-60 Counseling and Employment Services." The U. S. Employment Service should also be pressured to serve the elderly. Low-income elderly may be eligible to participate in various programs (which however only operate in some areas): Green Thumb and Green Light, Senior Aides, Foster Grandparents. Other federal programs such as VISTA and the Peace Corps (under ACTION) are not really set up to help the poor elderly but might be useful in any case, and particularly to skilled people who, out of need to contribute or because of loneliness, may be interested.

In some measure, so long as the Protestant ethic is so influential, older people are likely to seek "something to do" even when financial as well as other psychological and interpersonal considerations are not so crucial.

Therapy of body losses

Our efforts with respect to grief and restitution do not only apply to helping the dying in their grief and the survivors in theirs, but in dealing with the loss of people's body parts, organs, and functions. Help with feelings about limb amputation, mastectomy, and disfiguration is important. The loss of internal organs has still other psychological meanings and requires special help, as does the loss of sensory capacities—blindness and deafness. Losses of sexual capacities are especially poignant. Some 15 million persons over 65 suffer from serious chronic disease.

Suicide

Suicide cannot be treated; only prevented —Or can it? Suicide Prevention Centers have not had the impact of reducing suicide hoped for by Shneideman, Farberow, and others. The National Institute of Mental Health even closed down its Center for Studies of Suicide Prevention in 1972 (established in 1966). Old people did call the centers, but that mechanism has not been demonstrated to be a means of averting suicide. Telephone therapy by which most suicide centers operate may help people in other emotional crises, but not reduce suicide.

Immediate and supportive treatment when suicide has been attempted is of course indicated. For example, barbiturate poisoning, regardless of the dose taken, need not be fatal. Tracheotomy, peritoneal dialysis, active physiological treatment, and psychological support can save lives.

Should suicide always be prevented in old age? This is a difficult question; we already considered the "right to die" issue. In older persons, the desire for death may be refractory, persuasive, rational, and deliberate rather than irrational and precipitous. The absence of euthanasia may force some individuals to suicide.

We have more fully discussed potential suicide, including treatment, in Chapter 4 but wish to emphasize once again that depression-based suicide is perhaps the most preventable through treatment. There are a number of other motivations for self-destruction, which may not be easily amenable to therapy.

PARANOID STATES

Many paranoid individuals survive in the community throughout their lives. The situation of some paranoid patients worsens with age, as a result of the continuing contraction of their lives—further isolation through deaths of loved ones and acquaintances, with whom there may have been few contacts to begin with. When hostile paranoid feelings and/or delusions are specifically directed against other persons, hospitalization may be necessary, if only briefly. (This is the basis of the laws regarding the mentally ill where reference is made of "danger to others.")

It is an absolute necessity—and we purposely emphasize *absolute*—that one must be scrupulously honest with paranoid patients; one should be so with all patients, but the paranoid cannot accept our usual lapses. The therapist must be attentive, make reasonable suggestions, and be firm, combining warmth with detachment. The therapist must *not* "be nice," give out reassurances, or accept everything that is said. Nothing turns paranoids off more than to think they are being "buttered up." At various points there must be frank disagreements. If the patient and therapist never disagree, that too spells trouble. The therapist has to take issue with the patient or the latter ceases to believe in him. The therapist must have self-confidence and know what he is talking about (having listened long and hard). It is difficult to sustain a therapeutic relationship of trust with the paranoid patient; rapport is slow in building; work may be long-term.

Paranoid persons, having been deeply emotionally deprived, yearn for closeness and will not spurn it. They desire love despite their outward appearance of, for instance, withdrawn hostility. He or she has had years of "training" at recognizing phony talk. Irony and humor—referring to the universalities of the human condition—are valuable. The therapist must seek to get "behind the defenses" and understand the underlying anxiety. If he can obtain knowledge of when the symptom developed, he may be able to alter the equilibrium or eliminate the need for the symptom effectively without ever discussing the delusional systems. Environmental manipulation may be therapeutic but should be done openly.

Work with family can help only when the paranoid person is present. The therapist must help the older paranoid person with hearing impairments, through hearing aids. Tranquilizers, judiciously employed, may help somewhat when agitation is present.

RETIREMENT SYNDROME

A retired editor wrote "retirement will soon be the largest occupation in America." Many American men, reared in obeisance to the Protestant ethic of useful, lifelong, productive labor, find it painful to discover that they are not indispensable to their work or organization; then they must discover that work is not indispensable for their survival and happiness. They may need either to find new forms of "work" or new means of enjoying idleness.

There is undoubtedly much mythology in the notion of a "retirement syndrome." People who retire do not automatically develop declining mental and physical health. Streib and Schneider's* studies, like others, indicate any such generalization to be a fallacy. On the other hand, social scientists may inadvertently overlook those individuals for whom retirement is pathogenic. Reconciliation of clinical experience and social science data is often difficult because the individual gets buried within the larger data. Thus, although there may be no general retirement syndrome, clinical indications are that some individuals are badly affected. It is a function of economics, personality, and general health—in short, of the range of factors affecting an individual.

In 1971, 105,000 federal workers who could retire chose not to do so. In Streib and Schneider's work they found that "both men and women of higher income levels, higher educational attainments, and higher levels of occupational structure tend to work longer than their counterparts with lower socioeconomic status."

On the other hand, some groups cannot retire fast enough, usually those holding tedious, assembly line type or heavy labor type jobs. The latter, by the way, show some improvement, not decline, in health as a result of retirement, which is not so surprising. But this again illustrates how difficult it is to generalize from either the clinical or the social science perspective. What becomes clear, in our judgment, is the need for continuing specificity of research with careful, detailed studies of various categories (and not only socioeconomic classes and occupations) of people.

INSOMNIA

Sleep is a vital restorative in old age. It is myth to think the old need less sleep. They need more activity, meaningful and sensible, along with exercise and appropriate rest to support their activities. Early morning awakening is more common among the inactive,

*Streib, G. F., and Schneider, C. J.: Retirement in American society; impact and process, Ithaca, N. Y., 1971, Cornell University Press.

who retire early and take catnaps (sometimes steps toward serious day-night sleep reversal). This is not to say that a daily siesta is not valuable (Spanish men outlive American men!). Old people often need more sleep,* not less, because of the illnesses and degenerative diseases that create fatigue, headache, gastrointestinal complaints, aches, and pains.

Insomniacs fear sleep itself. With sleep, their defenses against anxiety, anger, and other emotions are down—which may have been functioning poorly enough while awake. Psychotherapy can help to understand the individual's basis for insomnia. The establishment of simple rituals is in order; warm tubs, well-made bed, bed boards for support, back massage, wine, warm Saki (Japanese rice beer) are all simple measures that should be tried before hypnotic drugs are used. There should be no "standing orders" on hypnotics. They should be reevaluated routinely. Active, pleasurable sexual activity, including masturbation, can be excellent sleep inducers.

In the elderly, arthritic pains and poor circulation lead to discomfort that provokes early awakening. Thus they do best with a hypnotic having slow onset and long duration of action. Analgesics such as salicylates may help.

Deep sleep (called delta sleep), the period of dreamless oblivion, lessens with, and may vanish, in old age. Moreover, REM (Rapid Eye Movements) periods decline with chronic brain syndrome (less dream time).†

PARKINSONISM (PARALYSIS AGITANS, THE SHAKING PALSY)

Persons who suffered with the 1919 influenza may develop parkinsonism in late life. But most cases are not understood (idiopathic is the term often used by physicians when that is the case). Arteriosclerosis is no longer believed to play a major role in parkinsonism. Of course, phenothiazines are often responsible.

The course of the disease is slow, characterized by rigidity of the whole body, "resting tremor," and slowness of movement. The tremor is notable for a "pill-rolling" movement of the fingers, accompanied by shaking head and shuffling gait (which are often all a source of embarrassment). The posture is usually stooped, with the head forward and elbows flexed. The facial expression is masked, lacking emotional expression, but the person is usually depressed. The disease affects men twice as frequently as women and rarely begins before 40 or after 65.

Emotional excitement and fatigue do appear to augment the tremor. A calm existence, if possible, is advisable—but not inactivity. A measured life is the disideratum. Massage and passive movement may help the rigidity. Drugs are invaluable. It is beyond the scope of this book to detail the various agents, including, most recently, L-dopa.* It is important for the therapist to deal with embarrassment and depression, to help in establishing a meaningful life, and to familiarize himself with the drugs the patient is taking so as to not misinterpret symptoms. The latter point, of course, is a crucial generalization; one should have the *Physicians' Desk Reference* handy to help assay drug effects.

STROKE

It is pitiful indeed when potentially rehabilitatable poststroke elderly patients are left dormant and bedridden. As many as

---

*Tiller, Philip M., Jr.: Bed rest, sleep, and symptoms. Study of older persons, Annals of International Medicine 61:98-105, 1964.

†Feinberg, Irwin, Koresko, Richard L., and Schaffner, Isabella R.: Sleep electroencephalographic and eye-movement patterns in patients with chronic brain syndrome, Journal of Psychiatric Research 3:11-26, 1965.

*Trihexyphenidyl HC1 or L-dopa (L-3, 4-dihydroxyphenylalanine) is found useful. Cotzins firmly established the clinical usefulness of L-dopa. It helps relieve the rigidity and akinesia, but has less effect upon the tremor. Side effects have included hallucinations, persistent vomiting, hypotension, and depression. See Cotzins, G. C., Van Woert, M. H., and Schiffer, I. M.: Aromatic amino acids and modifications of parkinsonism, New England Journal of Medicine 276:374-379, 1967.

75% have been estimated to have the capacity to ambulate successfully—with the assistance of a wheelchair, with crutches, canes, braces, or walkers, and even without assistance. Staff has to be trained to go beyond the provision of basic physical care. They must work against patient apathy by stimulating motivation, helping the person face his disability but not directly or subtly encouraging him to give up.

Patients who have been discharged from occupational and/or physical therapy as "having received maximum benefit" should not then be neglected and allowed to lapse back into inactivity. Staff members may do irreparable harm by "overnursing," providing full body care, grooming, bathing, and dressing, while the patient's previous gains in therapy disappear.

Psychologically, the stroke patient must come to some terms with his disability, and his inevitable depression must be treated. The difficult struggle of the person is sometimes interpreted as irritability and cantankerousness. Individual therapy is indicated if available, but group techniques can be quite useful.* Socialization can be coupled with exercise (e.g., use of exercise pulley for arms and access to parallel bars), games (such as throwing darts), exercise to music. Patients are also encouraged to eat and socialize together. Reading and discussion are valuable. Patient participation in the planning of therapy is beneficial.

HEARING AND VISUAL IMPAIRMENTS

Perceptual impairments are of great import to the elderly, most especially hearing loss. As we have stated over and over again, comprehensive evaluation is crucial.† When perceptual deficiencies are found, the mental health worker must consult with appropriate specialists in an endeavor to provide prosthetic help. Institutionalized older patients in mental hospitals and nursing homes are likely to be neglected in these respects. The attitude may be that "it hardly matters."

Those who are hard-of-hearing are often embarrassed, depressed, isolated, and suspicious—sometimes to the point of paranoid proportions. These feelings, trends, or states must be worked through. The deaf person is also frequently embarrassed over the hearing aid and this concern, too, must be resolved.

Both the hard-of-hearing and those with visual problems benefit from individual and group therapy. There are other special efforts that can be made—from the teaching of Braille for the totally blind to the provision of large-type newspapers (e.g., *The New York Times*) and cookbooks for the visually impaired. "Talking books" recorded on records or tape are useful. A sense of active aid and the elimination of isolation are key components in the care of those with perceptual deficits.

THOUGHTS ON NUTRITION

The most common causes of dietary inadequacy in the elderly are poor dietary habits, poverty, and complications of underlying disease states, including alcoholism and depression, with the latter an especially frequent contributor to malnutrition.

Other diseases or changes associated with aging that may affect nutrition and thus contribute to malnutrition include decreased gastric acidity, biliary tract and pancreatic diseases, fevers, especially if prolonged, and cancer.

In dealing with elderly patients, the physician will have to work with complex dietary prescriptions for various medical problems. He needs to know the practical limits of compliance by his patient, including how well-motivated the patient is and the patient's ability to shop for and prepare a special diet.

There is much remaining to be learned about nutrition for people of every age. It

---

*Bier, Ruth: The nurse's management of the aged dependent patient, ANA Regional Clinical Conference 6:16-23, 1965.

†Testing should be obtained at a local Hearing Society or be done by a specialist in otolaryngology. One must be careful of "testing" by hearing aid salesmen. Fraud is all too common. Both hearing and the hearing aid must be continuously checked.

is not enough for medical science to content itself with teaching the "basic five foods" to the public; a good deal of research needs to be done on the effects (both therapeutic and detrimental) of the many food substances and food elements on the human body and its health and its diseases. At present there appears to be "no compelling evidence" that the elderly require different nutrition than mature adults. But it must be remembered that in spite of much medical reassurance to the contrary, many mature adults are improperly nourished—whether out of necessity (inadequate income, etc.), habit, or lack of information. Cultural food habits (snack foods and "junk" foods, to name a few) chemical additives (preservatives, plant and animal growth stimulators, insecticides, pesticides, and herbicides), and food preparation (overcooking, overspicing—especially with salt—and the refining of flours and sugars) all contribute to a questionable national diet. An abundance of food should not be mistaken for high-quality food.

REFERENCES

Berezin, M. A., and Cath, S. H., editors: Geriatric psychiatry: grief, loss and emotional disorders in the aging process, New York, 1965, International Universities Press.

Bowlby, J.: Childhood mourning and its implications for psychiatry, American Journal of Psychiatry **118**:481-498, 1961.

Cameron, D. Ewen: Studies in senile nocturnal delirium, Psychiatric Quarterly **15**:47-53, 1941.

Carp, Frances, editor: Retirement, New York, 1972, Behavioral Publishers, Inc.

Eissler, Kurt: The psychiatrist and the dying patient, New York, 1955, International Universities Press.

Engel, George L.: Is grief a disease? A challenge for medical research, Psychosomatic Medicine **23**:18-22, 1961.

Engel, George L., and Romano, J.: Delirium: a syndrome of cerebral insufficiency, Journal of Chronic Diseases **9**:260-277, 1959.

Farberow, N. L., editor: Taboo topics, New York, 1963, Atherton Press.

Feifel, H.: Older persons look at death, Geriatrics **2**:127-130, 1956.

Glaser, B. G., and Strauss, A.: Awareness of dying, Chicago, 1965, Aldine Publishing Co.

Gorer, G.: Death, grief and mourning in contemporary Britain, London, 1965, Cresset Press.

Howell, Sandra, and Loeb, M.: Nutrition in aging: A monograph for practitioners, The Gerontologist **9**:1-122, 1969.

Kastenbaum, R.: The mental life of the dying geriatric patient, Proceedings of the International Congress of Gerontology, No. 842, Vienna, June 26 to July 7, 1966.

Kübler-Ross, Elisabeth: On death and dying, New York, 1969, The Macmillan Co.

Langer, Marian F.: Learning to live as a widow, New York, 1957, Gilbert Press, Inc.

Lindemann, Erich: Symptomatology and management of acute grief, American Journal of Psychiatry **101**:141-148, 1944.

Mitford, Jessica: The American way of death, New York, 1963, Simon & Schuster, Inc.

Munnichs, J. A. M.: Old age and finitude; a contribution to psychogerontology, White Plains, N. Y., 1966, Albert J. Phiebig Books.

Nagy, M. H.: The child's view of death. In Feifel, H., editor: The meaning of death, New York, 1959, McGraw-Hill Book Co., Inc.

Schoenberg, Barnard, Carr, Arthur C., Peretz, David, and Kutscher, Austin, editors: Loss and grief: psychological management in medical practice, New York, 1971, Columbia University Press.

Sheps, J.: Paranoid mechanisms in the aged, Psychiatry **21**:399-404, 1958.

Tichener, J., Zeverling, I., Gottschalk, L., and Levine, M.: Psychological reactions of the aged in surgery, Archives of Neurology and Psychiatry **79**:63-73, 1958.

Tolstoi, L.: The death of Ivan Ilych and other stories, New York, 1969, The New American Library of World Literature.

Talmon, Yenina: Aging II, Social aspects. In International encyclopedia of the social sciences, vol. 1, New York, 1968, The Macmillan Co.

Ullman, M.: Behavioral changes in patients following strokes, Springfield, Ill., 1962, Charles C Thomas, Publisher.

U. S. Department of Health, Education and Welfare. Strike back at stroke, U. S. Public Health Service Pub. No. 596. Washington, D. C., 1958, U. S. Government Printing Office.

U. S. Senate Special Committee on Aging: Hearings on hearing loss, hearing aids, and the elderly, Washington, D. C., 1968, U. S. Government, Printing Office.

Verwoerdt, A.: Communication with the fatally ill, Springfield, Ill., 1966, Charles C Thomas, Publisher.

Weinberg, Jack: Psychologic implication of the nutritional needs of the elderly, Journal of the American Dietetic Association **60**:293-296, April, 1972.

Wertenbaker, L. T.: Death of a man, New York, 1957, Random House, Inc.

15
OLD AGE AND THE FUTURE

Anyone who faces with older people the frequent and often intense struggles of their daily lives wonders how some of them keep alive the sense that new and good things can still happen. More remarkably, a number of the elderly maintain a capacity for creativity until very late in life, in spite of physical and emotional vicissitudes. Goya, who was deaf, is an example:

> . . . the longer he lived the more frightful did that world seem—the more frightful, that is to say, in the eyes of his rational self; for his animal high spirits went on bubbling up irrepressibly, whenever his body was free from pain or sickness, to the very end. As a young man in good health, with money and reputation, a fine position and as many women as he wanted, he had found the world a very agreeable place. Absurd, of course, and with enough of folly and roguery to furnish subject matter for innumerable satirical drawings, but eminently worth living in. Then all of a sudden came deafness; and, after the joyful dawn of the Revolution, Napoleon and French Imperialism and the atrocities of war; and when Napoleon's hordes were gone, the unspeakable Ferdinand VII and clerical reaction and the spectacle of Spaniards fighting among themselves; and all the time, like the drone of a bagpipe accompanying the louder noises of what is officially called history, the enormous stupidity of average men and women, the chronic squalor of their superstitions, the bestiality of their occasional violences and orgies.
>
> Realistically or in fantastic allegories, with a technical mastery that only increased as he grew older, Goya recorded it all. Not only the agonies endured by his people at the hands of the invaders, but also the follies and crimes committed by these same people in their dealings with one another. The great canvases of the Madrid massacres and executions, the incomparable etchings of War's Disasters, fill us with an indignant compassion.*

*From Huxley, Aldous: Foreword, the complete etchings of Goya, New York, 1943, Crown Publishers, p. 10.

> Goya once drew a picture of an ancient man tottering along under the burden of years, but with the accompanying caption, 'I'm still learning.' That old man was himself. To the end of a long life, he went on learning. As a very young man he paints like the feeble eclectics who were his masters. The first signs of power and freshness and originality appear in the cartoons for the tapestries of which the earliest were executed when he was thirty. As a portraitist, however, he achieves nothing of outstanding interest until he is almost forty. But by that time he really knows what he's after, and during the second forty years of his life he moves steadily forward towards the consummate technical achievements, in oils, of the *Pinturas Negras,* and in etching, of the *Desastres* and the *Disparates.* Goya's is a stylistic growth away from restraint and into freedom, away from timidity and into expressive boldness.*

Personal creativity is a little-understood but greatly admired (if recognized) phenomenon. But even though we do not know how to "produce" creative people or to provide "specific" conditions to nurture them, we are aware of the general amalgam of biology, personality, and culture that allows creativity to thrive. Goya, for example, was able to work in spite of his deafness but we can say with a high degree of surety that a chronic brain syndrome would have brought even his genius and determination to a halt. All humans, geniuses included, sustain themselves through tragedy, pain, and disabilities with varying but eventually limited degrees of success. There are individual threshold points beyond which persons can no longer function effectively and the accumulated losses of old age begin to take their toll. It is recognized that there can be

*Huxley, Aldous: Ibid., pp. 14-15.

great variations in personal reactions to any change, loss or disability, but if the impact of these events is severe, long-lasting, or chronic enough, individuality is erased and a fairly predictable response occurs.

Consequently the problem we are most interested in is not how to produce creative old people but rather how not to inhibit them. And our concern is not merely with genius but with the creative potential in each human being for a meaningful and satisfying life.

ABKHASIA—A SHANGRI-LA FOR THE ELDERLY?

We have available to us a few existent cultures that appear to have created conditions favorable for a desirable and extended old age. Natives in the village of Tamish and elsewhere in the Soviet Republic of Abkhasia are reported to live to 120 or 130 years, and even longer, in good health and with enjoyment.* Abkhasia is a subtropical land on its coast along the Black Sea, and alpine up to the main range of the Caucasus Mountains. The 100,000 Abkhasians, most of whom are farmers, have ancestors going back 1,000 years on the same soil. In 1954, according to Benet (the last year for which overall figures are available), 2.58% of the Abkhasians were over 90. Comparable figures for the USSR and the United States are 0.1% and 0.4%, respectively. There may be some question about these exact figures, but various studies support the general claim of greater longevity, lower prevalence of arteriosclerosis, and little cancer.

Abkhasians do not use euphemisms for old people (they are simply called long living); nor do they "retire." One does what one is capable of doing until the end, and that is often quite a surprising amount. Most work regularly and have good eyesight, good teeth, and an erect posture. Sexual potency and libido is retained by many of the men after age 70, and a number of women menstruate until age 55. They exercise regularly, with long walks and swimming in mountain streams. Work and diet are believed to be key elements in their longevity; they eat slowly, have a low caloric intake, eat relatively little meat and rarely eggs, salt, or sugar. Few smoke tobacco, and alcohol consumption is modest.

Benet was impressed by "the high degree of integration in their lives, the sense of group identity that gives each individual an unshaken feeling of personal security and continuity. The sense of continuity in both their personal and national lives is what anthropologists would call their spatial and temporal integration. . . Their spatial integration is in their kinship structure. . ." Old people are valued for their transmission of traditions, mediation of disputes, and knowledge of farming, among other things; and with increasing age comes increasing prestige.

Although the rural existence of Abkhasia appears like a flower under glass, protected by geography and circumstance from industrialization and change, we could well afford to benefit from their example in providing a truly healthy culture for the old. Indeed in our own country there are pockets of cultures where the elderly live well and proudly. Guttman describes the older Navajo men from the remote Rainbow Plateau and Navajo Mountain regions. "I found many Navajo of great ego integrity. . . . Typically, we found these men still on horseback, herding sheep and dry-farming their cornfields. Their faces are relatively unlined, their bodies tend to be lean, their manner is open and expansive and they tend to deny physical limitations. They often have much younger wives, and father children with them. . . . Longevity seems to go hand in hand with Navajo traditionalism and with . . . defiant refusal to accept a victim's fate. . . . The remote traditional society seems to breed a high proportion of these ageless veterans."*

*Benet, Sula: Abkhasia: the long living people of the Caucasus (to be published).

*From Guttman, David L.: The country of old men: cross cultural studies of the psychology of later life, Occasional Papers in Gerontology, vol. 5, Institute of Gerontology, Ann Arbor, 1969, University of Michigan–Wayne State University Press.

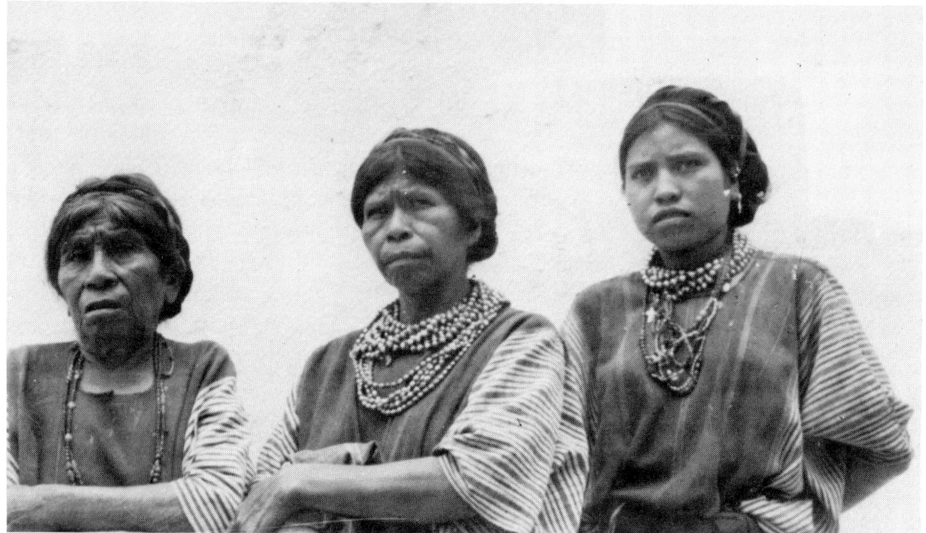

Three generations of women in a Guatemalan family.

Photo by Robert N. Butler.

Transcultural studies can teach both the universal aspects of the aging experience and the variations experienced by the elderly of each group. Already, in comparing our own national attitudes with the two cultures just mentioned, it is clear that we have not yet established roles of substance and purpose for the old. We isolate the realities of aging and death and deny ourselves the opportunity to build up the joyful, creative and generative aspects of human existence.* A major step forward would be the enhancement of age awareness—the creation of a sensibility that we are all enmeshed together in a complex life process with death as its end but with the potential for "life" all along the way.

PROBLEM OF HUMAN OBSOLESCENCE

The American social and economic system conspires to rigidify modern man's status and function in life. He is programmed and fixed early, and with advancing age—which means 45 on—he faces the possibilities of technological, intellectual, and social obsolescence, if not extinction. We must make bold moves so that our society can create a new flexibility within the individual and within the milieu in which he operates. Man must be able to change and grow throughout the course of his life, especially to keep pace with the rapidly changing twentieth century.

Retirement

Our present retirement practices emphasize the need for broad new socioeconomic arrangements. The cost of retirement, measured in dollars and cents alone, is enormous. In 1968 we paid out nearly $25 billion through Social Security and $2.1 billion to federal Civil Service retirees. This is only part of the total retirement bill of our nation. The human cost, in terms of personal indignity and loss of vital relations to one's community, is immeasurable. Retirement is based arbitrarily on age and not on competence, health, or desire except for a favored few professionals:

> Physicians do not tend to retire. Some should; more shouldn't. It depends upon their specialty and competence. Surgeons obviously should be monitored. If group practice grows it should be possible for group members to help assay a col-

*Martin, A. R.: Urgent need for a philosophy of leisure in an aging population, Journal of the American Geriatrics Society **10**:215-224, 1962.

league, help him or her with financial planning, utilizing experience if not direct activity. In 1971 there were 25,000 doctors over 65 in active practice and 6,000 of them over 75. Twenty-five percent of all practicing medical doctors and doctors of osteopathy are between 50 and 65. While others are forced to retire through arbitrary retirement systems, doctors may be forced out because they are refused malpractice insurance, or premiums are so high that part-time practice is not feasible. Moreover, doctors may stop referring, and remaining patients may be reluctant to see the older doctor. When the doctor is clearly competent, it is a tragic waste.

Social practices may be introduced into a society in response to emergency conditions; when the emergency is over, the practice continues. For example, in connection with the severe job scarcity of the thirties, labor unions pressed for earlier and earlier retirement to open up jobs for younger workers with families to support. Today with many more jobs available, early retirement still plagues us. Social practices are frequently inaugurated without an understanding of their fundamental long-range human consequences.

There should be a radical reshuffling of education, work, and leisure throughout the course of the life cycle. At present these activities are concentrated in the three distinct periods of childhood, middle life, and later life. Existing financial supports should be reallocated as required. Taking both ends of the life cycle as examples, youth could be given more job opportunities in coordination with their education, and older people could be given greater access to both education and jobs. The important and productive middle-aged group would especially benefit from continuing education and increased opportunities for leisure, relieving them of the pressures of constant work.

Although trends in these directions are evident, they clearly do not go far enough. In small ways the world of education, from public schools to universities, has moved beyond its traditional responsibilities to youth. Continuing education for professional people and for women in mid-life are two examples. Senior universities have been proposed for older people. New training and retraining for "middle starts" and "late starts" have been supported in some small measure under the Manpower Development and Training Act of 1962.

With respect to work and retirement, we are beginning to see shorter work weeks, 2½- and 3-day weekends, and expanded annual vacation periods. But these are small steps. There has been no major commitment by industry, government, or the universities to endeavor to meet the enormous problems of technological and personal obsolescence and the desire of many for a changed and less rigid life style.

Preparation for retirement

Postretirement seminars and counseling can often be more crucial than preretirement preparation. It is after being sent home with the gold watch that reality takes hold. The scheduled life is over. Income is halved. Man and wife are together for the first time (other than on vacations) on a 24-hour basis. This *is* retirement—whether arbitrary, voluntary, or forced by illness, plant shutdown, company merger, or reorganization. The work "grind" is over but the retirement "void" now begins. Individuals have not been taught to use their time on their own. Leisure is not one of the major subjects in school, since art, music and physical education are considered "soft" rather than substantial subjects.

With retirement one can turn to paid full-time, part-time, or seasonal work, either in the same line of work as one was engaged in previously or in a new area of interest. However, there are few available training programs for "new careers." One can also do volunteer work but will often be disappointed by assignment of tedious tasks such as stamp-licking and envelope-filling.

Poverty

First, to enjoy "leisurely retirement" one must have money, and some 50% of older people in 1972 had available $75 or *less* per week (often far less). So the monies needed to pursue hobbies, to travel, to visit children and grandchildren or exotic places are limited. Second, if the retiree does work, he will be penalized if he earns more than is "allowed" under the Social Security retirement "means test." (Those who clip coupons will not be punished, for stock dividends do not count as earned income.)

It is incredible to speak of retirement roles and activities until basic subsistence needs are met. Poverty in old age is extreme in America.* Official estimates in 1972 stated that one fourth of old people are poor. We regard the federal poverty threshold as most conservative. Poverty breeds mental illness in old age. It can cause the malnutrition and anemia that directly result in brain syndrome which, often unrecognized, becomes fixed. Poverty erodes the spirit. It makes visiting, jobs, and voluntary work difficult or impossible through lack of transportation.

A compulsory national security system financed through general revenues utilizing a graduated income tax (with no loopholes) should be one component of a retirement system. Built-in escalator clauses of two types should exist, one related to cost of living and the second to the general economic productivity of the nation. Supplementary to this should be a voluntary national personal-security system that is financed individually. For example, in 1962 the Self-Employed Individuals Retirement Plan was passed (the Keogh Plan). This permitted self-employed physicians, lawyers, businessmen, and others to put away up to $2,500 per year (in later amendments). Thus collective and individual providence would characterize income maintenance for the final period of life.

In early 1972 Senator Frank Church called upon the Congress and the Administration to seize a "historic opportunity to translate the recommendations of the White House Conference on Aging into action—immediate and long-range." The Chairman of the Special Committee on Aging of the U. S. Senate noted a few cost estimates on reforms that would help older Americans:

> "We could abolish poverty among the elderly for what it costs to run the war in Southeast Asia for just three months."
>
> "We could broaden Medicare coverage to include out-of-hospital prescription drugs for what we now spend for an aircraft carrier."
>
> "We could establish a comprehensive manpower program for older workers for the cost of one submarine."

RESEARCH ON THE QUALITY AND LENGTH OF HUMAN LIFE

Simply extending human life for more and more years is folly and even inhumane unless the quality of late life can be improved. Yet very little research in this nation concentrates either on the fundamental biological processes of aging or on the social and psychological supports for old age. Less than 1% of all the research monies of the National Institutes of Health is spent on research in aging. Even so, there are promising leads and challenging possibilities.

Numerous contemporary theories of aging represent the continuing efforts of humans to discover and retard the mysterious decline of the body over a span of years. Will one of these theories produce a significant clue? Collagen cross linking? Errors in protein synthesis? Autoimmunity? Gradual loss of information in the desoxynucleic acid (DNA) molecule? Decline in cell division? Free radical disruption of cell membrane structure and enzyme activity, with resulting formation of lipofuscin (the "age pigment")? Failure of hypothalamus in regulation of normal body rhythms and functions?

Progeria, an extraordinary rare disease that mimics in children the characteristics of aging, presents a compressed time-lapse motion picture of aging, which may give us clues.

The lipid (fat) peroxidation theory of aging is advocated by some: the unstable lipid portions of lipoprotein cell membranes

---

*"The golden years—the tarnished myth" was the result of one study called Project FIND. This was sponsored by the National Council on Aging (NCOA), funded by the Office of Economic Opportunities (OEO), and conceived and directed by Jack Ossofsky, NCOA Deputy Director.

are continuously undergoing spontaneous peroxidation through cosmic ray bombardment. Presumably, antioxidants such as the normally present antioxidant alpha-tocopherol or vitamin E retard peroxidation. Thus synthetic antioxidants are suggested as retardants to aging.

Research on specific diseases that affect the elderly also show signs of promise. As Seneca said, "Man doesn't die. He kills himself." Aging has yet to prove fatal, for man finds "natural diseases" to die from. The most common is arteriosclerosis, which in old age causes brain disorders and strokes as well as affecting such vital organs as the heart and kidneys.

In late December, 1971, a task force on arteriosclerosis* called for a major national effort against the "national epidemic" of heart disease. Cardiovascular disease causes the death of more than 1 million persons annually and disables many more. Successful efforts against arteriosclerosis will alter the picture of old age as we know it today—with the wrinkling, slowing, and other features associated with old age, which are partially due to reduced blood supply following upon "hardening of the arteries."

The task force sharply criticized current federal efforts in arteriosclerosis research as "totally inadequate" because of "sparse and discontinuous funding, a dearth of long-range planning, and uncoordinated programming." The group called for a permanent national commission to monitor progress against heart disease and to chart future directions of the efforts to combat it.

Significantly, the panel did not recommend a national population study of the relationship between diet and heart disease but did recommend dietary changes for the general public. ". . . it . . . would appear prudent for the American people to follow a diet aimed at lowering serum lipid concentrations. . . . This can be achieved by lowering intake of calories, cholesterol, and saturated fats."

*Appointed by Dr. Theodore Cooper, Director of the National Heart and Lung Institute.

Evidence implicating smoking as a factor in lung cancer, heart disease, and emphysema has been accumulating. There are data showing that heavy smoking is associated with skin wrinkling, probably because nicotine in cigarette smoke contracts small blood vessels in the skin.

In general, people of all ages should follow certain simple steps as a preventive measure against disease:

Eat foods low in saturated fats and cholesterol
Stop smoking cigarettes
Reduce if overweight
Exercise moderately, regularly
Control high blood pressure
Have a medical checkup periodically

Present research will bring both technological and social changes in the future. The following examples are illustrative:

> One happy spinoff from the National Aeronautics and Space Administration (NASA) can be the application of technology to prosthetics development. NASA's knowledge is useful in many areas, from the telemetry of human physiology across previous barriers of distance to the powering of robot arms for the limbless or paralyzed. (In the United States some 400,000 persons are permanently disabled by trauma and 519,000 are partially or totally paralyzed by stroke.)

• • •

> Religious thinkers joined social and physical scientists and physicians in the world's first institute organized to conduct research into the ethical and scientific aspects of human reproduction and development. The Joseph and Rose Kennedy Institute for the Study of Human Reproduction and Bioethics is located at Georgetown University Medical Center. One of the questions to which staff will devote attention, pertinent to gerontology, is whether the physician is obliged to keep an aged person alive when his condition is hopeless.

NEW LIFE STYLES AND LIVING ARRANGEMENTS

> Justice John Marshall Harlan insisted on constitutional and legal safeguards against intrusions on the home and the person to preserve "that spontaneity—reflected in frivolous, impetuous, sacrilegious and defiant discourse—that liberates daily life."

Older people need just such liberation in view of what one hears when one listens to old persons tell of their lives.* One senses immediately that much of human behavior is maladaptive. No one explains to the child that his life is the one and only life he has, that it is tender and short, that it must be carefully nurtured, that it is easy to "blow it." No one tells the child that he is a unique possibility, that no one else will ever duplicate him. No one helps prepare him to be resilient and resourceful. People enter friendships, marriages, and work essentially unguided and, once entered into, these "choices" tend to be fixed. Yet one's life need not be traced out with an indelible pencil. Too many lives have been wasteful in comparison to what they could be.

Newspapermen are fond of asking this question: "Would you like to live your life over?" Most old persons asked say no. Why do they say this? Is it that, as H. L. Mencken said, "No show is so good that it should last forever"? Is it too unbearable to consider seriously that one might have lived out one's life in another way(s)? Is it that, in many cases and even in the best of cases, no one wants to relive his life as it was lived? And indeed should anyone be content with his life?

It is striking to observe, in hearing the old speak, that those who have led open, evolving, and changing lives are few. Rather, people lead lives of fixed roles and enforced identities. They also try to escape. Many lives have an infrastructure—hidden, secret, parallel *infra-lives*—maintained often with enormous expenditures of energy. Underground living may be seen in the everyday bourgeois who becomes a weekend hippie. Some hold close a secret self that, because it is revealed to no one, leads to the elaboration of a richly fantasied other life. For some, extramarital relationship(s) may be more crucial than marriage, the avocation more salient than the vocation, the lives of one's children more highly valued than one's own.

A second form of escape is through *pseudolives*—barren, stark, empty, nonprogressing lives with retreats from danger, from risks. The identity is fraudulent. It is acting, role-playing. These are not even "lives of quiet desperation." The person who denies his sexual feelings, the person who continues to do what he no longer believes in, and those who pretend in order to preserve status and income are illustrative.

Third are those who do lead *"lives of quiet desperation,"* who usually do not have infra-lives, and who may be too honest or aware to allow themselves pseudolives.

Fourth are those who *disappear*. Some 100,000 middle-aged persons are said to disappear annually, not all permanently. Some try to start anew; some simply "cop out." And some old people disappear too.

To obviate the necessity for infra-lives, pseudolives, "lives of quiet desperation," or disappearance there must be greater freedom over and against identity—freedom to rebel against the freeze. Today, to leave or switch careers in mid-life, as trains switch tracks, or to cop out of the career ladder is regarded as "sick." The definition of "sickness" is critical to the evolution of social and personal "solutions." Yet with the threat associated with rapid and frequent social and technological changes, instead of an unfreezing of roles, tasks, and identities, there has been a greater intensification.

At the same time, however, there are experimenters, individuals who are playing with change and are likely to represent life styles of the future. Similarly, there are new, stable organizational forms and also anarchic, scattered, unstable forms. It is surprising how punitive society can be toward those who try out new life styles. It is almost as though they threaten society itself; in reality they lend stability, as an outlet for frustration and creativity. Some old people, like young people, are living in communes or out of wedlock. Some are simply lifelong rebels grown old.

*There are many programs that tape record the lives of older persons regardless of how well known such persons are. Such materials enrich knowledge and sense of history. Emerson said that history is collected biography.

January, 1972, found Jeannette Rankin of Missoula, Montana, 91, lifelong pacifist and activist, the first woman to win membership in the United States House of Representatives, living in a house with a dirt floor in her living room. She gave her money to the peace movement. She demonstrated what Emerson said of Thoreau, that he made himself rich by making his wants few. In 1968 at 87 she led the Jeannette Rankin Brigade of 5,000 women to Washington to protest the Vietnam war. She was quoted (*New York Times,* January, 1972) as saying that if she had her life to relive, "I'd be nastier."

The idea of man and technology as partners, not enemies, is important. Man must change at rates similar to his technology. He invented it, after all. We need not inhibit or destroy technology or oppose scientific development. However, we can respond more rationally by controlling such development. One notes man's apparent inability to be a decent housekeeper, to clean up after himself, and to leave the planet the way it was when he came—even if he cannot improve it. There is man's inability to feed and dress himself adequately. He cannot control his needs; he greedily devours his environment at the expense of his fellow man. He has not learned to limit his aggressiveness, his rapacity, and his violence. Nor has man regulated his sexual drive and his reproduction. A new kind of education, continuing throughout life, is necessary to keep pace with change and provide a humane and life-centered focus. A new kind of ethic—to the future, to posterity—is necessary to help, however weakly, to rectify the balance against individual man's exploitation of his brief visit on this planet.

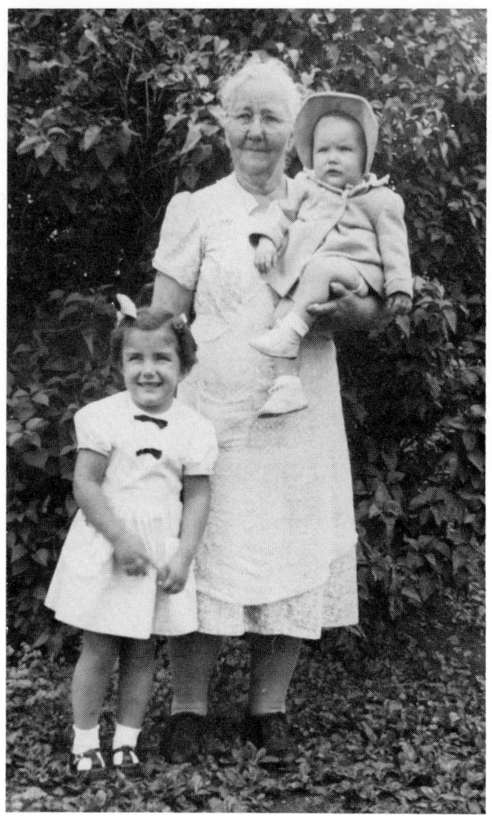

Grandparentage: part of an ethic toward the future.

Photo by Myrna I. Lewis.

Inevitable social and technological changes—sometimes euphorically called progress—have brought greater possibilities of choice, diversification of living styles, and options. People—old, young, and middle-aged—have suffered long enough from knowing all too well who they are and being afraid to change.

REFERENCES

Aries, P.: Centuries of childhood: a social history of family life, New York, 1962, Vintage Books.

Benedek, Theresa: Parenthood as a developmental phase, Psychoanalytic Quarterly **19**:1-27, 1950.

Bengston, V. L.: The generation gap, Youth and Society **2**:7-32, 1970.

Bernard, A.: The tragic plight of the aging physician, Medical Opinion **8**:38-43, Jan., 1972.

Binstock, R. H., and Lohmann, R. A.: Identity and power: the case of the aged. Paper presented at the 1971 annual meeting of the American Political Science Association, Chicago.

Birren, J. E.: A brief history on the psychology of aging, The Gerontologist **1**:127-234, 1961.

Bixby, Lenore E.: Income of people aged 65 and over, Social Security Bulletin **33**:3-34, 1970.

Blum, June E., Jarvik, Lissy F., and Clark, E. T.: Rate of change on selective tests of intelligence: a twenty-year longitudinal study of aging, Journal of Gerontology **25**:171-176, 1970.

Botwinick, J.: Cognitive processes in maturity and old age, New York, 1967, Springer Publishing Co., Inc.

Burgess, E. W.: Retirement preparation: Chicago plan. Case Study No. 5, Washington, D. C., 1961, U. S. Department of Health, Education and Welfare.

Burnstein, S. R.: Papers on the historical background of gerontology, Geriatrics **10**:189-193, 328-332, 536-540, 1955.

Butler, R. N.: Toward a psychiatry of the life cycle. Implications of socio-psychological studies of the aging process for policy in and practice of psychotherapy. In Simon, A., and Epstein, L. J., editors: Aging in modern society—Psychosocial and medical aspects, Washington, D. C., 1968, American Psychiatric Association.

Butler, R. N.: The burnt-out and the bored, The Washington Monthly **1**:58-60, 1969.

Butler, R. N.: Looking forward to what? The life review, legacy and excessive identity versus change, American Behavioral Scientist **14**:121-128, 1970.

Cain, L. D., Jr.: Age status and generational phenomena: the new old people in contemporary America, The Gerontologist **7**:83-92, 1967.

Carp, Frances, editor: The retirement process, U. S. Public Health Service Pub. No. 1778, Washington, D. C., 1968, U. S. Government Printing Office.

Carp, Frances, editor: Retirement, New York, 1972, Behavioral Publications, Inc.

Cohen, E. S.: The White House Conference on aging: will it fail? Aging and Human Development **1**:51-60, 1970.

Commission on History: Living history: program for the acquisition of tape-recorded memoirs of history, Washington, D. C., 1970, American Psychiatric Association.

Cottrell, W. F.: Governmental functions and the politics of age. In Tibbitts, C., editor: Handbook of social gerontology, Chicago, 1961, University of Chicago Press.

DeGrazia, S.: Of time, work and leisure, New York, 1964, Anchor Books.

Erikson, Erik H.: Childhood and society, ed. 2, New York, 1963, W. W. Norton & Co., Inc.

Gruman, G. S.: A history of ideas about the prolongation of life, Transactions of the American Philosophical Society **56**:1-102, 1966.

Havighurst, R. J., Munnichs, J. M. A., Neugarten, Bernice L., and Thomae, H., editors: Adjustment to retirement: a cross-national study, Assen, The Netherlands, 1969, Humanities Press, Inc.

Jung, Carl G.: The stages of life. In Modern man in search of a soul, New York, 1933, Harcourt, Brace & World, Inc.

Kreps, Juanita M.: Lifetime allocation of work and income—essays in the economics of aging, Durham, N. C., 1971, Duke University Press.

Levin, S., and Kahana, R., editors: Psychodynamic studies on aging: creativity, reminiscing and dying, New York, 1967, International Universities Press, Inc.

Maddox, G. L., Jr.: Disengagement theory: a critical evaluation, The Gerontologist **4**:80-82, 103, 1964.

Mitford, Jessica: The American way of death, New York, 1963, Simon & Schuster, Inc.

Munnichs, J. M. A.: A short history of psychogerontology, Human Development **9**:230-245, 1966.

Neugarten, Bernice, and Associates: Personality in middle and later life, New York, 1964, Atherton Press.

Neugarten, Bernice L., Havighurst, R. J., and Tobin, S. S.: The measurement of life satisfaction, Journal of Gerontology **16**:134-143, 1961.

Oriol, W. E.: Social policy priorities: age vs. youth; the federal government, The Gerontologist **10**:207-210, 1970.

Palmore, E., and Jeffers, Frances C.: Prediction of life span, Lexington, Mass., 1971, Heath Lexington Books.

Randall, Ollie: Some historical developments of social welfare aspects of aging, The Gerontologist **5**:40-49, 1965.

Riegel, K. F., Riegel, R. M., and Mayer, G.: A study of the dropout rates in longitudinal research on aging and the prediction of death, Journal of Personality and Social Psychology **5**:342-348, 1967.

Rosen, G. W.: Cross-cultural and historical approaches. In Hoch, P. H., and Zubin, J., editors: Psychopathology of aging, New York, 1961, Grune & Stratton, Inc.

Saveth, E.: Utilization of older scientific and professional personnel, New York, 1961, National Council on Aging.

Schaie, W., editor: Theory and methods of research on aging, Morgantown, W. Va., 1968, West Virginia University Press.

Shanas, Ethel, Townsend, P., Wedderburn, Dorothy, Friis, H., Milhoj, P., and Stehouwer, J.: Old people in three industrial societies, New York, 1968, Atherton Press.

Simmons, L. W.: The role of the aged in primitive society, New Haven, 1945, Yale University Press.

Social Security Administration: Social Security programs throughout the world 1971, Washington, D. C., 1972, U. S. Government Printing Office.

Sunderland, Jacqueline T.: Older Americans and the arts, Washington, D. C., 1972, National Council on the Aging.

Tibbitts, C.: Aging in the modern world: a book of readings, Ann Arbor, 1957, The University of Michigan Press.

U. S. Senate Special Committee on Aging: Hearings (December 5-6, 1967). Long-range program and research needs in aging and related fields. I. Survey, Washington, D. C., 1968, U. S. Government Printing Office.

U. S. Senate Special Committee on Aging: Economics of aging: toward a full share in abundance, Report, Washington, D. C., 1970, U. S. Government Printing Office.

U. S. Senate Special Subcommittee on Aging of the Committee on Labor and Public Welfare: Hearings on older Americans community service program, Washington, D. C.; Sept. 18-19, 1967, U. S. Government Printing Office.

VanGennep, A.: The rites of passage, Chicago, 1960, University of Chicago Press.

West, N.: A cool million or, The dismantling of Lemuel Pitkin (1934), New York, 1963, The Noonday Press.

Appendixes

APPENDIX **A**

SOURCES OF GERONTOLOGICAL AND GERIATRIC LITERATURE

1. Books

Shock, N. W.: A classified bibliography of gerontology and geriatrics, vol. I, 1900-1948; vol. II, 1949-1955; vol. III, 1956-1961, Stanford University Press, Stanford, Calif., 1951, 1957, and 1963, respectively.

Shock, N. W.: Index to current periodical literature, published quarterly in the Journal of Gerontology.

2. Periodicals

Administration on Aging, Department of Health, Education, and Welfare: Aging, Washington, D. C.

American Association of Retired Persons: Modern Maturity.

American Geriatrics Society: Journal of the American Geriatrics Society, New York.

American Nursing Home Association: Modern Nursing Homes. Hightstown, N. J.

American Nursing Home Association: Nursing Homes, Lake Forest, Ill.

Gerontological Society: The Gerontologist, St. Louis, Mo.

Gerontological Society: Journal of Gerontology, St. Louis, Mo.

Greenwood Periodicals: Aging and Human Development, Westport, Conn.

Institute of Gerontology, The University of Michigan–Wayne State University: Occasional papers in Gerontology, Ann Arbor, Mich.

International Universities Press: Journal of Geriatric Psychiatry, New York, N. Y.

G. F. Publications: Geriatric Focus, New York, N. Y.

Lancet Publications, Inc.: Geriatrics, Minneapolis, Minn.

National Association of Retired Federal Employees: Retirement Life, Washington, D. C.

National Council of Senior Citizens (NCSC): Senior Citizens News, Washington, D. C.

National Retired Teachers Association (NRTA): National Retired Teachers Association Journal.

Social Security Administration: Social Security Bulletin, Washington, D. C.

3. Pamphlets, bulletins, reports, etc.

Ciompi, L.: A comprehensive review of geronto-psychiatric literature in the postwar period: a review of the literature to January 1, 1965, U. S. Public Health Publication No. 1811, National Clearinghouse for Mental Health Information, Washington, D. C., 1969.

National Institute of Child Health and Human Development: International directory of gerontology, U. S. Government Printing Office, Washington, D. C., 1968. (Includes a list of persons specializing in geriatrics and gerontology by geographical area.)

United States Senate Special Committee on Aging: Hearings and task force reports, Washington, D. C.

United States Health, Education and Welfare Department. Directory, Medicare Providers and Suppliers of Service. Government Printing Office, Washington, D. C. 20402.

APPENDIX **B**

ORGANIZATIONS PERTAINING TO THE ELDERLY

American Aging Association
University of Nebraska Medical Center
Omaha, Neb.
Made up of scientists, it seeks to promote research in aging.

American Association of Homes for the Aging
529 14th St., N.W.
Washington, D. C. 20004
AAHA represents the nonprofit homes for the aging—religious, municipal, trust, fraternal.

American Association of Retired Persons
1225 Connecticut Ave., N.W.
Washington, D. C. 20036
Age 55 or above, retired to still-employed.

The American Geriatrics Society
10 Columbus Circle
New York, N. Y. 10019
The American Geriatrics Society, made up of physicians, has an annual meeting.

American Nurses' Association, Inc.
10 Columbus Circle
New York, N. Y. 10019

American Nursing Home Association
1025 Connecticut Ave., N.W.
Washington, D. C. 20036
ANHA represents the commercial nursing home industry.

American Occupational Therapy Association
251 Park Ave. South
New York, N. Y. 10010

American Physical Therapy Association
1740 Broadway
New York, N. Y. 10019

The Forum for Professionals and Executives
c/o The Washington School of Psychiatry
1610 New Hampshire Ave., N.W.
Washington, D. C. 20009

The interests of this group have ranged from contemplation to active examination of public issues, including those affecting the elderly.

The Gerontological Society
1 Dupont Circle
Washington, D. C. 20036
This professional society has an annual meeting and an international meeting every three years. It is made up of four components—Biological Sciences, Clinical Medicine, Psychological and Social Services and Social Research, Planning and Practice.

Gray Panthers
6342 Greene St.
Philadelphia, Pa. 19144
Activistic group of old people who resent "stereotyping."

The Institute of Retired Professionals
The New School of Social Research
60 West 12th St.
New York, N. Y.
This pioneering school also led the way in providing intellectual activities for retired professional people.

The Institutes of Lifetime Learning
These are educational services of the National Retired Teachers Association and the American Association of Retired Persons.

International Senior Citizens Association, Inc.
11753 Wilshire Blvd.
Los Angeles, Calif. 90025
Endeavors to reflect old people of many nations.

National Association of Retired Federal Employees
1909 Que St., N.W.
Washington, D. C. 20009
Represents and lobbies for needs of retired civil servants.

National Association of Social Workers
2 Park Ave.
New York, N. Y. 10016

National Council on the Aging
1828 L St., N.W., Suite 504
Washington, D. C. 20036
Research and services regarding the elderly.

National Council of Health Care Services

407 N St., S.W., Washington, D. C.
Represents commercial nursing home chains.

National Council for Homemaker Services

1790 Broadway
New York, N. Y. 10019

National Council of Senior Citizens

1911 K St., N.W., Room 202
Washington, D. C. 20005
Represents and lobbies for needs of the elderly. Membership at any age.

National Federation of Licensed Practical Nurses

250 W. 57th St.
New York, N. Y.
Educational Foundation.

National Retired Teachers Association

1225 Connecticut Ave., N.W.
Washington, D. C. 20036
Members once active in an educational system, public or private.

National Tenants Organization, Inc.

Suite 548
425 13th St., N.W.
Washington, D. C. 20004
Represents old people, among others, in public housing.

The Oliver Wendell Holmes Association

381 Park Ave., South
New York, N. Y. 10016
This group is interested in the expansion of the intellectual horizons of older people.

Retired Professionals Action Group

Suite 711
200 P St., N.W.
Washington, D. C.
This action group was organized through Nader. Its efforts include investigative reports and class-action cases.

Urban Elderly Coalition

c/o Office of Aging of New York City
250 Broadway, New York, N. Y.
Effort of municipal authorities to obtain funds for the urban elderly poor.

APPENDIX **C**

GOVERNMENT PROGRAMS FOR THE ELDERLY

VOLUNTEER/EMPLOYMENT PROGRAMS	SPONSOR	PURPOSE	ADDRESS
RSVP (Retired Senior Volunteer Program)	ACTION	Funds for volunteer programs in public and nonprofit institutions; volunteers reimbursed for travel and meal expenses	ACTION Washington, D. C. 20525
SCORE (Service Corps of Retired Executives)	ACTION, administered by Small Business Administration	Retired businessmen advising novices in business	ACTION Washington, D. C. 20525
VISTA (Volunteers in Service to America)	ACTION	Volunteers for one to two years in community projects in United States, with small salary to cover living expenses	ACTION Washington, D. C. 20525
Peace Corps	ACTION	Overseas service	ACTION Washington, D. C. 20525
IESC (International Executive Service Corps)	An independent organization supported by government and nongovernment funds	Overseas service by executives	International Executive Service Corps 545 Madison Ave. New York, N. Y. 10022

LOW-INCOME ELDERLY PROGRAMS*	SPONSOR	PURPOSE	ADDRESS
Foster Grandparents	ACTION	Provide relationship and care to orphans and mentally retarded children in institutions for 20 hours per week at $1.60 per hour	ACTION Washington, D. C. 20525
SOS (Senior Opportunities and Service programs)	OEO	Service in programs to meet needs of older people: nutrition, consumer education, outreach service	Office of Economic Opportunity Office of Program Review Washington, D. C.
Operation Mainstream programs			
1. Green Thumb (men) Green Light (women)	National Farmers Union Green Thumb/ Green Light 1012 14th St., N. W. Washington, D. C. 20005	Conservation and landscape (men) Community service (women)	Write sponsor or Manpower Administration Operation Mainstream Department of Labor Washington, D. C.
2. Senior Aides	National Council of Senior Citizens 1511 K St., N.W. Washington, D. C. 20005	Community service	Write sponsor
3. Senior Community Service Programs	National Council on the Aging 1828 L St., N.W. Washington D. C. 20036	Community service	Write sponsor
4. Senior Community Service Aides	National Retired Teachers Association Senior Community Service Aides Project 1225 Connecticut Ave., N.W. Washington, D. C. 20036	Community service	Write sponsor

*Only persons over 60 with incomes below OEO (Office of Economic Opportunities) guidelines are eligible.

APPENDIX **D**

GRANT PROGRAMS AND SOCIAL SERVICES

GRANT PROGRAMS CONCERNING AGING

The Older Americans Act of 1965, as amended, is carried out by the Administration on Aging within the Department of Health, Education, and Welfare, Washington, D. C. It provides funds for service, research, and training.

For community planning and for services

Title III of the Older Americans Act allots funds to states to strengthen state agencies on aging and to enable states to make grants to local public and private nonprofit agencies for projects that provide services to older people, for community services to older people, for community planning and coordination of programs, for demonstration programs, and for training of special personnel. Applications are made to the state agency on aging.

For research and demonstration

Title IV of the Act makes direct grants or contracts for research and demonstration projects of national or regional interest and value. Application is made to Research and Demonstration Grants Staff, Administration on Aging.

For training

Title V of the Act supports, through grants or contracts, specialized training of persons employed or preparing for employment in programs in aging. Application is made to Training Grants Staff, Administration on Aging.

NATIONAL INSTITUTE OF MENTAL HEALTH GRANT PROGRAMS*

Hospital staff development

The hospital staff development program is designed to improve the quality of patient care in public mental health hospitals included in state systems of care, through inservice training for personnel. It encourages hospitals to provide staff development programs at the subprofessional and professional levels through a variety of courses, such as orientation, refresher and continuation training, as well as through special courses for those who conduct the training.

Hospital improvement program

The hospital improvement program is directed toward improving the treatment, care, and rehabilitation of the mentally ill in the 302 eligible state-supported mental hospitals throughout the nation. It is specifically focused on use of current knowledge, in demonstrating improved services for patients, stimulation of the process of change, and development of relationships, with community mental health programs.

Research

The NIMH program of research in aging has as the following goals: the development of knowledge about human behavior and adjustment to the aging process; the increase of knowledge necessary for the understanding, treatment, and rehabilitation of the aged; and the evaluation of services resources designed to care for the aged. Within this context many subsidiary objectives are included, such as the effects of environmental conditions on aging in hospitals, nursing homes, and other settings; the effects of retirement; psychosocial studies of adjustment to aging; studies of the terminal stages of life; and experimentation with and evaluation of new methods of serving the aged in the community and in institutional settings. Through the support of basic behavioral science research, the program in aging encompasses studies in neuropsychology, personality and motivation, cognition and learning, and cultural variables that affect the aging process; these studies include such areas as tissue deterioration, biochemical change, perception, memory, and intelligence. Within the program of psychopharmacological research, studies are concerned with the use of psychoactive drugs with the aged and their effects on performance and memory. The program of clinical research supports studies relevant to aging.

*5600 Fishers Lane, Rockville, Md. 20852.

Training

At present the major portion of NIMH training funds concerned with aging is being used in support of training grants, including teaching costs and trainee stipends, fellowships, and research development awards. There is continued interest in the curricula of mental health professionals and in training new types of workers to care for the aged and provide preventive mental health services.

NATIONAL INSTITUTE OF CHILD HEALTH AND HUMAN DEVELOPMENT: ADULT DEVELOPMENT AND AGING BRANCH*

Research Grants and Contracts Management Branch for scientific studies of aging.

*Bethesda, Md. 20014.

Career Development Review Branch regarding training funds for professional and graduate schools, hospitals, and eligible clinics. Stipends for trainees.

SOCIAL SERVICES: SOCIAL SECURITY AUTHORIZATIONS

Under Titles I, IV, X, XIV, and XVI of the Social Security Act.

The National Council on the Aging: Funding social services in model cities. A guide to Title IV, Part A of the Social Security Act, 1971.

The National Council on the Aging, Community Development, National League of Cities—U. S. Conference of Mayors (Jane E. Bloom and R. H. Cohen) Social Services for the Elderly. Funding Projects in Model Cities through Titles I and XVI of the Social Security Act, 1972.

APPENDIX **E**

STAFF INSERVICE EDUCATION MATERIAL FOR WORK WITH OLDER PEOPLE

1a. Recommended fiction—concerning later life, memory, time, aging, disease, and death

In James Hilton's *Goodbye, Mr. Chips* (1934) the elderly protagonist reminisces in his room across from the school where he taught three generations of English boys.

Aldous Huxley's *After Many a Summer Dies the Swan* (1939) is a satiric novel. The hero is a California multimillionaire terrified of death. His physician is working on a theory of longevity. The novel ends in horror.

Georges Simenon's *The Bells of Bicetre* (English title: *The Patient*) portrays a powerful French newspaper owner who has a stroke that leaves him speechless and paralyzed. At first he is passive, with no wish to recover. His mind is clear; he views his wife, his doctor, and his own life with detachment. As his memories flow through his mind and he begins to recover his speech and movement, his mental attitude changes favorably.

In Muriel Spark's *Momento Mori* (1959) a woman's death and an anonymous phone caller who says "remember you must die" provoke a series of humorous adventures for a group of elderly English aristocrats.

Leo Tolstoi, in *The Death of Ivan Ilych* (1884), describes a Russian judge who learns that his wealth, status, and power are useless to him when he becomes ill. His painful disease and his death are merely inconveniences to his family and lifelong friends. A young peasant servant is his only comfort.

In John Updike's *The Poorhouse Fair* (1959) residents of an old folks' home put on their annual fair despite the well-intentioned mistakes of the new administrators and poor weather.

1b. Other fiction

Adams, S. H.: Grandfather stories, New York, 1947, Random House, Inc. (paperback).

Ashton-Warner, Sylvia: Spinster (1959), New York, 1961, Bantam Books (paperback).

Beckett, S.: Krapp's last tape (a drama) (1957), New York, 1958, Grove Press, Inc. (paperback).

Bromfield, Louis: Mrs. Parkington, New York, 1949, Harper & Brothers.

Cary, Joyce: To be a pilgrim, London, 1942, Michael Joseph, Ltd.

Hemingway, Ernest: The old man and the sea, New York, 1952, Charles Scribner's Sons.

James, Henry: The beast in the jungle (1903) in the short stories of Henry James (C. Fadiman, editor), New York, 1945, The Modern Library, Inc., pp. 548-602.

Lampedusa, G. di: The leopard, New York, 1960, Pantheon Books, Inc.

Mann, Thomas: The black swan, New York, 1954, Alfred A. Knopf, Inc.

Miller, Arthur: Death of a salesman, New York, 1949, The Viking Press.

Porter, Katherine Anne: The jilting of Granny Weatherall. In Flowering Judas, New York, 1930, Harcourt, Brace & World, Inc.

Proust, Marcel: Remembrance of things past (1913-1922), New York, 1934, Random House (two volumes).

Richter, C.: The waters of Kronos, New York, 1960, Alfred A. Knopf, Inc.

Romains, J.: The death of a nobody (1911), New York, 1961, Signet Book (paperback).

Shakespeare, William: King Lear (1608), Cambridge, England, 1960, Cambridge University Press (paperback).

Shaw, G. B.: Back to Methuselah (1921) (a drama), New York, 1947, Oxford University Press.

Trollope, A.: The fixed period, Tauchnitz editions of English authors, 1882, Leipzig.

Van Velde, Jacoba: The big ward, New York, 1960, Simon & Schuster, Inc.

Waugh, Evelyn: The loved one, Boston, 1948, Little, Brown & Co.

Wilde, Oscar: Picture of Dorian Gray (1906), New York, 1956, Dell Books (paperback); New York, Modern Library, Inc. (paperback).

2. Recommended films

Films are very important. Teaching films focus on diagnosis.* Certain movie films offer the subjective, human side of aging.

FILM	DIRECTOR	YEAR
The Last Laugh	F. W. Murnau	1924
The story of an old doorman demoted to washroom attendant.		
Umberto D.	Vittorio de Sica	1952
Concerns an aging impoverished pensioner who considers suicide.		
Tokyo Story	Yasujiro Ozu	1955
The story of an elderly couple's last visit to their children, its disappointments, its sadness.		
Wild Strawberries	Ingmar Bergman	1957
Concerns a 76-year-old physician who learns to love on the brink of eternity.		
The Leopard	Luchino Visconti	1965
Story of an aging Sicilian prince who realizes, "If one wants things to stay as they are, things have to change."		
The Two of Us	Claude Berri	1958
About a 75-year-old man and a 9-year-old boy.		
The Shameless Old Lady	Rene Allio	1969
Story of a 70-year-old French widow who, having spent her life serving others, serves herself in the last eighteen months of her life.		

*Miller, P. R., and Tupin, J. P.: Multimedia teaching of introductory psychiatry, American Journal of Psychiatry 128:1219-1222, 1972.

AUTHOR INDEX

SUBJECT INDEX

E

N

O

T